DON'T LET HEALTH CARE BANKRUPT AMERICA STRATEGIES FOR FINANCIAL SURVIVAL

George C. Halvorson

INTRODUCTION

We should not let health care costs undermine, weaken, and badly damage our economy. That would be a wrong, sad, and collectively incompetent thing for us to do. We are actually on that path today -- but we really do not need to allow significant levels of financial damage to happen to us.

We can do a lot better relative to health care costs. We can also do a lot better relative to the quality, safety, and effectiveness of health care. We are making some very bad and very expensive choices today that we should stop making. Health care costs are damaging both state and federal budgets and health care costs are making both care and coverage unaffordable for too many American families.

We spend three times as much money per capita on care as the rest of the world and we spend twice as much money on care as the other industrialized nations.[1] We need to understand why that is true. We need to be very honest with ourselves. Those other industrialized countries are not spending half as much money as we spend on care because those other countries are rationing care.

Many of those other countries get more care, faster care, better care and have better care outcomes than we do and they all spend a lot less money on care in the process.[2] This book shows both comparative care results and comparative care costs for us and several other countries. It is time for us to recognize the realities we face relative to health care costs.

We need to face those realities, and then we need to decide what we want to do about health care costs in this country.

It is time for us to use several of the very real opportunities we have to bring down the costs of care and to make both the quality of care and the outcomes of care in this country better in the process.

We are spending too much money today on care. We are incurring massive levels of unnecessary health care costs. That's bad enough. What is even more problematic and troubling is that instead of paying for all of those excessive costs today with our own current cash flow and today's money, we are using our federal debt as a key source for much of the cash we use to pay for today's costs of care.

Our Children Will Use Their Money To Pay for Our Care

That is not a good thing to do.

We should not be using a strategy of time-deferred financial accountability and debt-financed spending to deal with today's very high costs of care when we have alternative ways of actually reducing those spending levels so that we don't need to pay for government-financed care with debt.

That decision to use debt to pay for our current care is not good for our children and our grandchildren. They will live in a world where they will pay their taxes out of their hard earned paychecks and then the very first use of their tax dollars will be to pay for our long past, long gone, and long forgotten, currently incidental pieces of care.

By using debt financing to pay for today's care costs, we are using their money to buy our care and -- to add injury to injury -- we are using their money today to purchase the care we use now relatively badly. That is not a good situation. We are spending more money than we should be spending on care, and we aren't even spending our own money.

We Are Spending Badly Today

The truth is, if we made care more affordable now, we could fund today's care using today's dollars and we would not need to borrow money to buy that care.

Reducing the cost of care is a major premise of this book. We can get better care today and we can pay less money for that care if we are willing to take an honest, practical, results-focused, functionally adept and depoliticized look at the health care world we live in today and then make a few changes in the way we buy and deliver care that will make our care delivery world today both better and less expensive.

Rationing Is the Wrong Answer

Rationing absolutely is not the answer. Rationing is wrong. We do not need to ration care to afford care. Debt financing and economic deferral of today's excessive care costs into the future is one wrong answer to today's huge care costs. Rationing is another very wrong answer. We do not need to ration care. The food industry used to consume 40 percent of the total income of every American family and more than 30 percent of American workers were used and needed to produce food.[3]

Today, food costs take up less than 13 percent of the family budget, and food production uses less than two percent of our workforce. [4]

We did not deal with the cost problems for food by rationing food. Rationing was absolutely not the answer to American food costs. We have very simply reengineered both the production of food and the distribution of food -- and we have ended up with safer, more accessible, and much less expensive food. We need to reengineer -- not ration -- care.

We Need To Reengineer the Production and Distribution of Care

We need to apply that same thinking and functional strategy to health care. We need to reengineer both the production and the distribution of health care. We need patient-focused caregivers to deliver better care, safer care, more affordable care and more dependable care to American patients. We need to make a series of process improvement changes relatively quickly that can make care better and more affordable. We can do that work using tools that we already know how to use.

There are some obvious next steps we can take to make care better. We need to deliver better care to the people who use the most care dollars, for example. That can be done. We need to expand the tool kit we use to deliver care to create more flexible, more patient-focused and more affordable care. That also can be done. And we need to do some practical key interventions that will keep people healthy longer so we don't need as much care as we need today.

Those interventions in the progression of several major and very expensive diseases are entirely possible. We know now more than we have ever known about how to prevent disease. We actually now know how to trigger a couple of key behavior changes that can have a massive reduction impact on the burden of several of our most expensive debilitating diseases. We need to use that information in practical ways to reduce the disease burden for this country.

We Need Workable and Practical Solutions

This book is intended to help with that entire care improvement and care affordability agenda. This is very basically a book about the costs of care. This book is focused on the actual costs of care and on the practical and functional strategies that are needed to keep care costs both from bankrupting America and from transferring the excessive expenses that result from today's care to our future generations without their approval or their consent.

We Need To Expand the Care Support Tool Kit

We very much need to expand the tool kit we use to deliver care in ways that were not even dreamed of just a few years ago. We are building lovely new tools to support and enhance the delivery of care. If we use these tools well, we can make care better and we can bring down the costs of care. That should be our goal. We should pay for today's care costs with today's money and we should get better care in the process.

We Need To Focus on the People Who Create Most Care Costs

The book explains how we can design and refocus the business model we use to buy care to achieve those goals. Care delivery will change when the business model we use to buy care changes. Cash flow sculpts care delivery. This book makes that point repeatedly -- offering dozens of very real examples to prove that belief to be true. We clearly need to make a few well designed and strategically skillful changes in the way we buy care to get the care we want to buy.

To figure out what care we what to buy, we need to start by understanding several very real numbers that relate to health care costs.

Let's start with who is incurring care costs now.

Anyone who looks in practical and actionable ways at the real opportunities that exist to have a positive impact on the costs of care needs to begin by taking a very hard and clear look at which patients actually create most care costs in this country. We need to understand who these patients are and we need to clearly understand what those high cost patients need for optimal care.

The numbers are very clear. Chronic conditions win. Most care costs in this country come from patients with chronic conditions. Acute care problems like cancer, births, broken bones, infectious diseases, and accidents get a lot of media and public attention, but those very visible acute care problems actually do not drive most care costs in this country. Those acute care expenses represent about 25 percent of the care costs in this country.[5] Seventy-five percent of the health care dollars in this country are actually spent on patients with chronic conditions.[6] Diabetes, hypertension, heart failure and the other key chronic diseases create most care costs. Diabetes alone consumes over 40 percent of the total moneys that are spent by Medicare.[7] Eighty percent of those chronic care costs are spent on patients who have comorbidities -- patients who have multiple health conditions.[8]

So we need to follow the dollars.

We clearly need to focus our thinking on how to deliver affordable and effective care to our chronic care patients and on how we can actually prevent chronic conditions if we want to bring down the costs of care in this country.

We generally do a poor job in delivering and coordinating care today for far too many of those chronically ill patients. We do an even worse job providing care to the patients who have multiple health problems. We actually get care right -- according to current care protocols -- for many of our chronic care patients about half of the time.[9]

As this book points out in multiple places, we are extremely inconsistent in providing those very high cost patients with the right levels, the right pieces and the right packages of care. This book addresses many of those care delivery inconsistencies and quality related problems and discusses the huge opportunities that those shortcomings create in some detail. That focus on those conditions exists for this book because the opportunities to make care better for all patients really are huge. The savings that can result from fixing the current care delivery dysfunction for many of those patients are massive.

Our most expensive patients -- the patients who have with chronic conditions and comorbidities -- are at the top of the opportunity list for both better care and lower cost care.

We clearly need to deliver much better care for all of the very expensive patients who have multiple health conditions. Comorbidities offer a lot of care improvement opportunities. We clearly need much better strategies to treat chronic care patients much more effectively and to make patent-focused team care an expectation rather than an anomaly for those patients.

The final point made in the last chapter of this book goes beyond simply improving care. If we really want to bring health care costs down in this country, we also need to put in place very practical and achievable strategies that can prevent those high levels of chronic diseases from occurring in the first place.

Prevention needs to be a key strategy and a major component of our cost reduction agenda. We need to keep people from becoming victims of those diseases so that we don't have the high costs that inherently result from people having those diseases.

Chronic Diseases Create Over 75 Percent of Our Health Care Costs

That can be done. That isn't magical thinking or a pure economic wish list.

The good news is -- the chronic diseases that create over 75 percent[10] of our health care costs today actually can be prevented for most people. We already know how to do exactly that for most people. We are getting smarter every day on these topics. The medical science of prevention is becoming increasingly clear. We actually do know now how to significantly reduce the incidence of most common chronic conditions. We generally do that basic prevention work today both inconsistently and ineffectively, but we actually now do know what needs to be done to prevent those diseases.

Chronic Conditions Are Caused by Behaviors

We need to start that process with one powerful truth.

Behaviors cause most chronic conditions.

The useful piece of information and the lovely piece of medical wisdom that will allow us to do the needed work of reducing the growth of expensive chronic diseases in this country is that simple fact -- most chronic conditions are caused by a small set of human behaviors.

Type-two diabetes, for example, is now the fastest growing disease in America.[11] Over forty percent of all money spent by Medicare is now spent on patients with diabetes.[12] That is a lot of money. Diabetes creates a massive cost burden for Medicare. So the logic is clear. As is the math. Medicare expenses would go down by a lot if more people did not become diabetic.

That clearly, should be a major goal. We could save Medicare and we could bring Medicare costs down a lot if significantly fewer people became diabetic. We now know that type-two diabetes is caused by behaviors. We know that a couple of clearly defined behaviors hugely increase the risk of getting diabetes. That is the cold scientific, medical, physiological, and biological truth. We know that two basic behaviors create the diabetes explosion we are facing as a country and we know what those two behaviors are.

The chart below shows the explosion in the number of diabetics in this country.

There isn't a diabetes virus or a diabetes bacterium or any kind of biological diabetes-triggering contagious diabetes infection factor that has caused roughly 40 percent of all care dollars spent by Medicare[13] to be spent on the Medicare patients who have diabetes.

Figure I.1

Prevalence of diagnosed type 2 diabetes in the United States:

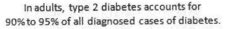

In adults, type 2 diabetes accounts for
90% to 95% of all diagnosed cases of diabetes.

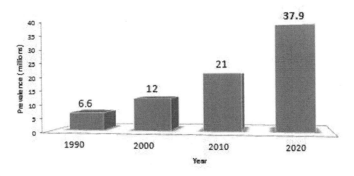

Inactivity and Obesity Are the Two Triggers for Diabetes

To be very specific about those triggering behaviors -- diabetes is caused by inactivity and diabetes is caused by obesity.[14] Inactivity and obesity are actually the twin terrors and twin towers of deteriorating chronic health status for America. Those twin terrors actually trigger multiple chronic conditions. The same exact two behaviors -- unhealthy eating and functional inactivity -- create a wide range of health problems and trigger multiple adverse health conditions. Heart disease, hypertension and a number of other very expensive chronic diseases and even a couple of key cancers are all very much increased by, caused by, aggregated by, exacerbated by, and triggered by the exact same two behaviors.[15]

Two Behaviors Cause Multiple Diseases

That is an amazingly useful piece of information. If you think in practical and functional ways about how we can actually have a major impact on multiple diseases, it is incredibly convenient to have multiple very expensive diseases all literally triggered by the same two behaviors.

That science about the full impact of those two behaviors wasn't well understood until relatively recently. It is now very well known. Those same two behavioral issues -- inactivity and obesity -- are the twin triggers for several very expensive conditions. The key chronic medical conditions that drive 75 percent of our health care costs in America -- along with some of the key cancer-related acute conditions and even some issues of mental health and neurological functioning -- are all activated, driven, supported, aggravated, and triggered very directly by the same two human behaviors -- obesity and inactivity.[16]

Activity -- by Itself -- Can Cut Diabetes by Half

That last chapter of this book explains how that intervention and behavior change processes can be done. Important work can be done and it can be done relatively quickly. Improving activity levels for people, all by itself, can have a huge impact on chronic disease growth. Activity actually has real and almost immediate impact. Most people do not appreciate the incredible medical and biological value of activity. Activity is -- all by itself -- a high leverage, very practical solution tool. Medical science only recently has learned the major value and positive impact that improved activity levels can have on people's health. Walking, alone, can transform health. If we can get people to walk 30 minutes a day, five days a week, we can cut the rate of new diabetics by half.[17] That same level of walking can cut the number of new senior citizen diabetics by nearly two-thirds.[18] Reducing the single most expensive current cost factor for Medicare by two thirds has obvious financial implications that we would be both stupid and inept not to utilize.

The human body is clearly made to walk -- and the human body is healthier when walking happens.

Walking that same amount of time -- 30 minutes a day -- also very significantly reduces hypertension, heart disease, and stroke.[19] Walking that same half an hour a day can alleviate the rate of Alzheimer's damage for patients at high genetic risk of Alzheimer's.[20] Walking that same half hour can directly impact depression.[21] Men who walk thirty minutes or more every day have a 50 percent lower risk of colon cancer.[22] Women with breast cancer who walk have a 40 percent reduction in the reoccurrence rate.[23] The new science of walking is both amazing and clear. The human body needs to walk. We need to recognize that reality. Chapter nine explains in practical ways what we can do to gain the benefits of walking for our communities, schools, and work sites. We need to focus on issues of obesity and healthy eating as well. Those issues are also included in chapter nine.

We Need To Make Care Better, More Efficient, More Effective -- More Affordable

The rest of the book deals with reducing the costs of care by making care better, more efficient and more effective and by changing the business model we use to buy care to reward caregivers for making care better and more affordable.

Costs are the focus of this book. Costs are the target of every chapter of this book. Using the business model of care to improve care by reengineering major aspects of care is the primary strategy embedded in this book relative to making care more affordable.

So this particular book is very much intended to have a positive impact on health care costs. I have written other books about health care reform, health care improvement, health care quality, and health care redesign. I have written articles, papers, essays, and books about the culture of health care and about the values that are and should be inherent in care delivery. Those elements are not excluded from this book -- but the overwhelming focus of this particular health care book is on cost. We obviously cannot afford the cost trajectory we are on now. We need to change that trajectory. We need to spend less money on care. We all know the numbers. Those costs of care for us as a country are unaffordable. It is time now to focus our attention on costs.

Health Care Costs Can Destroy Our Economic Future

Health care costs can badly damage our economic future. Health care costs can suck all of the resources out of our other essential governmental programs and leave too many important programs badly underfunded. We need to reduce the resources we are now wasting relative to excessive health care costs so we can use that health care money for our infrastructure, our public safety and for our entire array of education programs and services. Health care is stealing and spending the resources that those other key programs need.

Health care saves lives. That is true. That is wonderful. Health care can literally do wonders in restoring physical functionality. That is also wonderful. At the same time, health care costs can impair the financial functioning for the very lives that are saved. That is clearly not wonderful. It isn't right for care costs and health care expenses to financially destroy the lives that have been personally saved by the care.

This book points out in very specific ways how we can use the business model that we use to buy care to achieve a very wide range of safety, quality, and affordability goals. It is pretty basic stuff. As you will see when you read the book -- changing the business model approach works. It is actually the only thing that can work to make care more affordable.

Each Chapter Deals With a Major Point of the Solution Agenda

Each of the chapters of this book looks at a separate major piece of the health care cost situation, problem, and opportunity. The chapters are not brief, because the topics are both important and complex.

Far too many health care debates focus on just one piece of the total problem. Too many health care discussions look a lot like the classic fable of the blind men and the elephant. In that fable, several blind men are each touching a separate part of the elephant. The men who touches the side of the elephant believes the elephant is a wall. The man who touches the trunk believes the elephant is a snake. Far too many health care improvement discussions follow a similar pattern of partial, narrow, and incomplete focus -- with some people focused on the tail, some focused on the trunk, and some focused on various other parts that are equally misleading when we are trying to figure out what an elephant is in its entirety. This book is intended to put the entire elephant on the page -- in all of its charm and complexity. So the book has chapters that explain several of the elephant pieces with the intent of explaining how they all connect in the end to create what we have in this country for care delivery and care financing.

We Need To Fix the Mess We Are In

The first chapter of the book describes the mess we are in. That chapter talks about the massive costs of care. It also outlines and discusses some key flaws in care delivery -- including examples of sometimes highly unsafe care and the use of very weak and often inadequate tool kits and data flows to support the delivery of care. Chapter one also deals directly with some of the perverse consequences of the business model we use now to buy care. Chapter one looks at some key challenges and describes and addresses some of the key problems we currently face in care delivery. Chapter one is intended to help us understand why we need to change the business model we use to buy care to reduce many of those undesirable consequences.

We Need Optimal Care

Chapter two looks at care from the other end of the performance continuum. Chapter Two describes what should be the "right way" to deliver care. Chapter two is focused on the future of care delivery and outlines some real and very important opportunities we have to make care better. Chapter two is intended to describe what the ideal care system could and should do for us. This book believes that we need to restructure the business model we use to buy care in order to get better care. To do the needed reengineering of the purchasing model we use to buy care well, we need to first understand very clearly exactly what we want to buy. That is a very practical approach. Before changing the specific ways we buy care, we really need to understand clearly what we want the business model we use to buy care to actually purchase.

Chapter Two looks into the future and describes some of the key elements of care delivery and care functionality that should be included in the future core products of care. Chapter Two outlines and explains some of the basic care delivery capabilities that the new business model should incent and pay for. The chapter tees up what we should want to buy with our new business model for care. Having care delivery and care data flow both focused on the patient and not on the business units of care is, for example, one of the proposed end points for the way we buy care.

Having all doctors with real time access to current medical science that is directly relevant to their patients is another desired end point. Each of those goals is much more likely to happen if we set them up as clear goals and then build the cash flow of care and the business model of care to help make those approaches functional realities for actual care delivery.

We should not build our new business model and change our cash flow approach for buying care until we both define and understand the care we want to buy and until we are equally clear about the care we do not want to continue buying.

Prices Drive Costs in Too Many Settings

Chapter Three is about prices.

Chapter Three has been an unexpectedly painful chapter to read for many of the people who have read earlier drafts of this book.

Chapter Three outlines the prices that we pay for care in this country today. Prices obviously have a huge impact on both the cost and the production of care. Most health care books completely ignore prices as an area of focus -- either because the authors of those books don't understand the role that prices play in overall health care costs or because the authors want to avoid the political quicksand and the intense and often highly energized policy backlash that any focus on health care prices too often generates.

The primary public forum political debates on health care reform have consistently followed a deliberate path of pretending that prices do not exist as a relevant factor for American care costs.

Because almost everyone who writes or gives speeches about care costs has been ducking that politically volatile issue, this book offers an almost unique opportunity to look directly and clearly at prices as being part of the potential solution set for care costs in this country. I suspect chapter Three will shock quite a few readers of this book. It is by far the longest chapter of the book because the issue is so often ignored.

Health Care Is a Business

Chapter Four points out at a very basic and fundamental level that health care is a business. That chapter explains how the model and the approach we use to buy care influences the functional delivery of care.

The fourth chapter also gives several examples of how real changes in the business model of care can and do create significant changes in actual care delivery. Chapter Four explains how business model changes that have actually been made for some aspects of care have already made care significantly better and more affordable in some settings. Chapter four then describes additional ways that business model changes can make care better, safer and more affordable.

Someone Needs To Change the Business Model We Use To Buy Care

Chapter Five makes the equally basic and fundamental point that the business model we use to buy care cannot and will not change until someone changes it. It will not change on its own accord. People who talk about the need to change the business model of care usually do not include in their thinking the actual names of the real parties who can and should actually make those changes in the way we buy care.

Cash flow is obviously the key issue. We need to change the flow of cash. Only the buyers of care who are the actual sources of cash can make real changes in the flow of cash. That is an important point to understand. Neither wishful thinking or intellectual eloquence or well-intended but non-specific political rhetoric will actually change the flow of cash to American caregivers. Someone really needs to deliberately make any change that happens in the flow of cash happen.

Chapter Five outlines how each of the four key current sources of cash now used to buy care can and should be used to change the business model and cash flow for care. The four key sources of cash are known to us all. Chapter Five looks at each of those four sources -- consumers, employers, health insurers and the government -- in their role as current sources of cash and then explains the role each can play in improving the business model for care in the future.

Health Plan Premiums Need To Be Affordable

Chapter Six addresses the need for health plan premiums to be affordable. That is another key point that too often isn't clearly discussed in policy circles. Using health plans to be a primary element for achieving universal coverage in this country will fail as a strategy if health plan premiums are unaffordable or if health plans, themselves, fail as businesses. Chapter six outlines some key risks and concerns that exist today relative to both premium affordability and health plan stability. The consequences of possible risk pool deterioration issues that can result if only sick people buy health insurance are discussed in chapter six. We need the relevant risk pools of health insurers to contain a sufficient number of healthy people so that the average cost of care for insured people is low enough to make premiums affordable. Those issues are described in chapter six.

We Need To Improve Medicare and Medicaid

Chapters Seven and Eight are extremely important chapters. Those chapters deal with the government as a purchaser, and they focus on the huge financial challenges we now face as a country for both our Medicare and our Medicaid programs. Chapters seven and eight identify both problems and possible solution sets for both Medicare and Medicaid. Those chapters offer proposals explaining how we can and should cap the cost increases for both programs while improving care delivery for both programs at the same time.

The money we borrow from our kids to buy care today is basically spent on those programs. We owe it to our children to fix those problems. Fixing the cost problems for those two huge programs is at the top of the list of the cash flow issues we will need to resolve in order to keep care costs from bankrupting America and from continuing to defer payment for care to our children and grandchildren.

We need the courage, the skill, and the political dexterity to put a functional cap on Medicare and Medicaid costs -- without rationing care for the patients in either program.

We Need To Improve Health

Chapter nine focuses on how we can actually improve both individual and population health. Chapter nine explains how we can achieve that goal of better health by doing proactive things that have been proven to work in multiple settings. Chapter nine suggests real things we can do to keep people from getting the chronic diseases that create most costs of care in this country. Achieving all of the functional care delivery improvements and putting in place all of the care reengineering strategies that are described in the other chapters of this book but then not taking some key and important steps to improve actual health for large numbers of people would be a major mistake. We need to make care better and more affordable, and we also very much need to create a situation where fewer people actually need care.

That can be done. This book explains how to do it.

We Need To See the Entire Elephant

Enjoy the book. I do apologize for the fact that it is a complex, multilayered, and very long book that addresses a wide range of topics. I do believe the topics are all relevant and that they are all relevant in a shared context. Everything is -- as a world leader once said -- connected to everything else.

As noted above, we need to avoid the splintered thought processes that have resembled and echoed the inadequately narrow understanding levels that were experienced by the blind men with their elephant.

This book is an attempt to put a lot more of the elephant on display. At one point, this book was actually up to 700 pages. This is still a very long book -- but the goal is to help offer an overall context to the discussion that is more complete than the usual context of our health policy discussion. We have failed fairly badly as a country in trying to address and fix individual, out-of-context pieces of the health care cost and quality problems as separate solution agendas.

We really do need to address more of the big picture in order to fix the big problem. Things could improve a lot for health care if we make the right set of choices and then have the courage to do the things that need to be done to achieve the goals we need to achieve.

This book is intended to help with that process and to help create a dialogue about care that can get us to where we need to be and deserve to be. Enjoy the book. It is based on a long-time care system and care financing practitioner's front row perspective about how all of those pieces fit together and how they can all be fixed.

We have used political and politicized approaches to make care affordable and we have basically failed. Now we need an approach from the inside of care delivery, based on real strategies and approaches that have been field tested and proven to have value in the world.

This is not an academic exercise. It is a user's guide to health care.

Enjoy the book. I hope that at least parts of it are useful to you.

CHAPTER ONE

THE MESS WE ARE IN

Health care in America tends to be inconsistent, badly organized, often inefficient, inadequately supported by basic care improvement tools, too often both unsafe and operationally dysfunctional, deeply data deficient, and -- with all of those challenges and all of those functional problems -- far too expensive. We clearly need to improve the delivery of care in some important areas of care delivery in this country. We also need to spend less money on care.

Let's start with some macro numbers about health care costs in America.

We spend nearly 2.8 trillion dollars a year to buy health care in this country.[24]

That is a huge amount of money. If our health care economy was its own country, it would be the fifth largest country in the world.[25] We spend more taxpayer-generated dollars on health care than any other country in the world and then -- in addition -- we also spend far more money in private, non-governmental dollars to buy health care than any other country in the world[26] -- so we win twice.

Or we lose twice -- depending on how you feel about spending major amounts of money on health care.

That massive cash flow really is a mixed blessing.

Why is it mixed?

Health care is a very robust part of our economy. People in the health care portion of our economy tend to do well financially. Health care creates a lot of jobs[27] and almost all of those jobs are both local and well-paying. Health care paychecks flow into just about every local economy in America. Our hospitals alone are the largest non-governmental employers in the country.[28]

We also have a thriving American industry for the manufacture of medical equipment and supplies. We actually have a healthy and positive balance of trade for our medical technology sales. That is a good thing. We continue to be a world technology leader for care and that is a very good thing for our economy.[29]

We also lead the world in health care IT.[30] Our health care systems companies tend to be the largest health care systems companies in the world and those companies also generate both good local jobs and a positive balance of trade.

That Huge Cash Flow Is a Mixed Blessing

So health care -- from a pure economic perspective -- is clearly a mixed blessing. It creates great jobs and it destroys budgets. It saves lives, and it crushes people economically. The costs of care create great incomes for health care workers and for health care businesses and those same exact costs of care have eaten away the purchasing power of American families, crippled some state and local budgets, and bankrupted a lot of American patients. Surprisingly, there is no link between the cost of care and the quality of care -- and some of the most expensive care sites and some of the most expensive care procedures have the highest levels of patient damage and the highest rates of patient mortality.[31]

Sepsis care, for example, has been an area where the highest cost care sites have also -- far too often -- had the highest death rate for their patients. [32] That outcome alone, clearly tells us that we have a major opportunity to improve the business model we use to buy care in this country and it also tells us that we are spending too much money for significant aspects of care.

Overall, care costs are obviously very high, and going up for the country.

Health care premiums that are needed now to buy full benefit levels for a family of four in America already significantly exceed the total minimum wage for an American worker.[33] The pure new health care costs that have been channeled into our health insurance premium increases every year have literally more than offset the average worker's complete salary increases for more than a decade.

We Spend More Than Other Countries for Care

Other countries also spend a lot of money on care and have problems with their own growing costs of care, but we are very obviously a significant outlier when it comes to health care costs in any and all cost comparisons with the rest of the world.

Our health care spending now outstrips the rest of the world by significant margins. The chart below shows our health care spending measured as a percent of our GDP spent on care compared to the health care spending in the rest of the world for the past couple of decades. Our cost increases have clearly exceeded everyone else's health care cost increases...by a significant margin.

Likewise -- the premiums that are paid to buy health insurance in America clearly exceed the premiums paid in the other countries who also use private health insurers to pay for care for their people.[34]

We need to better understand health care premiums as we figure out our solutions in this country for care costs and care affordability. An amazing number of people in this country don't understand the basic cash flow factors and economic forces and the basic arithmetic realties that create health care premiums.

Figure 1.1

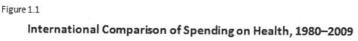

International Comparison of Spending on Health, 1980–2009

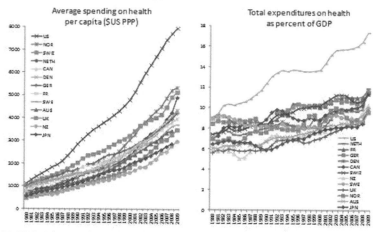

Note: PPP = Purchasing power parity—an estimate of the exchange rate required to equalize the purchasing power of different currencies, given the prices of goods and services in the countries concerned.
Source: OECD Health Data 2011 (Nov. 2011).

Health care premiums everywhere in the world where private health insurance plans are used to finance care are basically the average cost of care for a defined insured population.

Premiums Are Actually the Average Cost of Care

That's a very important point to know and remember. Premiums are -- very simply stated -- the average cost of care.

Premiums for health insurance coverage are calculated in every country by figuring out the total cost of care for an insured set of people and then dividing the total cost of care for those insured people by the number of people who buy the insurance. So when drug prices go up in a country, the price increase for the drug is paid by the insurer. That payment for that price increase directly adds to the average cost of care that is being paid by that insurer to buy care for their specific insured population. Since premiums for health insurance are based on the average cost of care, that means that premiums for health insurance go up with every prescription drug price increase.

Prices paid for pieces of care basically create the premium levels that are charged by health insurance everywhere -- including the U.S.

Other countries currently pay a lot less for the very same prescription drugs than we do -- as you will see in some details in Chapter Three of this book -- so their health insurance premiums are also a lot lower.

We currently pay more than anyone in the world for our prescription drugs.[35] That particular fact is relatively well known in health care policy circles. There have been a number of very public discussions about the fact that we pay more than other countries pay for prescription drugs.

Other Countries Spend Less for Pieces of Care

What many people do not know, however, is that the other industrialized countries also spend a lot less than we do for almost all other pieces of care. The average price charged for a CT scan in this country is $500.[36] Most other countries have an average cost for that same scan that exceeds $300.[37] The average cost of a day in the hospital in this country has now exceeded $3,000.[38] Other than Australia -- who now charges $1,400 a day -- most other industrialized countries have an average cost per day for hospital care that is below $1,500.[39] Almost all other industrialized countries charge less than $900 for a day in the hospital. We pay a lot more. Five percent of the U.S. prices actually exceeded $12,000 per day.[40] Those price differences for drug costs, scans and hospital days are not outlier price comparisons. Those are actually very typical price differences between us and everyone else. We pay a lot more for the same pieces of care compared to the prices paid for each piece of care in rest of the world.

As Chapter Three points out, we Americans spend more money on health care than any country in the world by a wide margin. We spend more by the patient, more by the piece, and we pay more by the condition than anyone on the planet.

Care Is Inconsistent and Can Be Dangerous

Those higher costs that are spent on care would arguably be less damaging and less painful as a total expense category for our country if our health care delivery approach wasn't so flawed and so dysfunctional in so many ways and places. Paying a lot of money for care would not be as big a problem if the care we bought with that large amount of money was consistently great care. Care is, unfortunately, not consistently good in far too many settings and it is also clearly not consistently safe across all care sites in this country. There is a lot of available research data that proves that statement about inconsistent and unsafe care in this country to be true. The Institute of Medicine Quality Chasm work needs to be read by anyone who believes that our care is consistently high quality or safe. Those comments about problematic care quality and inconsistent care safety in this country may make some people who read this book unhappy. We really do not want the data about unsafe care in this country to be true. We all want to believe that care everywhere in America is safe -- and we all want to believe that care everywhere in America is consistently based on best practices and current science.

Quite a few public speeches and presentations actually make that statement and say, definitively, that the best care in the world is here -- in this country.

A significant number of political speeches cite the "magnificence" of American health care as though those statements about the highest quality for care being delivered here was an irrefutable truth.

So what is actually true?

How safe and how good is our care?

There Are Wide Variations in Care Quality and Care Safety

The answer is a bit painful. What is actually, provably and measurably true is that there are wide variations in care quality and care outcomes in this country. Death -- everyone can agree -- is an important and relevant quality measure. Inside American health care today, death rates vary hugely. Multiple examples of differences mortality rates by care sites are described later in other chapter and at several other points in this book. Care outcomes vary, people die as a result. Care processes in this country are often flawed and processes are too often splintered and incomplete. One major shortcoming of American care delivery today -- a shortcoming that far too often results in poor care and damaging care outcomes -- is the fact that too much of the care delivery in this country tends to be uncoordinated, unconnected and functionally unlinked. Caregivers actually have a very hard time, in many settings, simply coordinating basic care. That in ability to coordinate care is true for far too many patients and too many care settings. We need to recognize the fact that there are woeful lacks of coordination and those deficiencies create particular problems for our many patients with multiple medical conditions who badly need coordinated care. We need to understand the reality of that situation. We also need to know why it happens. That lack of care coordination between our caregivers doesn't happen because our caregivers don't want to coordinate care. That weak performance level for care coordination in so many settings exists because we have a major tool deficit for that task. We need to understand that deficit. We need better tools for our caregivers. We simply don't have the very basic tools in place today that are needed to coordinate care for most patients who need care coordination. Our tool deficiency is a major functional problem that is addressed multiple times in this book. The current business model we use to buy care actually creates some of those tool deficiencies.

Seventy-five percent of the health care costs in this country actually come from our chronic care patients, and most of those costs come from patients who have co-morbidities -- multiple diagnosis and multiple diseases.[41] Those patients need their caregivers to work together and to be fully informed about the full array of care being received by each patient. The current business model we use to buy care does not pay for caregiver linkages, caregiver coordination, or the use of linkage tools by caregivers -- so those tools do not exist and they are not used.

We clearly need a business model for care, an economic reality for caregivers, and a robust care support tool kit that reflects that basic medical need for coordinated care for those patients and their caregivers.

Patients With Comorbidities Often Get Care from Unlinked Doctors

Because our care sites tend to be separate, stand-alone business units, patients in this country who have co-morbidities almost always get their care from multiple stand-alone doctors. Having separate doctors for each medical condition isn't inherently a problem -- as long as the doctors who share a patient can coordinate care and share information about the patient with one another. In this country, however, it is rare and often very difficult for those doctors to share information with each other about the patients they share simply because there are no tools or mechanisms to do that information-sharing work in most care settings.

Doctors in this country are also not paid money to coordinate care with each other in most care settings. No cash, no coordination. The fundamental truth about care delivery that is discussed in more detail later in this book is that we deliver the care that generates a payment. We do not deliver care that doesn't generate a payment. It is breathtakingly obvious that the caregivers and the care sites in this country tend not to do things that aren't listed on an approved fee schedule. The fourth chapter of this book deals in more detail with that issue and explains how the fee schedules we use to buy care actually dictate the delivery of care with some amazing leverage and impact.

We Also Have a Major Data Deficit

Data is also a problem. We also very clearly have a major data deficiency as well as a tool deficiency. That data deficit problem also seems hard to believe at this point in our history -- but it is also very true. We have amazingly poor and inadequate data about many aspects of care. Patients in this country have a very hard time making data-supported choices and data-supported decisions about both their personal, personal care and their personal caregivers.

Caregivers Also Have Data Deficiencies

That data deficiency problem isn't limited to patients. Caregivers in this country far too often do not personally know how well or how badly they, themselves, are doing as providers of care. The caregivers do not know how well they are doing because there is so little comparative data available at any level about care. We are almost data free in major areas of care where good data could help us improve both the quality and the affordability of care. Multiple studies that have been done have made that point very clear. This book gives a dozen important examples. Data can transform care. Data can save lives. But we do not have enough data about many aspects of care today. Care delivery data in this country tends to be inconsistent, incomplete, frequently inaccessible, and the thin and sometimes fragile layers of care related data that do exist in many care settings are far too often very sadly factually inaccurate, functionally inadequate and inconsistently available.

Quality Problems Are Far Too Common

Quality problems are far too common, as well in the current infrastructure of American care delivery. We don't have a deficit of quality problems. We have a surplus of quality issues. Look at the comparative quality data that does exist for several areas of care. Care quality varies a lot. That fact cannot be refuted. The variation in care quality today is significant and it is very relevant. As this book points out in multiple places, your personal likelihood of dying as a patient can increase by a factor of ten if you personally pick the wrong care site for your care.[42] Being ten times more likely to die based on your choices of caregiver or your choice of care site is something that a patient being treated for a disease or a health condition should know. You only get to die once. There are no redos and restarts and do-overs for actual death in the functional context of today's health care. Cryogenics isn't at the point where we can freeze dead people and then do a restart later when care gets better. So death is a relevant quality measure for care and we should look at what that very fundamental measure tells us. It tells us that death rates vary by a lot.

We Don't Use Mortality Information Often or Well

We know that to be true, but we don't use that information often or well. Those major variations in care quality and those often amazingly large variations in death rate that do exist are not on our current radar screen for either our governmental policy makers or for the purchasers of care.

For obvious functional, operational and primary logistical reasons, the twin problems of bad and inconsistent care outcomes and weak and inconsistently available care data are very much linked. It is very hard to make care better in any setting when even the caregivers who are directly providing that care far too often don't know that their own care is inadequate, dysfunctional problematic and or actually dangerous care. We need a robust set of data about care outcomes and about best practices for patients, and we need that data even more as a tool for the actual care delivery infrastructure. As noted above, the differences in outcomes between care sites and care approaches are very real. The death rate for heart surgery can vary by a factor of ten.[43] The death rate for sepsis can easily triple or quadruple between the best care sites and the least effective care sites[44] -- and the likelihood of being damaged for life by sepsis at least doubles at the worse care sites. The mortality rates for cancer patients can also double or triple depending on the care team and the care sites.[45] We know that those differences in that very basic outcome measure -- death – do exist -- but even that very basic piece of outcome data is far too often not available to either the patients or to the providers of care in any useful way.

Care Outcomes Vary Widely

These concerns are not speculation or idle theory.

We know for an absolute fact that the outcomes of care do vary significantly in key areas. So does care safety. This book makes multiple references to those outcome inconsistencies and those safety problems. That level of inconsistently in key areas is really unfortunate. When we spend $2.8 trillion dollars on care, safety should not be an issue. When we spend that much money on care, care should be safe. That is particularly true and particularly important because we actually do know how to functionally deliver safe care. It can be done. Doing better in those key care outcome performance areas isn't a theory or a pipedream or wishful thinking. We know that it actually is possible for care sites to do much better on safety and we know that to be true because there are some care sites that have directly targeted those issues and those care sites have addressed those performance shortcomings and safety malfunctions with care reengineering and with systematic care improvement approaches. The care sites in this country that do that care improvement work in a systematic way actually do have significantly lower mortality rates. Lives are being saved. Those care sites have lower infection rates. These sites and their care teams damage far fewer people. They kill fewer people. Care safety enhancement can be done. But the sad truth is that most care sites in this county have not gone down those paths. As noted earlier, data deficits are a huge part of the problem. Far too many care sites are data free in important areas of care performance.

So as a country, we have weak data and we have inconsistent care and we have often problematic care outcomes. As bad as these issues are, that isn't the full set of care deficiencies that we need to resolve.

It's Hard for Doctors To Be Current on Medical Science

We also, interestingly, far too often do not do a very good job of keeping up with best medical science. That is also both sad and unfortunate. Medical science changes and improves regularly. The unfortunate truth is that we and our caregivers both also tend to have inconsistent access to current medical science across American care sites and care settings.[46] Caregivers often can't keep up with medical science. That particular information deficit also surprises a lot of people.

Most people who get care have the comforting belief that their own personal caregiver is very much personally "keeping up" and is entirely current about the most relevant medical science relating to their personal care. That belief by patients about their caregiver "keeping up," unfortunately too often is not functionally accurate.

The science of medicine improves regularly. That is the good news. The bad news is that far too many caregivers in this country simply can't stay abreast of medical best practices or even with current medical science developments.

The IOM Is Studying Inconsistency

The Institute of Medicine -- the organization of senior medical and health care leaders, thinkers and researchers that has been charged by the U.S. government with taking an ongoing overview look at American health care performance and health care operations -- has been deeply concerned about these issues and has studied those medical science "keeping up" issues relative to care delivery in this country quite a bit in recent years. The results have been sobering. As noted earlier, the IOM has concluded in a couple of key reports that care in America is too often inconsistent.[47] The IOM has also concluded that care delivery in this country is far too often dangerous.[48] More recently, the IOM has also reported that care delivery in this country is far too often not consistently based on the most current science about either care delivery or care processes.[49] The IOM studies on these issues are cited in the endnotes to this book. They are clearly worth reading if you have any doubts about whether those problems about best use of medical science exist in this country.

The IOM has a taskforce set up right now to help the country figure out how to keep care scientifically based across all American care sites. The clearly defined goal of the current IOM task force is to have 90 percent of health care in this country based on medical science by the year 2020.[50]

Is Ninety Percent Science-Based Too Little or Too Hard?

That is a fascinating number.

Ninety percent is a very clear goal. It is worth thinking, however, about what that ninety-percent goal for the IOM task force really means and what that goal tells us about the current state of science relative to American health care. To some people, a goal to have 90 percent of the care delivered in this country based on medical science by the year 2020 seems both very low and very slow. Some people believe that specific 90 percentage target is programmatically weak and unacceptably inadequate to be a primary performance goal for medical science applicability and the use of science by the caregivers of our country. But the task force that is doing the work on that issue actually felt that 90 percent goal was both ambitious and aggressive. They believe that goal was aggressive and even optimistic because the research that was looked at by the taskforce to learn how well we actually do today in keeping up with medical science and with medical research showed that major portions of the care we deliver and receive every day in this country does not meet that science-based standard now. The number of care decisions and care procedures today that do not meet that science-based care delivery standard is far less than that 90 percentage goal that was set by the IOM task force.[51]

That fact shocks a lot of people. It alarms patients when patients learn that those medical science-related problems might exist.

We all want best care. We all want and need our care teams to be scientifically current. If we want to solve that problem, we need to first recognize that being current is a problem in many care settings today.

Why Isn't Care Based On Best Science?

Why isn't care consistently based on best science now?

Why are so many caregivers challenged relative to keeping up with the most current medical science?

That question is worth asking and answering at this point in this book.

The answer is pretty simple.

We haven't made that "keeping up" goal either a priority or a requirement for either delivering care or paying for care. Being current and following best science clearly is not rewarded or incented by the business model we usually use today to buy care. Because keeping up is hard to do -- and because it isn't part of the business model we use to buy care -- it is relatively inconsistently done.

We Don't Have Good Tools for Keeping Up

Again, we have a significant tool deficit.

We simply have not built and implemented the basic mechanisms and tools that we need to make keeping up easy to do. Our caregivers who do want to keep up with current medical science and with current best practices frankly usually don't even have access to the basic tools that are needed to be current about the full range of scientific and functional developments in the science and delivery of care.

That seems hard to believe, but it is true. It is another basic functionality deficit. It is another missing tool. It is another failure that results from the business model we use to buy care. We clearly have another major tool deficiency relative to having basic tools in place that can help caregivers simply keep up with current medical science.

That keeping up deficit should be unacceptable to us all. It should be unacceptable because it does not need to exist. There is no good reason today at this point in our history and at this point in the world of technology -- with all of the technological functionality that is now available to create systems related and systems supported toolkits -- with an ever expanding availability of a wide array of electronic communication and electronic data access tools -- for us not to have a robust set of "keeping up" tools easily available for use by all health care practitioners. The internet is now at our disposal everywhere. There is no good reason today not to have fully functional, easy to access electronic medical libraries that are made available to all caregivers when our caregivers need current and best care information for any patients or care related issue or decision.

That access to current information can be done. A few large and well organized care delivery teams have shown that it can be done and that the tools to do the work can help caregivers be current in the science of care. But we have not chosen to put those tools in place for all of our caregivers and care quality in this country suffers in too many instances as a result.

We Have a Tool Gap, a Data Gap and a Science Gap

We have a tool gap. We have a data gap. We have a medical science gap. And we have a significant business model deficit relative to the use and the existence of several badly needed health care connectivity tools. Money is clearly at the root of each of basic gap problems. Rather -- the lack of focused money is at the root of those particular problems. We simply have not put those needed care improvement tools in place for our caregivers in most care settings because no one pays for those tools to exist and no one pays for them to be used.

In settings where the cash flow we use to buy care actually pays for those tools, they exist -- and they help transform care. Examples later in this book explain how the death rate for HIV patients was cut in half using team care and connectivity tools. The death rate for stroke patients was cut 40 percent using team care and connectivity tools.[52] Broken bones in seniors were reduced by over a third using team care and connectivity tools. [53] Team care can do some amazing things relative to better patient outcomes. So can data-supported care. We need to make data-supported care a goal of business model we use to buy care. The benefits of data-supported care are particularly evident when the data is electronic. When the data about care is not electronic -- but simply stored in paper medical records -- all of the gaps listed above are exacerbated by that inadequate data source.

Paper Medical Records Are Dangerous and Dysfunctional and Bad

The truth is -- paper kills. A number of care strategists use that phrase to discuss the health care dark problems. Why do those experts say that paper kills?

They say that because most medical records in this country are still maintained purely on paper...and care suffers as a result.

We still use paper medical records in most medical care sites.

Very functional and well-designed computerized medical record systems exist and these systems are widely used -- but most medical information in this country is still stored in paper files.

That seems hard to believe, but it is true. That isn't good at multiple levels. Paper medical records are a communications and logistical nightmare. Information about patients that is kept in paper file folders is isolated, insulated, inaccessible, sometimes illegible and almost always significantly incomplete.

We Need Patient Data To Be Patient-Centered and Electronic

One of the very best government investments that has been made by our government over the past decade has been to subside funding of the actual implementation of electronic medical records in a growing number of care sites. That funding was included in the economic recovery funding legislation in 2009. That funding approach requires the care sites to computerize care information and then use the information in a "meaningful" way. That electronic medical record tool legislation was a very smart thing for the government to fund. We very much need care data to be on the computer. We really can't make care better in many ways until we have better data about care and until we can share the electronic data for each patient when that information needed by a caregiver to deliver patient focused care.

Improving the level of consistent data availability and making health care data electronic will have the same kinds of positive impact on health care data flow that railroad tracks and interstate highways have had on transportation infrastructure and traffic flow in this country. Putting care data in a computer does not somehow -- all by itself -- magically improve care -- but having electronic data gives us tools and the essential information flow tracks that we can use to improve care. That electronic medical record support and expansion agenda for this country points us in a very good direction, and it gives us badly needed tool we can use to get important things done in care delivery. It isn't enough, however, to simply have health care data on the computer. We also need the computers to share data with one another. We need to be very sure the electronic data is sufficiently connected so that it can be used by the caregivers when it is needed for patient care.

Isolated Electronic Files Are As Bad As Isolated Paper Files

Having isolated electronic files for patients is just as bad and dys-functional as having isolated paper files. But when the data about patients is both computerized and made available in an intercon-nected, patient-focused way to all of the caregivers who deliver care to a given patient, care can get better very quickly. Having data on the computer and then creating access to that data allows us to create mechanisms that we can use to track and improve care outcomes and care processes in ways that paper-based data files could never hope to do.

So we are moving in the right direction relative to the avail-ability of electronic data. But most medical files are still on paper and that is a bad thing. Far too often, inadequate, incomplete and dysfunctional patient care results from care supported only by paper files.

MultiSpecialty Medical Groups Lead in Patient Data Sharing

Most care sites today can't share data about patients they share. Some care sites, however, can and do share their patient data now. It can be done.

The various multispecialty physician group practices that exist across the country have almost universally addressed those data linking issues long ago. The multispecialty medical groups basically solved those data access problems by creating tools that both computerize the data and make it available to the entire care team when needed to provide care.

Doctors who practice today in large multispecialty medical groups can usually share data and information about the patients they share. Those multispecialty groups have always appreciated the scientific advantage that results from shared data. Most of the multispecialty groups in this country have entirely eliminated their paper medical records. The larger and more complex medical groups now almost all use computerized medical records to both share information and to keep their patient information current and constantly available.

However, that level of electronic data sharing between doctors who share patients is still only true in a minority of American care settings. So that lack of that data sharing is another major tool deficit. Most doctors who share patients today cannot easily share information about their patients with other doctors and care suffers as a result.

Most patients in this country generally do not know that particular sad fact about our care information linkage and our data-sharing gaps and communications deficits to be true until the patients, themselves, need shared care. Then the data gaps between caregivers often loom large in a very negative way. Most patients don't discover or understand that data link problem until they, themselves, actually need care from multiple caregivers. What that happens patients usually learn both directly and quickly that their own individual care information from their multiple caregivers is painfully and dysfunctionally unlinked and unconnected.

Horror stories about American caregivers who can't get even their most basic levels of information shared for the patients they share are far too common. We have all heard those horror stories from patients and we have heard them from their families. Most people who are patients who have serious medical problems and who have multiple doctors often have an urgent need for data sharing by their caregivers and those patients far too often suffer from that dysfunctional non-system of data storing. Patients often end up carrying armloads of their own paper medical records from care site to care site -- and they too often find that the care site that they give their data to are often badly equipped to actually use that data from the other care sites when patients carry it to them.

We Need Better Care Connectivity

We clearly can do better in these areas. It is silly and wrong for us -- in this day of easy computer connectivity and massive electronic databases -- to accept and simply continue those connectivity inadequacies as a functional reality of American care delivery. Our payers -- the entities that purchase health care in America -- need to collectively insist that the care sites of this county install the right set of connectivity tools so we can make care safer, more effective, more connected and more affordable. Major health plans and government agencies should facilitate that data sharing and support it financially. The good news is, as we stated earlier, that we actually do have the tools to do that work now. We just don't use those tools in most care settings. In the care setting where they exist, care gets better.

We Have an Informed Choice Deficit

We need to solve the data deficits, the connectivity deficits, and the ongoing access to medical science deficits -- and then we need to put in place processes that will allow patients to make their own care choices based on key performance factors relating to care.

We also very clearly have an informed choice deficit. We don't have good processes in place to help patients make informed choices about their own care options. Those tools exist. Some are wonderful. Those patient-choice facilitation tools aren't used in most care sites. We have a tool deficit for patients in that regard. We have an equivalent parallel deficit relative to caregivers knowing both the most current medical science and how well they are doing as caregivers relative to the outcomes and the comparative consequences of the care they deliver.

All of those performance challenges -- weak data, bad care linkages, inconsistent science, and business models that don't pay for patient-focused team care -- create major suboptimal consequences for care delivery and create care problems for patients. The consequences are that care delivery does not perform at a consistently high level -- and our care infrastructure does not achieve the same results in all settings. The bad news is -- some care results vary highly.

We have a very serious information deficit about those life-threatening variations in care outcomes.

Death Rates Vary

A noted above, death is a good and relevant measure of care outcomes and care effectiveness.

We need people to understand the fact that the death rates for various categories of care vary from care site to care site and from care team to care team. So do other key care outcomes.

If we were delivering care in the most responsible way, we would expect that both patients and care teams knew that those differences exist and knew what the differences are.

Both patients and caregivers today tend to have the belief that all care delivered by licensed caregivers or by licensed care sites is roughly of equal value and equal effectiveness. People also tend to believe that their own personal caregiver is likely to be one of the care delivery resources who is most likely to produce an optimal care outcome for them as a patient. Most data-free caregivers tend to have very similar positive opinions about their own skill sets and their personal care delivery effectiveness. That is human nature for both patients and caregivers. People generally have a very strong tendency to trust their own caregiver and to believe that the care that is being delivered at their care site is among the best possible set of care delivery processes and approaches.

In our current non-system of care, the truth is that care outcomes actually vary widely and sometimes wildly from site to site and from caregiver to caregiver. We need to understand that reality. Care will actually not get better in any consistent way until we face that reality. We need to have the individual insight, the collective political courage and the functional capability to look clearly at a wide range of key issues relative to care performance variation and that will not happen until we begin with basic data about care performance.

To look clearly at the truth about the variable consequences of care, we need to know the truth about that variation.

If we do decide to look at those issues of significant variation in care outcomes and care functionality, where should we start?

Mortality Rates Are a Good Place To Focus

As noted above, death is a good place to start. Mortality rates have been mentioned several times in this book already.

We need to start with some relevant measurements -- and there are several good reasons why mortality rates give us a very workable foundation to begin the process of making comparisons relative to care performance levels.

For starters, we can measure death. There are several other measurable levels of relative care delivery performance data that can be very useful -- but death is an important and a highly relevant care outcome. Death rates do vary enough in a number of areas of care that measuring death rates can tell us a lot about the quality of care in various care sites and care teams.

The differences in mortality rates are not insignificant.

Your chance of dying from heart surgery literally increases by a factor of ten if you get your care at a higher risk surgery site compared to having your surgery done at a lower risk, better performing surgery site.[54]

Ten times is a lot.

Making a care site decision that increases your personal risk of dying from a major surgery by a factor of ten might not be a good thing for a patient to do. Patients should have information about these relative death rates, and that information should be required by the people who buy care. Chapter Four looks at those issues in more detail.

Likewise, sepsis is the number one cause of death in American hospitals. Sepsis kills more patients in hospitals than stroke, heart disease, or cancer.[55] The least effective hospitals have almost one in three sepsis patients die. The best hospitals lose less than one in ten of their sepsis patients.

Sepsis is the largest single one cause of death in American hospitals, so those are very relevant differences in sepsis mortality rates. Those are also differences that you should know if you are choosing a hospital for your care. You should know that the hospitals with the worst death rates for sepsis also have the highest percentage of patients who are damaged for life by that condition.

Sepsis performance levels clearly belong on a patient choice scorecard. Those issues are discussed more fully in Chapter Four of this book.

Infection rates are another very good area where comparative performance measurement makes sense. Nearly two million people get a hospital acquired infection every year in an American hospital.[56] Pressure ulcers happen to quite a few patients. Your personal chance as a patient in a hospital setting of getting a damaging, disfiguring and potentially fatal pressure ulcer varies by more than ten times depending on which hospital you choose for your care.[57] That variation in your likelihood of being damaged or even killed by a pressure ulcer happens based simply and purely on the hospital site you have chosen for your hospital care. In the very worst performing sites, your risk of getting those horrible ulcers and being damaged, disfigured, crippled or killed by them actually increases by a factor of ten compared to the performance of the best sites.[58]

The second chapter of this book has charts that show differences in heart surgery deaths rates and sepsis outcomes between care sites. As a patient, those levels of performance differences should matter when you chose your care site.

Cancer Survival Rates Vary As Well

Right now, that kind of information is almost invisible to patients. People don't ask for that data because people believe that all care sites have about the same success levels. That is not true. All care is not the same. Success rates vary. Your personal cancer survival rates actually vary hugely depending on the site and the care team you chose for your care. Hardly anyone knows that these differences exist. The very best care teams now achieve a breast cancer survival rate upwards of 95 percent. The average care sites have survival rates for their breast cancer patients that run under 90 percent. Some of the lower performing breast cancer success programs actually run closer to 80 percent survival rates.[59] There are entire regions of the country where the average survival rate for all breast cancer patients is close to 80 percent. [60] So your personal chance of dying of breast cancer also more than quadruples depending on the cancer site you chose for your care. Only a very small number of cancer patients get any data from anyone telling the patient what those relative performance levels are.

Quite a few cancer care sites now participate in the SEER cancer care reporting process. Being part of the SEER reporting agenda is a major step forward for both care improvement and care site accountability. The SEER data shows us that there are major differences in mortality rates between care sites for a number of cancers. The variation in survival rates are probably even greater in all of the cancer treatment sites that do not participate in the SEER reporting process. The cancer sites that don't participate in SEER may often be the sites that do not have the best cure rates. In any case, these measurable differences in cancer survival rates based on the care team and the site of care are an important fact for cancer patients to know. Not all care is equal. Care approaches matter. Care teams matter. Cancer is a treatment area where the care approaches vary quite a bit, and the care outcomes for cancer patients can vary by a lot. If you are personally a cancer patient, important pieces of data about relative care outcomes can be very relevant. The next few charts show several variations in the cancer death rates that are reported to SEER by various care sites for several categories of cancer. The differences are real and significant. What is fascinating -- and not entirely unexpected -- is that care patterns and care outcomes for cancer care not only vary by care sites -- they even vary by states and by geographic regions within states.

Figure 1.2

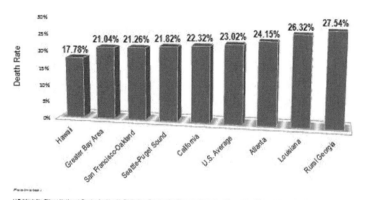

**SEER Female Breast Cancer Death Rates, 2005-2009
By Registry, All-Ages**

Footnotes:

U.S. Mortality Files, National Center for Health Statistics, Centers for Disease Control and Prevention. Rates are per 100,000 and are age-adjusted to the 2000 U.S. Std Population (19 age groups - Census P25-1130).

The SEER 9 areas are San Francisco, Connecticut, Detroit, Hawaii, Iowa, New Mexico, Seattle, Utah and Atlanta.
The SEER 11 areas comprise the SEER 9 areas plus San Jose-Monterey and Los Angeles.
The SEER 13 areas comprise the SEER 11 areas plus the Alaska Native Registry and Rural Georgia.
The SEER 13 areas comprise the SEER 13 areas plus California excluding SF/SJM/LA, Kentucky, Louisiana, New Jersey and Georgia excluding ATL/RG.

That next chart shows the variation in average death rates for several states for breast cancer. Most people have no clue that cancer survival rates not only differ from care team to care team -- the survival rates also differ significantly from state to state. Different states actually have very different average mortality rates for that condition.

Those variations in death rates would not exist between those areas if all cancer caregivers in this country were following similar or identical best practices for their cancer care. The point made earlier about the value of the Institute of Medicine work that is being done to help create care consistency around medical best practices is reinforced by that amazing variation in death rates for various types of cancer. Some of those geographic areas clearly need better collective access to the most current science and to best practices relative to cancer care.

As hard as it is for patients to believe, care patterns are sometimes based more on regional care cultures then they are based on pure and current medical science. That particular piece of information can be both startling and disconcerting for patients. The truth is geographic care culture differences do happen. Look again at the last chart. Only 17 percent of the patients in Hawaii die from breast cancer. In rural Georgia, the death rates from that same exact cancer currently averages 27 percent. The differences are even greater when you look at the comparative results from some of the individual care teams and the caregiving organizations. At the well-organized, scientifically current, fully multispecialty integrated care systems like Kaiser Permanente, the Mayo Clinic, and the Cleveland Clinic, the death rates for patients with that particular cancer now run lower than 10 percent.[61] The death rate from that cancer at the Kaiser Permanente care sites is less than half of the Hawaii death rate -- based on last year's SEER data.

So there are obvious differences in the survival rate for various cancers by care site, and there are even very real differences in survival rates by state. We need to recognize that those difference exist and then we need to collectively look very closely at the sobering fact that none of those significant differences in care outcomes or in survival rates is relevant in any way to the business model we use today to buy care. We do not buy care well.

We don't base our payment for cancer care today in any way on the outcomes of that care. In fact -- the relationship between the cost of that care and the outcomes is sometimes absolutely the reverse of what you would want to see in a well-designed business model for care. Some of the highest cost care sites have life expectancies for cancer treatment that are clearly inferior to some of the lower cost sites. The business model we use to buy care would not survive in any other industry. We don't pay for cure. We buy cancer care by the piece and we pay for procedures. We currently pay the cancer care businesses cash by the piece to do procedures -- and we do not pay to save lives. We pay for services -- not results. And we don't even reward better results when they do exist. Some of the procedures that are used by some of the lower performing care sites are clearly more effective in creating cash flow for the business site than in creating cures for the care site. That is obviously a flawed, inferior, and dysfunctional way to purchase cancer care.

If you personally have cancer of some kind, and if you want to survive, information about the success levels of various caregivers can be highly relevant to your life. You should look to getting cancer car from care teams that continuously improve their cancer care. You may actually improve your chances of survival by moving to a state with better cancer outcomes. Care results differ by care site, the state where you receive care, and the results even differ by region within a state.

In the state of Georgia, for example, the patients in rural Georgia and the patients in the city of Atlanta, have very different mortality rates.

The next chart shows the death rates by states from two other cancers -- with mortality levels and life expectancy data shown, again, for several geographic areas. Prostate cancer and colorectal cancers are among the most common cancers in the country.

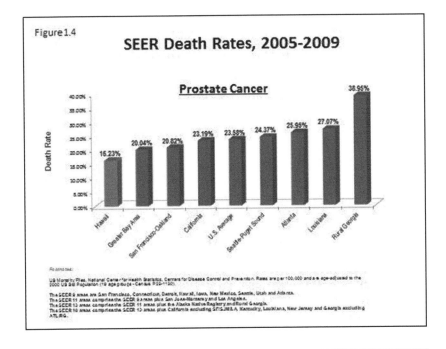

Figure 1.4

SEER Death Rates, 2005-2009

Prostate Cancer

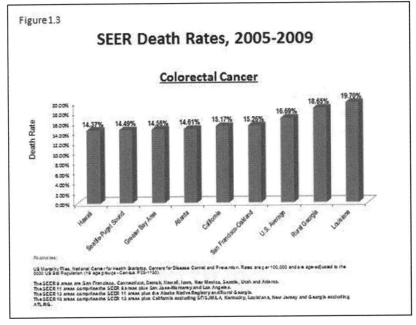

Figure 1.3

SEER Death Rates, 2005-2009

Colorectal Cancer

Those charts also show the mortality results for those cancers that are achieved by some of the best care sites in the SEER database. As was the case with breast cancer, the death rates for those same cancers in the best performing SEER sites are significantly lower than the national average survival rate for the cancers.

One of the things we can conclude from all of that data is that when care is delivered in a systematic and science-based way by an integrated care system like Kaiser Permanente, or the Mayo Clinic, results for these care teams tend to be significantly better than the results from the average community cancer sites.

A SEER-format study done of the cancer death rates for Kaiser Permanente for Southern California, for example, showed a mortality rate of under 10 percent for prostate cancer. That is a number far below the national average. [62]

So why would a care team like the caregivers of Kaiser Permanente have better cancer survival rates? Early detection and best science are both more likely to happen in a care team setting.

Kaiser Permanente is an integrated care system that has medical best practices embedded into its care support systems. Kaiser Permanente has one of the largest electronic medical record support systems in the world and the Kaiser Permanente care team places a very high priority on early detection of cancers. Kaiser Permanente also places a very high priority on using the best care protocols to cure the cancers once they are detected. The results of that early detection and that best practice medical approach are shown on the following charts for prostate and colorectal cancer. Focused care improvement strategies have their obvious positive results. Systematic cancer care detection and treatment in that integrated care context clearly results in a death rate in that particular care system that is significantly lower than the national average for those cancers.

So, major differences in outcomes exist for the care of basic cancers. Unfortunately, that information about differences in death rates is invisible to cancer patients it is also invisible and to most care sites that treat cancer patients. That information also isn't part of the business model that we use in this country for purchasing cancer care.

Cancer isn't alone in having variable care outcomes.

That same level of mortality rate variation that exists for cancer care happens for other areas like heart care, diabetes care, and stroke related care. Your personal chances of dying from a stroke or a heart attack or an amputation are all significantly higher if you go to one of the higher risk care sites for your care. Again, your personal risk of dying from a stroke can literally double depending on your site of care.

Better Care Isn't Accidental -- It Is Intentional

An important thing for us all to remember is that better care isn't accidental. Better care is also not simple serendipity or blind luck. Better care is very deliberate and intentional. The best care sites not only have better survival rates for those key conditions -- the caregivers at those best sites work to continuously improve their survival levels. The best care teams use data, process engineering, best science, and process reengineering approaches in a very deliberate and intentional way to make care better. Stroke death rates have gone down consistently at the best care sites...and that has happened because those sites are committed to continuously improving their care. Those death rates have decreased because those intentional, deliberate, and organized care sites use a combination of data, care tracking, and care improvement to make care better.

At many other care sites, the stroke death rate hasn't dropped at all over the past few years. Some sites have gotten worse. In a very perverse and unfortunate way, the business model we usually use to buy care in this country tends to generate more cash flow to the care sites that deliver the worst care. Death rates vary and those variances can be very perversely rewarded from the perspective of creating cash flow for caregivers.

The worst sites can often charge the most money for care because the patients in those settings generally need care longer and because those patients in the least effective sites spend more time in the most intensive care settings.

Both Patients and Caregivers Need Data

So, unfortunately, patients do not have enough information today to make good care site choices, and the care sites, themselves, are also almost data-free. Poorly performing care sites often have no clue at any level that their care results are suboptimal. In fact, the most data-free care sites in this country tend to have a very consistent belief that they are all delivering best care. That isn't intentional deception or even willful self-deception. Caregivers are all very well intentioned people. Too many data-free caregivers tend to believe that being well intentioned is the functional equivalent of being an optimal, high-performing care site. Those care sites beliefs about the relative quality of the care they are producing is often completely and even tragically wrong –- but those beliefs die very hard in those care settings without data.

So we need key pieces of data. We need to know mortality rates. We need to know sepsis cure rates and stroke survival rates. We need to know five-year cancer survival rates. We need to know that information by the site of care and by the care teams so that care sites and care teams that do not have the best results initially can make the changes needed to subsequently achieve the very best results.

We will have that data if we change the way we buy care. Ideally, the market model for care should pay the best providers more money for better outcomes and safer care and the business model we use to buy care should channel larger numbers of patients to the care sites with the best outcomes.

Our Current Business Model Rewards Failure and Bad Outcomes

The truth is -- the business model we use to pay for care in this country doesn't work at all to reduce and improve those deadly variations in the mortality rate and in the quality of care. This point was made earlier, but it bears repeating. The hard truth is, caregivers in this country generally make more collective money as an infrastructure when care goes wrong. Bad care can be very profitable. Look again at the quality data variation levels that are known today about care delivery.

Pressure ulcers are a perfect example of the perverse way we pay for care today. Seven percent of the hospital patients, on average, end up with a pressure ulcer in American hospitals.[63] The best hospital care sites in this country now have less than one percent of their patients getting pressure ulcers. The very worst care sites have upwards of ten percent of their patients getting pressure ulcers.[64]

Ten percent ought to be regarded as an unforgivable number. Seven percent should also not be an acceptable percentage by hospital care teams.

Some of the very best hospital care sites have managed to go for more than a year without one single stage-two or higher pressure ulcer.[65] Not one. That is amazing patient-centered, patient-focused care.

Patients who get those ulcers are often in great pain. Some are damaged for life. Some are badly disfigured. Some die. Getting a pressure ulcer is not a good thing for a hospital patient.

So how does the business model we use now to pay for care deal with those major differences in performance for care sites relative to pressure ulcers?

Very badly or very well — depending on whether you are paying for those ulcers or charging fees to treat these ulcers.

Care actually costs a lot more at the worst care sites. Those sites get paid more money because they deliver bad care. A lot more cash flows to the very worst care sites. Patients are individually damaged at those worst care sites and the way we buy care today, the sad truth is that the cash flow for those poorly performing care sites increases significantly as their care deteriorates.

More Patients Survive at the Best Sites

By contrast -- a lot less money is spent at the best sites, and more patients survive at those best sites. The surviving patients in those best care sites also tend to suffer significantly less damage from their ulcers when those kinds of ulcers do occur. Those patients suffer less permanent damage because the care teams at those best sites do much faster and more competent interventions when ulcers happen. Care is better, faster, more focused, and much safer.

The best hospitals have care teams who intervene before the new ulcers deteriorate. So the best hospitals have patients who are much less likely to have those ulcers, and the best hospitals also have patients who are much more likely to both survive the ulcer and have full physical recovery -- suffering less lifetime damage, crippling, and scarring from their ulcers.

As noted above, those best hospitals also make a lot less money from each ulcer patient and from pressure ulcers, overall. Based on the way we buy care today in this country, the reward for doing well is to get paid less.

We actually pay the worst care sites far more money per patient. A bad pressure ulcer can add from $20,000 to $100,000 to a hospital bill. The average bill is now close to $40,000.[66] A bad pressure ulcer can result in multiple additional therapies, additional treatments, and extended recovery programs and -- relatively often -- the patients who survive really bad ulcers then also need expensive and purely remedial plastic surgery.

What is particularly frustrating for the very best care systems is that the very best care not only results in lower hospital use, it also involves doing multiple very important very specific things for their patients that are not reimbursed by a standard insurance piecework payment fee schedule.

This book has a couple of sections that explain the dysfunctional consequences and the perverse and rigid patterns of care that can result from buying care entirely by the piece -- when the pieces of care that are paid for are defined by a fixed insurer-developed and approved fee schedule. Buying care only by the piece rewards volumes of pieces. That payment approach doesn't reward care outcomes or care improvement. It simply rewards care volume. When care is purchased by the piece, it tends to be delivered by the piece and it is designed and structured to be delivered by the piece.

When care is purchased entirely by the piece, doing smart things to reengineer the delivery of care is often penalized. How is doing something smart penalized? Only the pieces of care that are defined by the fee schedule and have a "CPT" code tend to happen in the real world of care. Because that is time, the caregivers who are paid by the piece tend not to improve care by redesigning any of the basic processes of care.

Why is that issue relevant to pressure ulcers?

The work that is done in those best hospitals to keep patients from getting pressure ulcers is almost obsessive work. It is very hard work relative to screening, protecting, and responding quickly to the potential care needs of hospitalized patients. The work of preventing pressure ulcers involves multiple care steps and is very intense. None of those patient-focused intensive care steps have a billing code and are paid for by a Medicare or insurance fee schedule.

Not one of the steps involved in scanning patients, screening patients, replacing bedding for patients, or applying ointments and medications to patients at exactly the right time show up as source of payment on any of those insurance fee schedules. Those key and essential steps do not count as billable work. So the hospitals that actually do that work who are paid only by the piece for their care receive no money from their insurers or from the government for doing that work.

By contrast, if that work is not done or if it is not done well and if a hospitalized patient gets one of those ulcers, the payers who use the insurance fee schedules to define the care they pay for will cough up an average of $40,000 in fees to the care site for each pressure ulcer patient.

The perversity of being paid nothing for perfect care and being paid a lot of money for crippling, disfiguring, damaging, painful and sometimes fatal care is really obvious once people realize how badly we actually buy most care in this country today and how dysfunctional that fee code process is relative to buying care.

We get what we pay for. We also do not -- most of the time -- get what we do not pay for. A few great care sites have shown what can be done to reengineer care to get better results in a number of areas of care improvement. As we pay for care today, the number of sites who do that care improvement work is not very large.

The piecework way we pay for care today encourages care complexity. The way we pay for care discourages care both process optimization and efficiency-focused care redesign. The way we buy care also discourages care teams or care sites making significant improvements in care outcomes in multiple areas of care.

We almost always buy care in this country by the piece. That's our basic business model for care. We use a piecework payment model. Buying by the piece is often a very perverse way to pay for care. Each and every remedial procedure needed for an ulcer patient who already has an ulcer creates a billable event and significant cash flow is triggered for the current infrastructure of care based on that piecework payment model. Doing all the things needed to keep those ulcers from happening are not accepted as billable sources by the fee schedule that is usually used to pay for approved care -- so very few fee-based care sites do that preventive work.

Health Care Is Built Around Billable Events

Billable events are the key point to understand. Chapter Four of this book discusses that in greater detail. Health care, delivery, infrastructure and performance in any fee-based payment system are all very directly built around billable events. People who deliver care know that to be true. Billable events have immense power. Billable events sculpt and even dictate the behaviors, the functions, the structure, the infrastructure, and the operational model that creates the financial and economic realities of American health care.

More Than 1.7 Million Patients Get Infections

Bad care pays well. That isn't just true of pressure ulcers. It is true of just about every category of hospital acquired infections. It is also true of asthma crises, congestive heart failure crises, and heart attacks. Bad outcomes actually increase cash flow.

The truth is, more than 1.7 million Americans enter hospitals every year and then get an infection that they did not have on the day they entered the hospital.[67] Many of these patients die. All suffer. Many are damaged. Some are crippled for life.

Those are not good infections. They are really hard on people. They happen a lot. We know how often this happens. They happen to one point seven million people every year.

How does the American system of care purchasing deal with all of the infections that are acquired at those care sites?

Perversely.

It's the same reality as the cash flow that is triggered by heart attacks, strokes, and congestive heart failures. Bad outcomes generate revenue. Infections create cash flow. Infections, in fact, usually pay really well.

No Hospital Deliberately Infects Anyone

No hospital in America would ever intentionally infect a patient. That absolutely does not happen. That will not happen. No one needs to fear that anything of that sort will ever happen in any American hospital. The ethics of basic care delivery in this country are far too strong and the morality levels of our caregivers are too high for any intentional damage or any intentional infections to ever happen in any American care site. American hospitals never intentionally damage any patients.

However -- it is also true that more than one and half million Americans actually did get those hospital acquired infections in American hospitals last year.[68] Those patients literally did not have those infections the day they were admitted to the hospital. They happened in the hospital. So the question we need to ask is -- are those infections inevitable?

Are those infections simply something that we all need to live with as an inherent functional reality of hospital care?

The answer is -- No.

We know for a fact that the very best care sites can and do take steps to both bring down the rate of those infections and to alleviate the damage to the patients when they do occur. The very best care sites now intervene much more effectively and quickly to decrease the damage done by those infections when they do happen. Hospitals can -- with the right processes -- make those infections very rare. Some of the best hospitals have managed to eliminate some of those infections for months at a time. In some cases, the very best sites can eliminate some of those infections for entire years.

It is possible to achieve very aggressive infection reduction goals -- and yet the reality is that relatively few hospitals actually do the fully dedicated, intense, process-focused infection prevention work that is needed to make those infections disappear. That work by the hospitals can have a huge positive impact that reduces both care costs and patient damage -- but it is not the consistent level of care that exists everywhere in American hospitals today.

In some cases -- like sepsis -- the germ that causes the infection is usually acquired outside the hospital and the main job of the hospital is to diagnose the sepsis infection very quickly when it occurs and then treat the sepsis patients at warp speed. That work, to improve sepsis care, really needs to be done at hospitals all across the country.

The Number One Cause of Hospital Death -- Sepsis -- Is Often Not an Operational Focus for Hospitals

Sepsis is actually the number one cause of death in American hospitals today.[69] Sepsis kills. As noted earlier, sepsis infections of the bloodstream kill more patients in American hospitals than cancer, heart disease or stroke.[70] A Californian study showed that one in five seniors who died in California hospitals actually died of sepsis.[71]

So sepsis is a huge and widespread problem. It kills a lot of people. It damages and cripples many more. The key is to respond to the infection quickly and well. The very best sepsis response programs in hospitals can cut the death rate significantly. Those sites can reduce the death rate from nearly 30 percent to under 10 percent and can also reduce the lifetime damage done to sepsis patients by major amounts.[72] So how does the business model we use today to buy care in this country deal with sepsis?

Very poorly. We don't reward good sepsis care in any way. We also don't penalize bad sepsis care. With only a few notable exceptions, we don't insist on best practices being in place for sepsis care. Sepsis generates a lot of cash flow for hospitals. Just like the pressure ulcers. Each patient with a bad case of sepsis can end up with a bill that is a multiple of the normal cost expected for that patient based on their original admission diagnosis and disease. A five thousand dollar patient can become a fifty thousand dollar patient or even a hundred thousand dollar patient if the sepsis infection for that patient is diagnosed slowly and if the treatment for the patient is delayed.

The Sepsis Death Rate Can Be Cut in Half

So what can be done about sepsis? At least half of the sepsis deaths can be prevented.

Speed is the key. As noted earlier, the key issue for sepsis actually isn't prevention. The issue for sepsis is immediate intervention.

The very best care sites know that sepsis responds really well to rapid diagnosis, rapid response and rapid care. Sepsis experts refer to the "golden hour" when sepsis death rates can be cut in half with the right care.[73]

This is an area where process engineering and process reengineering can be magical and extremely effective.

The right care for sepsis patients involves setting up the work flow in the hospital so that the laboratory processes in the hospital run the needed sepsis tests for each suspected patient in minutes, rather than hours. The right care involves having the right medicines ready for use immediately for sepsis patients -- instead of having the pharmacies in each hospital simply putting those medicines together in a reactive way for each sepsis patient after the fact when a sepsis diagnosis has been made for the patient. In hospitals where the needed medication isn't prepackaged, the pharmacists are too often only filling those life-saving sepsis care prescriptions and medication kits as part of their normal work flow for all current pharmacy requests in their hospital. When you need to treat a sepsis patient inside of an hour to save the patient's life and when the hospital's pharmacy normal response time to fill a normal medication request from a doctor is two to four hours, that normal response time frame in the pharmacy clearly isn't optimal for the sepsis patients who need the right life-saving medication in their body immediately. The science is clear. The biology is well known. The very best hospitals very much know that speedy response is needed and so the very best hospitals simply prepackage the needed supplies for their sepsis patients to have the medication ready for each patient in minutes rather than hours.

Basic Process Engineering Saves a Lot of Lives

It isn't rocket science. That is very basic process engineering. It is basic process engineering targeted at significantly reducing the impact of the number one cause of death in American hospitals.

That sepsis quick-response reengineering approach works really well. It should be done everywhere in the world where patients get hospital care and need to be treated for sepsis. The state of New York is doing some important primary work in requiring sepsis care improvements. Other states should study their approach.

As the number one killer in American hospitals, sepsis obviously deserves special treatment by each hospital care team. Doing care right for sepsis patients literally drops the death rate from upwards of 30 percent of those patients in the most challenged hospitals to under 10 percent in the best hospitals.[74]

As noted earlier, the business model we use now to pay for care pays the hospitals with the worst sepsis survival rate the most money. Those hospitals are expensive and deadly.

Most hospitals today do not have those very basic life-saving care processes in place for the number one cause of death in hospitals. That is clearly not good for all of the patients who do get sepsis in those hospitals. Hospitals have very different outcome levels for their sepsis patients. Again -- as is true for cancer mortality rates and for heart surgery survival rates -- the death rate from sepsis varies a lot based on the care site you choose.[75]

We Make Five Million Prescription Mistakes As Well

We also make other medical mistakes in our care infrastructure. Some experts estimate that our total health care infrastructure squanders about 30 cents of every dollar spent by delivering inappropriate care. If that is true, that would be $750 billion that the American public now spends every year without getting better care.[76]

In addition to the problems of inappropriate care -- we have an amazingly large and undebatable problem with functional and operational screwups and mistakes. Care appropriateness can be an issue where multiple opinions are legitimate. Care screwups have no legitimate defenders.

In the real world of care delivery, operational mistakes happen at an amazing level. Studies have said that there are more than 5,000,000 prescription drug mistakes made in the delivery of care in this country each year.[77] Five million is a big number. Patients are damaged by many of the mistakes. Again -- as with weak sepsis care and bad heart care -- the cash flow for the overall infrastructure of care increases when those mistakes are made.

People would like to believe that those problems do not exist. Pretending will not make them go away.

The Joint Commission's National Patient Safety committee -- a well-intentioned organization studying these issues -- now estimates that the damage level done to patients actually runs about 25 damaging events for every 100 admissions in our current infrastructure of care.

We clearly can do better. This is not the level of care delivery we should be getting when we spend two point seven trillion dollars to buy care. We need safer care, more consistent care, better coordinated care, and we absolutely need more affordable care. This book is about the cost of care... and -- as the examples above point out fairly clearly -- the really good news is that better care usually costs less.

Care is clearly less affordable for everyone when we reward bad outcomes with additional money. Care is obviously less affordable and less valuable when we reward care delivery errors with a rich flow of cash.

How can we make a difference in those areas?

We Need To Improve the Data Flow for Care

This chapter is intended to point out some of the issues that we need to address as problems for care delivery in this country.

The next chapter outlines some of the functionality and successes that we should expect and receive from the care delivery infrastructure of this country.

Before going to the chapter on how care delivery should function, we need to be very clear on one very important problem area. Data.

We have massive data deficits in our care delivery today. Data and quality are linked. Data is a basic, fundamental tool that we need to improve processes and products in any industry. Health care is no exception.

As this chapter noted earlier, we now have painfully inadequate data about care performance in far too many areas of performance. The good news is, when the right data exists, that data can have a very powerful impact on care delivery. The chart below shows the drop in the death rate from sepsis in an array of hospitals that put rapid response teams in place and spent time to put a continuous improvement process in place to refine sepsis care and make it better over time.

They started with data.

The numbers shown on the chart are the results for all of the hospitals in that care system. The care system actually tracked performance sequentially on sepsis death rates for each of the three dozen hospitals. The initial numbers for the sepsis death rate showed a variation between hospitals that more than doubled the success difference between the best and the lowest performing hospitals.

No one in that entire hospital system knew that the level of variation existed before the data was collected. All the hospitals on that chart believed they were doing great work on sepsis care. They were all extremely well-intentioned people, and everyone believed they were doing great work because they were doing what they knew how to do and doing it with good intentions.

Good intentions, it turns out, was not as useful as good data. That data about relative death rates was a golden gift for the lowest performing hospitals because it woke them up to very real and immediate opportunities that existed for saving lives. Caregivers like to save lives. People become caregivers to save lives. That comparative data helped those hospitals and those caregivers accomplish that goal at a level they could not have attained without data.

The data was needed by each hospital. Data was the key. That really is an important point to understand -- and it extends to a great many areas of care performance. People are well-intentioned everywhere. Being well-intentioned is not enough.

Figure 1.5

FOR ILLUSTRATIVE PURPOSES ONLY

Sepsis Mortality Rates

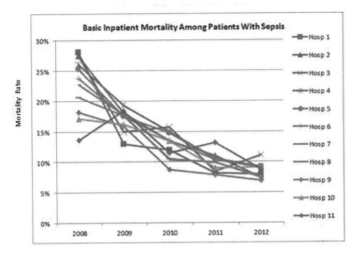

Each of the hospitals in that care system who improved sepsis care year by year could not begin to do that work until they had real data about their own sepsis death rates and then put together real data about each step of the sepsis related care process inside the hospital.

Those hospitals now know exactly how many minutes it took -- on average -- to get the lab test for sepsis care for each of the care units. Those hospitals know -- in minutes -- the average time it took to get the needed medications to each patient. Real processes are being measured and real processes are being continuously improved.

Care got a lot better when that total package of data-supported work was done. Lives were saved. Data anchored that process. Without honest and competent data, that work would have been impossible, and those lives would not have been saved.

Most care sites do not have that kind of data. Most care sites also don't keep track of performance for their asthma patients and their congestive heart failure patients. Most care sites do not have the ability to have the entire data about each patient or the ability to have comparative date about all patients.

Aggregate data saves lives. Patient-centered, complete data saves even more lives. Caregivers can deliver better care when caregivers are better informed. We have major deficits relative to the tool kits needed to do that work. We need to use the business model for care to help bring these tools into care delivery.

We Need To Improve Population Health

The business model we use to buy care also does an extremely weak job of dealing with issues of population health. The introduction to this book described that problem briefly. It is a major deficiency. We are facing an explosion of obesity in this country.[78] Inactivity levels are also increasing and, the sad truth is, inactivity levels are now at life-threatening high levels.[79]

The next chart shows the increase in the number of diabetics in America. As the introduction to this book pointed out, people with diabetes now use more than 40 percent of the total care dollars spent by Medicare.[80]

Good research tells us that -- on average -- only 25 percent of all people with diabetes are getting the full care agenda they need.[81] Diabetes is the number one cause of kidney failure, amputation and blindness in America[82] -- and the sad truth is that we get care right for Americans diabetic patients less than half of the time across the full infrastructure of care in America.[83]

Getting care right for diabetics should be a high priority. And -- if we really want to do the right thing at the most effective level for both diabetes costs and overall care costs in America -- we obviously also should be taking very specific steps that can go upstream in the disease development process to successfully prevent the disease. We need fewer people to become diabetic. That is possible. We can and should do very important things that could reduce the number of new diabetics in this country by half or more.

Figure 1.6

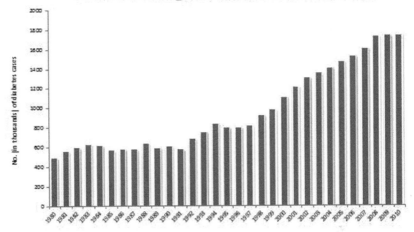

Annual Number of U.S. Adults Aged 18-79 Years with Diagnosed Diabetes, 1980-2010

Source: Centers for Disease Control and Prevention (CDC), http://www.cdc.gov/diabetes/statistics/incidence/fig1.htm

Prevention Can Have Short-Term Rewards

This point isn't theoretical or hypothetical or ideological. It is very practical work that should be done more broadly very soon. Contrary to the belief of many people, prevention is not a long-term strategy that has no short-term benefit. People used to believe that prevention interactions with patient populations would only have a payback and a positive financial return years down the road. Those people are now wrong. That long-term payback scenario was true for some earlier levels of population health improvements, but that benefit time frame isn't true for the strategies we are building today. We now know that we can actually do some short-term behavior change work and we can achieve significant reductions in both disease levels and disease costs that happen fairly quickly because that work was done.

We now know that several basic behavioral changes can have major impact and those basic changes can result in positive financial paybacks in weeks and months -- not just in years or even decades.

Diabetes itself can actually be reversed for some patients -- just by increasing activity levels for those patients. That is extremely important information to know -- particularly in the face of another belief system that said diabetes was permanent as a health status for all type-two diabetic patients and that any positive impacts of behavior changes for prediabetic patients happened over decades and not months.

The final chapter of this book addresses several very practical strategies we can use to achieve a set of important health improvement goals.

Some very important people in Washington, D.C., are beginning to put some important programs in place to help this country deal with both the issues of inactivity and the issues of obesity. When the first draft of this book was written, those programs did not exist.

Today, they are in existence and growing in both scope and effectiveness. We will have a deficit as a country relative to improving our population health, but we are beginning to address those issue. There is reason for optimism that we will address those issues a county with an increasing level of commitment and competency.

We Need a Better Business Model for Buying Care

Overall -- looking at all the issues addressed in this chapter -- we clearly need to change the business model we use to buy care to achieve the goals we want to achieve in care delivery. We will not do better, and we will not get better until we recognize clearly and explicitly how challenged we are today in many areas of care delivery. We need to stop pretending that all care is good care and that all American care is automatically the best care.

This chapter had pointed out major differences in care outcomes and care delivery success levels. This chapter has also pointed out that care can too often be both unsafe and destructive.

We need to deal very directly with those issues.

So what should we do? We need to fix the business model of care so that we can buy what we want to buy in care delivery and spend less money in the process.

We also need to change the business model we use to buy care so caregivers can take advantage of all of the opportunities to improve care without being financially penalized for their functionalized successes.

Caregivers all tend to be good and ethical people. The people who run the major care organizations all tend to be good and ethical people. We need to remember that reality as we change the way we buy care.

We Need a Better Model for Buying Care

The people who lead all of the health care organizations and who deliver care to all our people do not underperform because they want to underperform. They underperform because the business model we use to buy care pays well for the underperformance and it actually penalizes best care in far too many ways. It is possible to cut the number of broken bones, the number of heart attacks, and the number of stokes significantly. To make the point one more time, those successes are not rewarded by the way we buy care most of the time today. Cutting the number of strokes in half is great for patients, but that reduction in strokes creates massive revenues losses for the care sites who treat stoke patients.

We need to buy care in a way that incents the best care sites to cut the number of strokes in half and then also cuts the death rate and the damage levels for the people who have strokes in half. That level of care improvement is possible. The truth is, caregivers would love to be able to deliver that care -- so we need financial models that can free the health care infrastructure and the business unit of care to do that work without being financially damaged.

Our strategy needs to be to make some very basic changes in the business model and the cash flow for care to empower and reward caregivers for giving us the care outcomes and the care costs that we need.

What Would an Optimal Care Delivery Approach Look Like?

Before proposing any changes in the business model to address the problems that have been outlined in this chapter, it clearly makes sense to achieve some clarity about what we will actually want the new business model of care to achieve.

We need to begin with the end in mind. To be really smart purchasers of care, it is a good idea to have some clarity about what care we want to purchase. That thinking about what we want to achieve needs to be done first at a macro level. What are our macro goals for care delivery? And then we need to look at more immediate level of care delivery. We need to look at both macro care issues and micro care issues. How do we want care delivery to function at the individual level for care? What are our micro goals? What do we want care to do and look like for each individual patient?

We Can Build a Model To Buy Care When We Know What Care We Want To Buy

When we get clarity on both those micro and macro points, then it becomes a lot easier to define a design a business model that buys care in a way that causes the infrastructure of care and individual caregivers to meet those goals. Let's start with a sense of how good care could be if we got all of this right.

The next chapter outlines a set of tools, processes and commitments we might want to make an embedded part of care delivery that results from the business model we use to buy care in America.

So what should the care delivery infrastructure of the future of care look like?

We need to start by focusing on the patient.

Chapter Two

THE OPTIMAL CARE SYSTEM SHOULD BE THE GOAL OF THE BUSINESS MODEL WE USE TO BUY CARE

The most effective way of changing care delivery is to change the business model we use to buy care. We get what we pay for -- so if we want better, safer, more effective and more affordable care, we need to put in a place a business model that pays for better, safer, more effective and more affordable care.

Before we put in place any new business models to actually buy health care in this country, it's a good idea to think about what care we want to buy. We need to be very clear about what we want to achieve through the care delivery process before we change the way we buy care.

Clarity is a good thing for any buyer in any industry. Health care is a complex topic, so it is a particularly good idea to achieve some clarity about the overall care we want to buy before we start making either incremental or massive changes in the way we buy care.

Several macro purchasing goals are actually relatively easy to identify. Those purchasing goals can create a context that can help us think about all of the various elements and tools and products we can put in place to achieve those goals.

We Need Patient Focus and Continuous Improvement as Care Goals

For starters, we clearly need our care delivery to be more patient-focused. We also need care delivery to be safer, better coordinated, data-supported, and continuously improving. As the first chapter of this book pointed out, we should insist on continuous improvement as a foundational philosophy, skill set, and business model for American health care. We will only continuously improve care delivery if we consciously make continuous improvement a foundational goal of the business model we use to buy care and if we actually pay caregivers to continuously improve.

We also need to make affordability a major goal. The current market models obviously do not support or create affordability. We need affordability to be a key part of the thought process and the financial reality for caregivers. We need to very consciously make affordability a key component of the way we buy care in the future and we need to reward caregivers who provide affordable care.

The first chapter of this book outlined how dysfunctional, unsafe and inefficient that current care delivery reality often is. If we want better, superior, and more affordable results for the money we spend, then we need to be much more skillful in using the cash flow of care financing to make those better results happen.

Understanding, articulating and then clarifying the overall goals before building the basic set of tools to achieve those goals is a philosophy that has been learned, developed and field tested over three decades of direct experience being the CEO of one care system or another. The experience of the author in managing complex organizations for quite a few years has led to the deeply held belief that random change is rarely a good thing to do in any organizational setting. Piecework and incidental solutions can far too easily end up with unintended and dysfunctional consequences. Even the best intentioned piecework perspectives and unlinked and isolated solutions to subsets of complex situations can easily end up being unintentionally counterproductive and even equally unintentionally perverse relative to the processes we need to improve and the problems we need to solve.

First, We Need To Define the Goals

We need to look at the goals before we look at tools. It is amazingly easy to focus initially on tools instead of focusing on goals. Tools are fun. Tools seem to be easy to understand. Some of the most intriguing tools have their own seductive pull. There are some lovely and handy tools –- but if we focus just on tools instead of goals, we are likely to find ourselves with less than a complete solution set, and we can have a tool create its own momentum that may achieve some marginal benefit but not help us address in a systematic way the issues we need to resolve.

Far too many health care reform strategies today start purely with pieces of the solution set in mind and with specific tools instead of beginning the planning process by setting overall goals for optional care delivery and then figuring out what tools are needed to achieve these goals. People far too often focus on just one favorite tool and then believe that tool will be a magical solution for major portions of the health care problems we face.

Some people believe that the real problems of care delivery would be solved, for example, if we just had more primary care doctors. That point of view has a lot of supporters.

Other people believe with great passion that the problems of care in this country would be solved if we just had better electronic medical records in all of our care sites. Some very well intended people very strongly see having electronic data about care to be an end in itself. A few people believe that some of the new care monitoring portable tools and computer apps can fix care by improving specific pieces of care delivery.

The truth is, we could add quite a few primary care doctors to our total infrastructure of care and creating that additional primary care medical resource might solve absolutely nothing of any significance if we did not also change any of the key processes of care delivery and if we did not use that new resource well. Likewise, we clearly could computerize all care-related data, and we could then just as easily have that new computerized electronic care data functionality be useless -- either because that newly electronic data literally isn't used or because that new electronic data is not used well.

The new computer applications could give us a nice set of targeted data then -- but if it isn't linked to a care plan and care team of some kind, it can be just another interesting data silo.

Primary care doctors, electronic medical records and new care apps are each just care improvement tools. They are not endpoints or solutions in their own right. We need to understand our real endpoints in order to solve the issues we need to solve in health care. We need to understand and clearly define our actual fundamental care delivery goals and then we can figure out how both electronic medical records and primary physicians and a broad array of other highly useful tools can all combine in some important, strategic and functional ways to help us to achieve that clearly defined set of care improvement goals.

The Patient Needs To Be the Center of the Care System

So what should we want to achieve with the care system in this country and what tools do we need to put in place to make that improved care system a reality?

Let's start with the patient.

As our very first priority, the patient should be at the core and the center of our care delivery system. The patient needs to be at the center of the reform thought process and at the center of basic care delivery functionality. Being patient-centered should be a key first priority of our planning process and our business model for care.

When you look at the good things we want to accomplish, with the care delivery in this country, we obviously need patient-centered care to anchor that agenda. We don't have patient-centered care today. Care today is focused far too often on the business needs of caregivers. Care delivery is centered on the infrastructure functionalities and the operational realities of the caregiver business units. That is the wrong focus. That focus gives us far too many of the dysfunctional processes that are embedded in the current delivery mechanisms for care.

The basic premise of this chapter and this book is that we need to start with the patient as both the center of our planning process and as the strategic focus for functional care delivery. We need to design the sites of care and the tools we use to support care very clearly around the patients who will be receiving care.

That seems obvious -- but it isn't the way we usually set up processes and care sites and data flow today.

It would be a mistake to simply perpetuate a care infrastructure that is built primarily around provider cash flow. We also don't want to continue to support a care infrastructure that is structured most heavily around the convenience or the functionally of caregiver business entities.

Patient-centered care should center our thought processes.

Being patient centered is not an idealistic, theoretical, ideological, rhetorical, or even a politically correct top priority goal for health care delivery planning. It is common sense. Patient-centering is actually a highly practical and extremely functional operational anchor for care design. Speaking from decades of experience in designing and implementing care delivery processes, the author knows that building on that patient-centered focus is extremely useful in very productive terms in putting together the tool kits and the data flows that are needed to support care. Centering the care we create on the patient is actually a highly functional and practical way to think about the processes of care. That focus and priority creates and sets up a very practical operational context for figuring out what to do and how to do it in the functional delivery of care. With that patient-focused goal in mind, we can design both the processes and the key tools that are needed for patient-focused care delivery. It is very much the right focus and the right first priority to center our planning on the patients.

That should be an easily understood goal and it can be very useful as we figure out the rest of the key elements we need to enhance in care delivery.

Care Should Be About Patients

Care is, of course, inherently about patients. To improve care delivery, we need to understand and focus on the needs of the patient as the rightful center of the care processes we build and use. Care happens to patients and care is done to patients. Care meets the needs of patients. The tools that are made available to caregivers should improve the ability of the caregivers to meet patient needs.

Our data collection should follow that exact same top priority -- with a clear focus for our data on the patient.

Data Should Be Patient-Focused

We need the data base planning and the operational reality for care delivery to be focused on the absolutely clear goal of having all of the data about each patient available to the patient's caregivers in convenient and usable ways at the point of care when it is needed for the patient's care. Care is much better when caregivers have all of the information about their patients at the time of care. Mortality rates improve when caregivers have a high level of patient-centered data. We need to design our care support tools with that goal in mind. Our data flow between all of the electronic storage sites for care data should be set up and designed to achieve that goal of patient-centered care -- with the data flow set up to optimize the care delivered to individual patients.

Patient-Centered Care Isn't Our Usual Organizations Model

The key operational unit in any combination of care delivery processes and care delivery data flows should be the patient who is receiving the care. That guideline seems obvious and even simplistic -- but it actually is not how we usually organize care data or care in this country today. The bad, dysfunctional, wasteful, disrespectful, ineffective, inefficient and sometimes counterproductive care delivery processes we see far too often in far too many places in health care delivery are usually the processes that have been built around the care delivery business units and not around the patient. Patients are often badly served, inconvenienced, and even sometimes insulted and demeaned at a basic, human level by some of the existing procedures and by a number of the care-related processes that are functionally focused on caregiver business units instead of on patients. Good processes should be centered on patients and good processes should have the care delivery infrastructure able to support the needs of each patient. To make that focus successful, the flow of data should be set up so that the data follows the patient and is available to the caregivers at the point of care.

Today, most of the time -- when patients get care, their caregivers have incomplete data about the patient's full set of medical information. That problem of incomplete data exists because health care data today is not patient-centered. Health care data is care site-centered. That data availability model is not the best way to use data to improve care.

The business model we use to buy care should help make both that patient focus by the care teams and that patient-centered data flow happen.

So being patient-centered should be a key first priority for our planning processes and for the new business model we use to buy care. When anyone purposes any changes in the way we deliver care, ask the simple question -- will the data that results from this piece of care flow in practical and usable way to a data tool that will allow that data to be accessed the next time this patient receives care? If the answer to that question is no, then the process should be improved until the answer is yes.

Care Delivery Should Benefit Financially By Meeting Patients Needs

The second priority of the new business model we use to buy care should be to enable caregivers to benefit financially by meeting the needs of their patients for continuously improving and hugely affordable care. That goal of having care providers benefit financially from the new approaches is an absolute necessity if we want any significant new approach to succeed. We need to incorporate the explicit goal of having caregivers benefit from both continuous improvement and affordability into our business model redesign or the redesign will fail. That approach can be done. If we set the new business model up correctly, the caregivers will profit from doing intelligent care redesign. If we set the model up well, our caregivers will also benefit financially from skillfully using and optimizing the amazing new tool kit of care support tools that are coming into existence to support the delivery of care. We have wonderful opportunities in front of us to improve access to care and to improve care delivery functionality in patient-friendly ways. New tools are being developed every day. We will have wonderful opportunities to use those new care support tools to make care more affordable. As you will read later in this chapter, there are some very impressive and existing new care support tools coming into existence. Unfortunately, because of the piecework approach we use to buy care today, the current business model of care delivery actually tends to resist those tools. The current caregivers far too often create both significant barriers and sometimes crippling impediments to the use of those new care support tools.

In-home monitoring tools, electronic medical visits with physicians and nurses, remote diagnosis support tools and electronically connected care follow up processes all can make huge sense for patients. A whole generation of those tools is emerging daily. That's the good news. The bad news is that the effective use of far too many of those new care support tools and approaches can be crippled, detoured, and even stifled by the way we buy care. We need to set up a financial model that encourages and rewards our care providers for using those tools and using them well -- instead of using a financial model to buy care that penalizes our caregivers when those tools are used.

The Patient Focus Should Drive Decision Making

With that patient focus as our goal for both care and caregivers, we need a cash flow for care and a model of care that has the patient as the focus of a fully functioning and continuously improving care system.

As part of that strategy, we need to free the key care sites from their current financial addiction to piecework fees. Multiple studies have shown that current care delivery is motivated and activated far too often more by the existence of a billable technology than by the actual patient need for that technology. There was an all too familiar scandal last year when Medicare discovered it had a lot of hospitals doing double CT scans for all of their

Medicare patients.[84] Those double scans were clearly incented by revenue stream goals for the care sites rather than the care needs of the patients. Horror stories about unneeded and even dangerous care approaches exist and abound. Horror stories about unnecessary surgery, useless and expensive procedures, and care delivery activity volumes that create no improvement in patient care can be found in multiple books and reports. We don't need to repeat those horror stories about unnecessary and sometimes dangerous care in this book. Other books have written clearly about those problems. The Institute of Medicine has published a couple of very powerful books that clearly address those issues.

As we build a new business model that we can use to buy care, we need to embed in that model the fact that patients need data-supported care. We also need to embed in that model very direct support for team care. Most care costs in this country come from patients who have chronic conditions and multiple care needs. We know very clearly that the patients who have both chronic conditions and comorbidities very much need data-supported team care. We clearly do not want a business model for care that continues to create real barriers to team care, coordinated care, and to care that is well supported by the next generation of innovative and flexible care support tools. Instead, we need a business model for care that reaches out and effectively uses the various technological improvements in the way we distribute care that are becoming available to us. We want optimal, patient-focused, continuously improving processes for care…with patient needs trumping care business unit billing priorities.

We Need Patient-Centered Data

Data will be a key tool to achieve those goals. Having the right levels of data about care delivery also needs to be a top priority for the way we buy care. We need to be very clear and very insistent that the right flow of data happens and that the data that is collected is used to improve care.

The last chapter outlined a number of process engineered care improvements that have saved many lives and kept people from a lifetime of damage and harm. Those systematic care improvement programs succeeded because those care sites had key pieces of data. Those successes could not have happened without that data. We need both outcomes-based care data and we need patient-centered data so we can create and enhance patient-centered care.

Those two data collection goals should clearly dictate our design of both data-gathering approaches and data flow to a very large degree. We need to start the care improvement process with patient data. We need all of the information about each patient flowing from site to site with full care-related information about each patient available in real time when that information about each patient is needed by the care team that is delivering care to each patient.

Caregivers can do a much better job in taking care of patients when all of the care information about a given patients is available to the caregiver at the point of care. Having that kind of shared information created a tool kit that has dropped the HIV death rates for one huge care team to half the national average.[85] That level of shared information has simultaneously cut the number of broken bones in seniors treated by that care team by over a third.[86] Those care improvements happened in a large integrated care setting and they were possible because those caregivers have a fully functioning electronic medical record in place. The medical record for that care team has all of that data for each patient and their systems make that data about each patient available in real time to support their caregivers. The approach works. Lives are saved. Care is better because the caregivers have better information and have it in real time.

We need to be very clear about the need to achieve that same data availability goal and tool kit for each patient in all of our care settings in this country. That level of data-supported care should not be limited to a small number of virtually limited care settings.

We need to set a national goal to make that level of care support possible for all of our caregivers and all of our patients.

That need for an available care database and the value that tool kit creates when it is ready for use for each patient by caregivers at the point of care seems painfully obvious when you understand functionally and operationally how to deliver the best care and how to use those tools to actually improve care. But that organizational approach to data flow is currently not how either databases or data flows exist in most care sites in this country today. We still accept data isolation as a reality in too many settings. That is clearly an area where we need to make some significant improvements.

Paper Medical Records Are Dangerous and Dysfunctional

We also, as a key priority for the future functionality of care delivery, need to be very clear about the need to move way from having major portions of the health care data base stored on paper. In this day and age, it seems almost a little odd to have to make that point in a book chapter about the future delivery model for health care functionality. The need to move away from the paper storage of data to electronic data storage seems to be almost too obvious to need to be mentioned in this chapter. But the sad truth is that most medical information in this country is still stored on paper rather than being stored in computers.

We need to change that data storage reality.

The care delivery system of the future needs interactive data about patients to deliver best care. Paper –- for obvious reasons -- has a very hard time being interactive.

When medical records are all on pieces of paper, then each of those pieces of paper and each data piece is inherently inert. The logistics of data isolation in a paper-based non-system are clear. Pieces of paper can't link with each other, and pieces of paper can't exchange data with each other. Paper medical records create a huge barrier to data sharing between caregivers. Paper records also make basic tracking of care quality and care outcomes extremely difficult.

At this point in our history, as the first chapter of this book pointed out, there is no excuse for that kind of data isolation and for that level of information segregation. Medical records can easily be electronic. Those are some great electronic medical records systems in use today in many sites and those tools are continuously improving. The data for each patient and each piece of care can easily be connected electronically when connectivity is part of the basic agenda -- when systems are put in place in the right ways, basic patient information should be able to flow to each and every other relevant care site for any given patient in real time. The technology exists to do that work today. The next generation of patient data files should be designed to be very much patient-centric and those data designs should be focused on creating care support tools that are built around the care needs of each patient.

Data Should Be Continuously Available

The new business model we use to buy care should demand -- as a basic condition of paying providers for the delivery of care -- that shared data be both available and actually shared. Any data isolation that exists for any reasons other than protecting patient confidentiality should be penalized -- not rewarded -- by the business model we use to buy care.

Data Should Be Built Around the Patient

As noted above, the patient needs to be the focus of our overall data strategy.

Data for the next generation of care obviously should be built around each patient -- so that we can meet the care needs of each patient in the most fully informed way.

Caregiver teams for each patient who needs caregiver teams should have easy, fully confidential and fully protected access to complete medical data about each patient that can be used to support their care.

That goal should be embedded in the business model we use to buy care. It is the right thing to buy. As noted earlier, some of the best computer-supported care sites in this country that already have that kind of patient-centered complete access to data have cut stroke deaths by nearly half.[87] Those care sites that have that level of available data and computerized care support tools sites have literally cut HIV deaths to half of the national average.[88] They also have fewer heart attacks, and lower rates of diabetic complications. Some of the best equipped and most patient-focused care teams have even reduced broken bones in seniors by over a third[89] by having and using patient-centered databases that anchor and support patient-focused team care in those settings. That work can be done. It isn't a theoretical or hypothetical set of objectives. The goal of having patient-centered data for all patients in this country is an important functional goal that we know is entirely realistic and achievable because it is being done well in some settings now. The value of being able to provide full data about their patient to caregivers at the point of care is being proven every day. Lives are saved. Damage is being averted. Care can be both safer and more affordable when the outcomes of care are improved by access to care data about each patient in real time at the point of care.

We Need Computerized and Accessible Medical Libraries

Doctors need more than just complete patient-centered care data. Doctors also need complete data about medical science. That issue was discussed in Chapter One. We very much need our caregivers to deliver the best care to our patients. To deliver best care consistently and well, caregivers need complete data about the most current medical science for the patients' conditions. To deliver best care, our caregivers also need easy access to data about the current set of medical best practices for multiple health conditions.

Knowledge is a wonderful thing. Knowledge about current medical science should be a standard care expectation, not a rare exception.

We very much need easy and convenient access for our caregivers to the medical knowledge and to the medical science that is directly needed by each caregiver for each patient's care. The unfortunate problem we have in this country of too many caregivers not being able to consistently keep up with current medical science was mentioned in some detail in Chapter One. That "inability to keep up" with current science and with current best practices by our caregivers should not be acceptable to us as a nation. We will soon spend nearly three trillion dollars for care. We should expect that we are getting the best care for that money. Easy access by each caregiver to the best levels of current medical science should clearly be both a basic requirement and an explicit goal of the business model we use to buy care.

This is, unfortunately another area where we fail to deliver a very basic care supporting tool to our caregivers for far too many patients. The truth is -- as Chapter One described in some detail -- most caregivers in this country do not have access to a good tool that can be used to do that work. As a result, of that tool deficit we fail to meet that basic goal of full access to current science in far too many care settings in this country today.

One important IOM Task Force recently filed a well written report that concluded clearly that far too often American caregivers today do not have current knowledge about many relevant developments in the science of care.[90]

The Logistical Barriers to Medical Science Data Distribution Are Clear

Again -- as we look at how we should be delivering optimal levels of care, we need to recognize that the logistical issues and the functional challenges and barriers that exist today to easy access by caregivers to current medical knowledge are obvious and clear. There is no shortage of new science. There is a lot of new research being done for multiple medical issues. Absolutely wonderful learning about the science of care is happening in multiple settings. That is the good news. That is also the bad news. Multiple settings are involved. Tens of thousands of medical journals are published every year.[91] The ability of any solo caregiver or of any solo care site to keep up with all of those current scientific developments is clearly frequently inadequate. The keeping up processes are often extremely difficult, and the data flow about new science is often dysfunctional to the point of creating what are sometimes dangerous levels of knowledge impairment relative to particular points of care delivery and current medical science by individual caregivers.

Knowledge Deficiency Is Not a Good Foundation for Care

We should not accept that too frequent knowledge deficiency -- even partial knowledge impairment -- as the foundational status for medical knowledge for our country's caregivers.

So how can we achieve a much better level of consistent and accessible information sharing about best care for all caregivers?

The answer is amazingly simple. The last chapter also made this point. We need a very basic information access tool made available to all caregivers.

Doctors Need Electronic Medical Libraries

Electronic medical libraries are a key part of that information availability answer.

Our caregivers all should be able to use robust and current electronic medical libraries that are consistently available and very easy to both access and use. As part of the business model we use for buying care, we simply need to insist that -- in order to be paid fully for delivering care -- each care site should certify that it has access to real-time electronic care library information. As a practical issue, we don't need to have any caregivers certify that the information that is in whatever library is available to them will be used for each patient and for each piece of care. We don't want to monitor the library's level of use or do patient-specific oversight of any kind. The doctors should know and will know based on their own judgment when they each need to reach into the library for pieces of information. We don't need to mandate consistent use of that library. We definitely should, however, mandate absolutely consistent access to that level of information by every key caregiver. We should simply have all licensed caregivers certify that a full scope information access tool exists in their practice and that current medical science is actually available to that caregiver in their care site at the point of care.

Urgent Information Should Be Distributed Quickly

If we really want the best care outcomes for a wide range of patients, we need to be able to communicate important new information to the infrastructure of caregivers quickly and well.

We actually need new medical science made available to caregivers at a couple of levels. We need a passive sort of information-sharing system -- a library that simply allows all caregivers to scroll through new and old medical science easily by topic. We also need a more proactive communications tool set. We need a process that identifies urgent new care science and care delivery information and then makes that urgent information available very quickly to care settings where that piece of information can change care and save lives.

An example of a need for very rapid information distribution to caregivers might happen when a prescription drug is found to be dangerous and is recalled. Likewise, there are times when pieces of medical technology are found to be dangerous and also need to be recalled.

Both hip implants and heart implants have had recent situations where new science has shown that some types of existing implant technology have been discovered to be harmful and even dangerous.[92] That new set of information about the danger levels should result in those implants or those devices to be either recalled or closely monitored. In each of the instances that have occurred to date, we have seen that those care sites that now have electronic care data about each and every patient and each and every implant have been able to learn about the alert and then sort through their full array of relevant data in hours or -- at worst -- days to figure out which of their patients might be affected. The best EMR-supported care sites can usually do that work overnight or even faster.

By contrast, the care sites that still use paper records for all of their patient data can take months to figure those issues out. It can take months or even years in a paper-based system to simply get a sense of which patients might be affected by the bad technology. In some cases, and in some settings, literally no one is accountable to conduct that search process through those paper record files to find any patients who might be affected by that information.

In the current non-system, there have some situations where recalls or major product warnings have happened and many of the patients who should have been contacted or supported by their care team fall between the data flow cracks and never learn of their risk -- until the device actually fails and they are damaged. That level of inadequate information availability about the key patient care issues should be unacceptable. We clearly need the kind of patient-centered dataset that can add huge positive ability for caregivers to do that work on behalf of patients.

It Can Take Months or Years To Share New Learning Without Electronic Support

When medical research or various safety learnings identify better ways of delivering care, it can be a very hard -- even impossible -- thing to make all relevant caregivers aware of that care improvement opportunity. Systematic notifications about those new learnings usually do not happen today. Several studies have shown that an important new medical learning can take years to have on an impact on care for most care settings. There are no mechanisms in most care sites to even disperse and distribute key new pieces of information to relevant caregivers and there are almost no systems anywhere to track to see if important new information was ever used by the caregivers.

There is a better way. If we design the information and care support systems well, we can use support processes embedded in our care sites to do that work and to do it well.

The Death Rate for Stroke Doubled Without the Drug – And No One Knew

As one real-world example of how computer support tools can improve care, we should look at some recent work that was done to figure out the impact of statins on the death rate for stroke patients. That piece of research was done by Kaiser Permanente researchers using the new Kaiser Permanente expanded electronic medical record database. The researchers looked at stroke patient hospital care and they focused on stroke patient survival rates. The study actually looked at a computerized database for millions of patients for three full years. They drifted down to look specifically at patients who had been hospitalized for stroke. The data search in the electronic medical records for those patients was a gold mine. The EMR-based study learned that stroke patients who received statins while they are hospitalized for stroke had an average 6 percent mortality rate.[93] That same research showed that the stroke patients who did not receive those same statins while they were in the hospital being treated for their stroke had an average 11 percent mortality rate.[94] That is a much higher death rate. Eleven is nearly double six. That is a huge difference in the rate of stroke patients dying. The data showed that the major difference in the death rate for those stroke patients was based on the differential use or non-use of just one medication -- a medication that is easily available to all hospitals.

That difference in overall death rates wasn't even the most dramatic finding that resulted from that particular research, however. The same study also learned that if the hospital stroke patients had been taking statins prior to admission and if their statin medication was continued for the patient in the hospital -- the death rate actually dropped to five percent.[95] That's a great outcome. But the researchers also learned that if that same medication was being used by the patient before the stroke and the use was discontinued while the patients were in the hospital, the death rate for those discontinued patients who didn't get the statins jumped to 23 percent.[96]

So the death rate for stroke patients who went down one treatment path is one in four patients and the death rate for stroke patients who went down the other treatment path is only one in twenty patients.

Figure 2.1

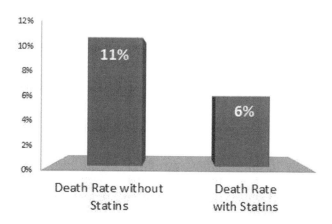

Overall Stroke Mortality Rate

Source: Inpatient statin use predicts improved ischemic stroke discharge disposition. Kano O, Iwamoto K, Ikeda K, Iwasaki Y. Neurology. 2012 Dec 4; 79(23):2294.

Figure 2.2

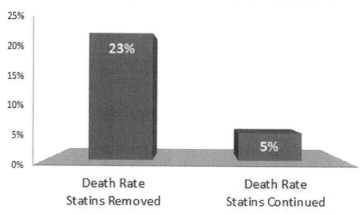

Stroke Mortality Rate -- Prior Statins Users

Source: Inpatient statin use predicts improved ischemic stroke discharge disposition. Kano O, Iwamoto K, Ikeda K, Iwasaki Y. Neurology. 2012 Dec 4; 79(23):2294.

That is obviously extremely important information. A lot of people have strokes. Likewise, a lot of people are taking statins.

The researchers learned that the death rate for stroke patients literarily doubled or quadrupled based on the care choices made by their care team about the use of statins.

So why is that example of important medical research included in this book chapter about optimal care delivery approaches?

It's important to understand what was done with that care-changing new information. In an optimal medical science information distribution situation, patients would hope that all hospitals and all physicians in the world who treat stroke patients would actually know about those important care results relative to statins and stroke patients.

That universal learning did not happen in the real world. Learning did happen. That information was shared through "normal" channels with the rest of the health care world. And the sharing process largely failed.

The point about how difficult it is for caregivers across the county to "keep up" is very relevant to this story. Unfortunately, there is literally no systematic approach that can be used for knowledge sharing about important new scientific discoveries for care sites across the planet today.

That particular set of information about stroke death was shared through the normal channels that exist. That new science about stroke deaths went into the usual distribution process that we use for new medical science. That particular piece of research was published in a highly respected medical journal. Anyone who read that particular journal that month might have learned about those results. That journal and that piece and research are on file.

So that very important piece of information about major differences in the death rates for stroke patients was shared with the health care world in the usual way that medical information is functionally shared with the health care world. It went to a "refereed journal." Publishing new science in a refereed medical journal is a very good thing to do. The steps that are involved in a refereed journal screening process include having objective experts on any given topic read the information that is proposed for inclusion in a research paper and those experts gave as judges and evaluators before the information is actually accepted and then published.

These steps can add real value. It creates a lovely intellectual rigor for the information. It improves the science and gives readers and the journal the comfort of knowing that objective experts have looked at the materials and the data in the paper. It is a good process.

On its own, it is also a functionally inadequate process. Unfortunately, the facts are that the pure publication of that kind of information in a refereed journal isn't enough to get that important new information to all relevant caregivers. In this case, that journal publication obviously did not and could not get that information to all doctors and all hospitals that are treating stroke patients.

The journal that actually published that research had important and relevant readers -- but that article also was one of tens of thousands of refereed journal research articles that were published that same year.[97]

The truth is, for any given article on any given care topic, most caregivers who treat patients in America will never read any particular single study or any single report. Publishing new medical science in refereed medical journals is clearly a good thing to do. A very good thing. But it isn't enough. Publishing something really important about patient care in a journal that 90 percent to 95 percent of our relevant caregivers will never see and will not read is not an optimal or even a functionally adequate way of sharing really important new key information about improving care with all of the people who should learn that information.

We Need A Mechanism To Trigger Alerts About Important Learning

What would a more optimal approach to sharing that kind of information look like?

Because every individual caregiver can't possibly read tens of thousands of medical journals every year, there needs to be a resource put in place that has appropriate, well- qualified care experts very intentionally and consistently scanning through all of that medical research information. That expert-reader scanning process needs to look for breakthrough ideas as well as looking for key pieces of research that can either point care in a new direction or reaffirm the validity of old and in-place care approaches and directions. Patients deserve to have that scanning resource in place and functioning for the use of their caregivers.

Caregivers who want to keep up with current medical science also need to have a resource of that nature up and functioning to do that work for them. That resource should scan the new learning in health care and should make key pieces of information available in a systematic and convenient way to caregivers. Ideally, there should be both a prioritization process and a functioning mechanism that can be used to get that key information in front of the front line care practitioners.

If that kind of resource had existed and if it had been in place last year when the stroke death rate research was done and published, the set of objective medical experts who did the screening of all research studies could have read the article, appreciated the huge importance of that particular discovery, and they could have both flagged that piece of research and given it a high priority for distribution and teaching for all relevant care teams and caregivers.

That is not an unreasonable expectation for either patients or caregivers. The right information distribution model for new medical science could have highlighted that piece of critical research and then the distribution model could have ensured that all caregivers who treat those patients would have easy access to that piece of information.

Only The Internet Can Easily Distribute That Information

This is another key area where the internet can be a lovely resource to enhance the provision of care. Ideally, that kind of lifesaving information should flow electronically to all relevant caregivers. It is clear at a very basic logistical level that only the electronic distribution of that kind of information can achieve the very best results. Mailing a hard copy of a printed journal to thousands or even tens of thousands of people is obviously not going to reach all the people who need to be reached with that information.

Electronic versions of the journal could reach more people — but electronic versions of those Journals only reach the caregivers who pay to subscribe to the Journal. Simply adding that information — and other information like it--to an electronic medical library would be a very good thing to do. That would be a far superior mechanism for sharing that information with all caregivers. But even inserting the information entirely into an electronic medical library would probably not have been adequate to create targeted sharing if important new information of that magnitude.

For the most important pieces of new medical information, we need to go a couple of steps further on down the distribution road to create prioritized information sharing. In an optimal care delivery information support world, there should also be reminders and prompts available for the relevant caregivers and those reminders should be embedded in the actual computer systems that are used by each of the caregivers at the point of care.

Real-time reminders about that particular piece of stroke treatment information could be extremely useful to the caregivers. When the death rate quadruples if the doctors choose the wrong treatment path, then information about the right treatment path should be prompted and available for the caregiver at the point of care.

We need actual electronic reminders given to caregivers about that new science and those reminders should happen at the actual point and time of care could remind each relevant caregiver to do the right things for their stroke patients. The findings from that particular study literally create an issue of life and death for patients. A lot of people die from strokes. A lot of people have prescriptions for statins.

We also know from other data that the stroke mortality rates actually vary significantly now from hospital to hospital. Death rates for strokes vary from care setting to care setting. Some of that unnecessary variation in the percentage of people dying from stroke could be ended or reduced if there were consistent reminder mechanisms in place to remind the relevant caregivers at the point of care in each hospital what the very best current medical practices are for their stroke patients.

Electronic Reminders Only Exist in Some Settings Today

That work can be done. That is not a hypothetical or theoretical suggestion. Those processes exist in some care sites now. It is entirely possible to insert electronic prompts and automated reminders about key points into care processes -- but that particular tool can only be done at the point of care if the care site treating the patient actually has an electronic care support tool kit and electronic medical record support system in place that can do that work at the point of care.

It Is Entirely Possible To Give Caregivers That Tool Now

That piece of information is relevant to a chapter that is describing what the providers of healthcare should build into their purchasing specifications for care delivery. These tools should be included those specifications. That ability to do electronic information sharing with care team members about important medical science and about best practices for medical conditions actually exists today in most of the large multispecialty group practices.

The ability to do that level of care support can also be found in a number of hospitals who have implemented well designed electronic medical records. Those reminders can be in place when those particular hospitals use their computerized record systems well. Those electronic reminder systems can and should remind caregivers very consistently at the point of care when the right thing should be done for a given patient.

At Kaiser Permanente -- the care site where that actual original piece of stroke mortality research was done -- the research, document itself, was included in the comprehensive Kaiser Permanente Electronic Clinical Library. That Kaiser Permanente electronic medical library is available to all KP physicians and caregivers in real time...wherever they may be. That library contains all basic medical text books and journals.

So that piece of refereed journal-published research actually was included in the KP electronic library. In addition to sharing the actual research paper electronically, the care support team at Kaiser Permanente also built that important piece of science into the set of recommended care protocols that are developed and undated regularly for Kaiser Permanente caregivers.

There are currently 2,500 care protocols in the Kaiser Permanente electronic medical library.[98] Those protocols are developed by medical experts using current medical science. That recommendation to add that particular medication to the treatment plans of every relevant stroke patient was very quickly added to the recommended Kaiser Permanente care protocol in place for stroke patients.

Make the Right Thing Easy To Do

That was not the end of the information distribution process at Kaiser Permanente for that stroke research.

Most importantly -- and most effectively -- that life-saving piece of information about stroke patients was also very carefully and systematically made available in all Kaiser Permanente-owned hospitals to doctors at the point of care.

The basic mantra of the Kaiser Permanente care team is to make the right thing easy to do. That guideline of "Making the Right Thing Easy To Do," is used at Kaiser Permanente for both caregivers and patients. In this instance, the right thing to do is to provide statins to the stroke patients. To make that piece of advice easy to do, the care support team at Kaiser Permanente also embedded that information into the computerized recommended order set for stroke patients that pop up on the computer at the point of care for stroke a patient. The order sets are not mandatory -- but they are very convenient and they have great utility as a care support tool.

So that recommendation to the physician to use that medication was simply added to the set of real-time electronic care "prompts" and it was added to the onscreen suggested "order set" for the computer support systems that the doctors in Kaiser Permanente hospitals use at the point of care for their stroke patients.

The point-of-care real-time order set is an extremely important care improvement tool. Adding that particular drug suggestion to the suggested "order set" that appears on the screen for the doctor at the point of care in the hospital ensures that those key information elements will be available in a very convenient way for the relevant doctor at the most useful, convenient and relevant time for that information to appear. Making the right thing easy to do is a very good thing to do. The death rate from stroke for Kaiser Permanente patients has dropped by over 40 percent over the past few years.[99] The full set of care support tools -- combined with Kaiser Permanente's extremely successful and also computer supported highly patient-focused hypertension reduction agendas -- have combined to achieve those results.

Most Hospital Do Not Offer Reminders of Best Practices at the Point of Care

Sadly, most hospital care sites do not have that tool kit. Most hospitals and physicians do not have an electronic medical library. Very few caregivers or care systems have care reminder prompts or even recommended treatment order sets in place. Some patients die and many are damaged for life because that took kit doesn't exist in their hospitals. Being damaged for life is a very sad care outcome.

The full set of problems that too often results from suboptimal care is bigger than just the difference between hospitals in their stroke patient death rate. Strokes kill people and strokes also create damage in many of the people who survive them. For stroke patients, the likelihood of the patient going home and achieving high levels of recovery after their stay in the hospital instead of having to go to a nursing home from the hospital with permanent damage after their inpatient stroke care is over is significantly better in Kaiser Permanente hospitals as a result of those interventions. The likelihood of going home without damage is higher because that set of automated care reminders exists in those hospitals and because the patients in those hospitals who receive that treatment approach are not -- on average -- damaged as badly by their strokes.

All Hospitals Need Better Care Support Tools

These care reminders are a lovely care support tool. That kind of support system for physicians should not just be a feature and function of care in Kaiser Permanente hospitals or other major care systems. All hospitals should use those tools. It is important to recognize that the employers and the government agencies who buy care can help make that tool kit happen. Chapter Five explains how using better care-related purchasing specifications can help improve care in those directions in many settings. The organizations that pay for care -- the employers who buy insurance coverage for their workers, the government agencies that pay for care for their beneficiaries and the private health plans that serve as our primary care-purchasing mechanism for care in this country -- should all insist that the hospitals they pay for care for stroke patients should have those kinds of basic functional electronic care support tools in place for their physicians at the point of care in order to be paid in full for hospital care. If the care sites do not have these care support tools in place, they should give payers a timeframe for when the tools will be installed and used.

Care can get a lot better -- and care will be cheaper -- when patients get best care and when caregivers have all of the information they need to provide each patients care.

The chapter of this book that deals with the changes we should make in the business model we use to buy care deals with those issues. For the purpose of this chapter, it's good just to point out that we need our care delivery infrastructure to have both easy access to best medical science and easy access to useful care support tools. That is particularly true in the hospitals for patients who need best care because those patients are clearly in need of care or they wouldn't be in a hospital.

We Do Not Want Computers To Dictate Care

That recommendation to have computer-triggered care prompts and care reminders does not mean that we want computers to practice medicine. That would be both incorrect and wrong.

We absolutely do not want the computers or the people who run computers to dictate care. Computers should never dictate care. We do, however, want the computers that are used in each care setting to offer easily accessible data and easily accessible medical science. We also want computers to offer easily accessible information about best care to the appropriate caregivers in real time. We very much want the computers to sometimes trigger or flag key pieces of information and we even want our computers to sometimes ask questions to the relevant caregiver about some aspects of care when that questioning and that reminder process could improve care and possibly help save lives.

The good news is, we do not need to invent that whole array of next generation care support tools.

Those tool kits exist. Prompts and reminders happen in some care sites today. As noted above, they are used now in some systems-supported care settings. Those tools actually work. We need to use them when appropriate for all patients and we need all caregivers to have easy access to the right information about best care. We pay $2.8 trillion for care in this country today.[100] We should be buying the right care and we should be buying the right processes of care when we are spending that much money on care.

We Very Much Do Not Want Anyone Dictating Care Approaches

This is very much not, however, a suggestion that we should have someone or anyone dictating care protocols to our caregivers. We absolutely do not want computers practicing medicine and we also do not want mandatory care protocols imposed by outside agencies or outside parties dictating care. Having the government impose specific and detailed delivery care mandates should not be a function of either our business model for care or a function of our regulatory model for care. This is not a suggestion that specific care protocols or specific approaches should somehow be determined, defined, and then dictated by outside parties. That level of care-related dictation by outside parties would be a mistake.

Why would that be a mistake?

Care would suffer if that happened.

Why would care suffer?

Continuous Improvement Needs To Be Our Goal

Continuous improvement is our goal. Continuous improvement should be our mantra. We need continuous improvement. Continuous improvement should be a core philosophy in our infrastructure for care. We will only optimize the delivery of care in this country if we are committed to a process of continuously improving care and then actually continuously improve.

We want and need care to be continuously improving. We need to nurture and support and encourage and protect continuous improvement as a philosophy, a commitment, a strategy, and a skill set. Continuous improvement done in a systematic and consistent way is needed for care to get continuously better. That is why we should not mandate specific protocols. Continuous improvement requires continuous flexibility. Mandates can create rigidity. Mandated specific protocols have an inherent rigidity that is created by their mandate. Rigidity is bad. Rigidity and continuous improvement are a bad and non-functional combination. One kills, impedes, or impairs the other. We obviously very much do want care protocols for care delivery and we very much want medical best practices but -- with very rare exceptions -- we do not want anyone external to the care process dictating the specific care protocols we all use. Rigid, mandatory, regulation-based very specific and detailed care delivery rule sets and process mandates can and will stifle continuous improvement processes in operational care sites.

Continuous improvement should be our goal -- almost our obsession -- so we should not allow the use of rigid rules about processes that lock specific care delivery processes into place.

Continuous Improvement Should Anchor Our Thinking

Continuous improvement is a good thing.

We need patient-centered care that continuously improves.

We definitely do want continuous improvement to become a core mantra and a basic priority for the entire infrastructure of American health care. We need an industrial revolution for care delivery that is firmly anchored in continuous improvement. Continuous improvement needs to be a major part of our tool kit. Our business model and our regulatory model should both reflect the fact that we need continuous improvement for our care infrastructure. We clearly have huge opportunities to make care better. Care today tends to be badly organized, unconnected and many aspects of the care information are entirely unintentional -- driven by revenue streams rather than by patient needs. Care does not get better in that dysfunctional context. We want care to continuously improve. We can make care safer, more efficient, and more affordable when we look in a systematic way at entire processes of care delivery and then repeatedly engineer and reengineer care around the patient in a continuous improvement context and approach.

Care Can Be Best Engineered in Packages -- Not Pieces

Most health care in America is sold by the piece. This book discussed that issue in several places. We currently have a piecework cash flow that funds care. That piecework approach and cash flow makes reengineering care very difficult.

When care is sold entirely by the piece, then the cash flow for the caregivers is obviously dependent on not losing any of the billable pieces of care from the overall process of care. Asthma care that is sold by the piece generates a flood of cash that is triggered when patients have an asthma crisis. Asthma care that is sold by the piece also experiences a direct, immediate, and major dearth of cash flow when those asthma crises do not occur. Dearths can discourage care improvement.

A cash flow dearth is -- for obvious reasons -- not good for the financial health of caregiver business units. Anyone with enough intelligence to get though medical school or through health care administrator training knows that dearths of cash are hard to use to keep a business intact and alive. Dearths don't bank well. So when asthma care is purchased entirely by the piece, we generally don't see caregivers spending time and energy putting in place various care approaches that will keep asthma attacks from happening and that will cause asthma billable events to shrink.

This chapter isn't intended to explain the specifics of how the business model we use to buy care needs to change in order to allow caregivers to sell asthma care as a package and not just sell asthma care by the piece. Chapters Four and Five both deal with those issues. But this chapter does have the task of pointing out how the different the consequences of the two approaches are.

Patient-Focused Asthma Care Creates Fewer Crises

When asthma care in any care setting is sold as a package and not just by the piece, asthma care becomes much more patient-focused. When caregivers have a direct cash flow that can support prevention and when caregivers are not dependent on each asthma crisis to make money, the care delivery perspective changes. The total care approach for the asthma patients generally gets much better when that cash flow change happens. Patient-focused asthma care involves and includes proactive interventions, quick response times and effective and timely patient education. In the right business model for asthma care, the thought process about that care for those patients is focused with real energy on reducing both the number and the severity of asthma attacks... not just responding after-the-fact on a piecework basis to each incidental but revenue-rich asthma crisis. Those are two very different approaches to care. It is a very different business model for care.

The normal functionally and the standard care patterns for each asthma patient today in our piecework care model generally involves the business sites of care waiting for an asthma crisis and then doing expensive (and profitable) and usually entirely reactive things to and for each patient in each situational setting to help resolve each situational care crisis.

The Care Sites With a Different Business Model Build Patient-Centered Care

Some care sites today already do have a different business model where they currently do sell care by the package and not by the piece. Those sites who sell an entire package of care today can and do look at asthma care at the patient level rather than just reacting at the incident level to each asthma crisis triggered "moment of care." When the payment model works well, the sites that sell care by the package can actually benefit financially by averting asthma crises rather than literally losing money when an asthma attack is prevented. In the package care model, the caregivers also benefit financially when the asthma care needs of patients are handled so well that the care team response to an asthma issue doesn't always become a full medical crisis. That is much better care for asthma patients. The thought processes for each of the two approaches are fundamentally different.

The care sites and care teams that have a total package of care focus for asthma care tend to develop an early intervention plan for each asthma patient. Prevention becomes a top priority when the cash flow model changes. That is a good thing. Prevention works. The number of asthma crises for those patients are reduced. The truth is, nearly 75 percent of today's hospital-admission triggering asthma care crisis -- in many care settings -- are preventable.[101] Care is better and life is better for the patients who are not going through those crises. Patient-focused, proactive asthma care is far superior to crisis focused, fee-fed asthma care. The caregivers can afford to reengineer the procedures of care when the caregivers are prepaid and when the caregivers can benefit from the reengineering. Without that very basic change in the cash flow, for caregivers, reengineering simply changes provider revenue in an adverse way. As this book says several time -- no industry ever reengineers against its own self- interest. That is true of any other industry and it is very true of health care. So we need to make care reengineering in the best interest of the care industry and reengineering will quickly happen.

Asthma obviously, isn't alone in offering us a universe of opportunity for better care that is anchored on a better business model and reengineered processes of care.

Congestive Heart Failure Care Is Also Better as a Package

For patients with chronic conditions -- and particularly for patients with multiple conditions -- we really need proactive and intervention-focused, process-based thinking to make care better and more affordable.

Congestive heart failure (CHF) is another good example of an area of care delivery where looking at the total care needs of each patient in a proactive way creates far better -- and less expensive -- care than a care delivery approach that is focused entirely on responding on a piecework basis to CHF crises after they occur.

Multiple settings have shown that care is much better for those patients when their personal CHF crisis are reduced or prevented. A congestive heart failure crisis can be pretty grim for patients. Those crises are really not pleasant experiences for patients. When patients have a congestive heart failure crisis, they are often drowning in their own fluids. Those CHF crises can be horrible, terrifying, painful, frightening, demoralizing and deeply unpleasant experiences for the patient.

They are actually very much like a typical asthma crisis. And -- like the asthma crisis -- most of those terrible and painful CHF crises do not need to happen for most of those patients. Hugely competent, proactive patient-focused, well organized care approaches for each congestive heart failure patient can use systematic intervention processes to cut those horrible crises by half or more.[102]

Patients' lives are obviously significantly better when that happens. Cutting the number of CHF crises in half also reduces the cost of care for those very expensive patients by almost half. So care is better and care also costs less when it is delivered in a proactive patient-focused package rather than simply being sold to the patient after the fact entirely by the piece. Continuous improvement can also happen once the care is set up as care processes instead of being trigged as purely reactionary incidents of care.

Once caregivers begin looking at these issues through the lens of continuous improvement and not through the lens of piece-work-billing volume, creativity can flourish and care finally can get continuously better.

Proactive Care Needs To Be Incented by the Business Model for Care

The sheer value of patient-focused care and of proactive care and interventional care strategies as the basis for our new continuously improving business model for care is obvious. This isn't a theoretical or ideological or philosophical insight or aspiration. It is an entirely practical and highly functional aspiration. The functional ability of care teams to actually do proactive patient-focused care clearly exists. We know that is true because in some care settings whose business model already incents and rewards those approaches, care teams are doing that level of proactive intervention care now and they are doing it well. People have significantly fewer asthma and significantly fewer CHF crises in those care settings. So we clearly would be well served to put the tools and the financial models in place to make that kind of purchasing and care process improvement happen in more places for more medical conditions.

Most Care Costs Come From Patients With Comorbidities

Another major focus of the new business model we should be using to buy care should be to put programs and tools in place to help achieve team care. We need care to be data based and we need care to continuously improve. We need process reengineering to maximize the effectiveness of our ability proactively to reduce care crises. We also need a care delivery business model that incents team care.

Why do we need team care?

We want health care costs in this country to go down and team care is a great tool for achieving that goal.

We need to recognize the very powerful reality that most health care costs today come from patients with chronic conditions and comorbidities -- multiple health conditions. We know from multiple studies and we each tend to know as patients from our own care experiences that most of the patients in this country who have comorbidities have badly coordinated care today. Their care is badly coordinated because we haven't built any care coordination processes and we have not implemented any care coordination tools in most care settings. We don't support team care financially and we don't support it functionally with team care tools. We very much need to improve the processes of team care for those patients who have multiple health conditions if we are going to reduce costs for those patients. We need to do that work as a conscious strategy rather than hoping that somehow the infrastructure of care will spontaneously and magically improve in a number of key areas. The opportunities for better care based on care teamwork are huge and they are very real. We actually can cut the needed hospital days by half or more for many of those patients with multiple health conditions if those patients get great care and if they -- as a result of better care -- have both fewer direct crises and fewer complications. To do that care coordination job for those patients well, we need the caregivers who share that patient to be able to function as a team.

We Need Care Coordination Tools

For our caregivers to function as a team, there are a few very basic sets of logistical issues and operational realities that need to be addressed. Tools are the first issue. We need tools. Chapter One talked about our tool deficits and our tool gaps. They are very real. Tools are essential. Most caregivers do not have the right set of care coordination and care support tools today. We need to build the right tool kit to support team care and coordinated care and then we need to put that tool kit in place and use it.

What will those particular tools do? Information sharing is a key functional need. Minimally, we need all of the caregivers who collectively treat patients who have comorbidities to be able to share current information about each patient they share. That data sharing need is particularly important for all of the patients who have comorbidities. That tool to share knowledge is actually equally useful in many respects for many other patients who have serious single illnesses. That tools is needed for the patients because many of the patients who have very serious single primary illnesses often have multiple doctors as well who can't easily share information. We clearly need a care delivery infrastructure and care delivery tool kits that allow our caregivers to share information as needed for each shared patient -- with a focus on information sharing for the patients who have comorbidities and complex medical conditions.

Team Care Is Wonderful

We clearly need to build business models for care that will both create care teams and make it possible for patients to have easy access to those teams.

We clearly need to support and facilitate team care if we want to achieve the goal of improving care and reducing the costs of care. We need doctors, nurses, pharmacists, lab techs and various categories of therapists working together for each patient in ways that their collective and joint care is focused on their patients and not just on the cash flow and the operational convenience needs of various provider business units.

Patients and Caregivers Need Data About Care Consequences

Chapter One talked about the extreme variation in care outcomes and even mortality rates that can happen between care sites and care approaches today. Far too often, those significant performance differences exist and they are invisible both to the caregivers and to the people receiving care. We also should do much better in regard to sharing data about care performance levels with both patients and caregivers.

Both patients and caregivers will benefit.

Patients should be able to know what the likely outcomes are for various medical procedures and patients should be able to compare performance for various care sites and care teams.

Care sites very much need comparative data about their own performance in key areas. The chart below was referenced in Chapter One. It shows the sepsis death rate in a number of individual hospitals as it occurred over several years at a major American hospital system. That comparative data helped those care sites improve care. That death rate chart shows why data is so important to caregivers. Having the data very clearly and directly helped bring the death rate down for those care sites. A decade ago, no one even measured outcomes like sepsis death rates at the caregiver level. For the hospitals on this chart, data on that topic was not gathered, collected, received, or even considered ten years ago. As noted earlier, sepsis is actually the number one cause of death in American hospitals -- killing more patients than stroke, heart disease or even cancer.[103] Sepsis is the single biggest cause of death in hospitals and most hospitals do not even collect the level of data that is shown on those charts.

Hospitals Didn't Believe That Data Was Needed

People who run hospitals very much want to do the right thing. Until fairly recently, however, the people who run hospitals believed that doing the right thing actually did not require using a lot of data.

For the hospitals on this chart -- before the initial data set was collected -- everyone in each care site believed that their own hospital was doing a great job on sepsis care. People at those same data-free care sites also believed they were doing a great job on all of the other care-related infections for their patients. All of the care sites shown on this chart believed they were using best practices and all of the care sites believed that their outcomes for patients were as good as or better than the outcomes at other care sites. Then the first actual measurements were done at the hospitals. The hospitals that did that initial measuring of their own performance and then built their first level of data comparison capabilities actually learned very quickly there actually were major differences in death rates between hospitals. Sepsis turned out to be an area of significant performance variation. The hospitals learned in a very powerful way that everyone in the hospital world was not delivering great sepsis care. Results were inconsistent. Some very good people who had believed very sincerely and honestly that their own hospital care was the best available hospital care on the planet learned after looking at real data about sepsis outcomes that their results for that condition were actually worse than the results in other hospitals in the comparison group.

That was unexpected. And it was shocking to many people.

That data was golden. It was honest. Some of that data was painful. Overall -- having that data was, in total, wonderful.

That data has saved a lot of lives.

Because that comparative data finally existed and also because the data was made available, accessible, and transparent to the care teams at each hospital, all of the care sites in that hospital system began the process improvement work that was needed to bring down the death rate from sepsis at their hospital. The next chart shows very clearly the reduction in overall death rate for all of those hospitals as a group over a couple of years of continuously improving care.

The mortality rate in those hospitals is now far below the national average death rate in American hospitals for sepsis. Lives are being saved every day in those hospitals that would be dead in most other care settings. There is no possible way that those absolutely impressive levels of performance improvement in all of those hospitals could have happened without that data.

Figure 1.5   FOR ILLUSTRATIVE PURPOSES ONLY

Sepsis Mortality Rates

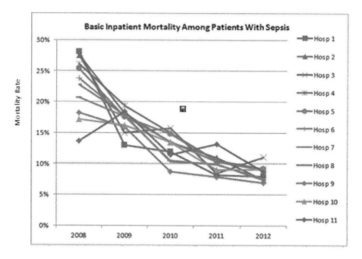

So why did these hospitals manage to achieve those reductions in the sepsis death rate while other hospitals here made a

Other Hospitals Need To Collect That Data

What does that example have to do with the data elements that we want to build into the future business model of care? We should want all other hospitals in this country to do down similar paths of data-based continuous process improvement for multiple important areas of care. It is possible to do. Buyers can help make that happen, as Chapter Five explains. We need to buy care in a way that will incent and reward a continuous improvement process approach that will make the outcomes in all American hospitals in key areas get better every year.

So why did these hospitals manage to achieve those reductions in the sepsis death rate while other hospitals here made a lot less progress? The business model used to buy care was relevant. Those hospitals on this chart actually benefited financially by improving sepsis care because these hospitals are already selling care by the package and not selling care by the piece. Those hospitals do not lose revenue when sepsis patients are quickly cured. For other hospitals that sell care entirely by the piece, an equivalent improvement in sepsis care results could have reduced revenue by many millions of dollars per hospital. The business model of selling hospital care as a full package instead of selling that care purely by the piece enabled that stunning level of care improvement to happen. And allowed all of those lives to be saved.

Hospitals Need a Business Model That Rewards Better Care

Those sepsis results show why we need to change the business model for other hospitals in a couple of key ways -- to stop paying more money when care is bad and paying even more money when care is worse.

We need that same commitment to continuous improvement to be true in other hospitals as a core financial and operational reality that allows those hospitals to benefit when sepsis response minimize damage to sepsis patients.

In a nutshell, we need to put American hospitals into a financial reality where better care creates financial rewards rather than creating financial penalties. This book addresses some new ways of compensating hospitals that can work toward these goals -- including having hospitals functioning as part of the new Accountable Care Organizations' approaches to care delivery that are described in Chapter Four and Five. Quite a few care organizations are trying to set up Accountable Care Organizations as a way of creating team care and changing the business model to reward proactive care instead of penalizing it.

The new ACO models for care delivery and care financing that are being built have the potential to create a new financial reality and a new cash flow model for hospitals and care teams that will incent and deliver better sepsis care rather than penalize it. The ACOs that sell care by the package will also have the potential to incent better asthma care and better congestive heart failure care. That ACO strategy is discussed in both Chapters Four and Five. For this chapter, the point to be made is that care can get a lot better when the business model we use to buy care rewards better care. We need business models that allow and incent better and safer care to be the norm rather than the exception.

Consumers deserve safe care. The business model we use to buy care and the care support tools we use to deliver care need to support safety, and patients need to know which care sites create the most risk for them as patients.

Patients Should Know Which Care Sites Are Safe

In the new health care world we are building, patients should have much better data about care delivery performance and care outcomes. Having access to key pieces of needed data about care outcomes and care safety is an area where one very effective tool we might want to use to improve the business model of care might be the law, itself. Laws create their own business reality. Business models can be created by the marketplace -- and business realities can also can be created by regulatory edict. In some cases, laws clearly have a role to play in making care better. Laws about care delivery very much create their own business reality about care delivery for care sites. When something specific is required by the law, care sites tend to invest the resources needed to do whatever is required by the law in order to stay in business or avoid regulatory penalties.

We May Need Regulations About Care Outcome Reporting

Laws are a clumsy and potentially damaging tool to use to structure specific aspects and care delivery, but laws can create a context for data availability that can be extremely useful for caregivers, patients, and buyers. We may actually want to set up a few additional regulations about care data reporting that will require care sites to gather and report a whole array of outcomes-related data about specific aspects of care.

In the best of all worlds, that data about care quality could be voluntarily reported. That voluntary reporting approach for care outcomes has not happened in most care settings, however. Some care sites already do that data gathering work and they do it well -- but the sad truth is that too many sites will not gather or report significant levels of outcome data voluntarily. That lack of outcomes data for care delivery isn't good, if our primary goal is to improve the quality of care and also -- in the process -- allow patients to make informed choices about care sites based on comparative performance and safety data. We need to use a combination of market forces and regulatory oversight to make appropriate levels of safety data available to consumers and caregivers.

Safety Is a Key Issue

Safety is a good place to start when we are looking at areas where data transparency can be useful and meaningful.

Patients should know which care sites are safe. The business model we use to buy care should make safety a priority and the specifications used by key buyers should make public data about safety levels a mandate. As the last chapter of this book pointed out, the death rate triples and quadruples for several categories of care if you go to the wrong hospital or to the wrong care team.

The next four charts show some graphic and powerful differences in care outcomes by hospitals. The National Health Grades Report rated an array of hospitals in this country.[104] The Health Grades teams looked at available performance and operational data and then they assigned from one star to five stars to each hospital based on the quality improvement and the continuous improvement programs that are in place at each hospital.

What did they learn?

Figure 2.4

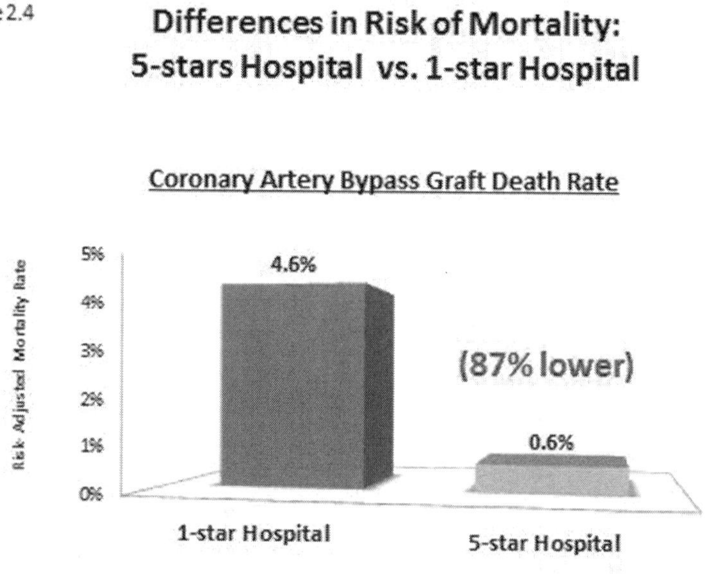

Differences in Risk of Mortality: 5-stars Hospital vs. 1-star Hospital

Coronary Artery Bypass Graft Death Rate

Risk Adjusted Mortality Rate	1-star Hospital	5-star Hospital
	4.6%	0.6%

(87% lower)

Source: 2012 Health Grades Report

They learned that the existence or the lack of existence of very basic data based quality programs in each measured hospital had a huge impact on saving people's lives in each hospital setting.

The hospitals that were given five stars were hospitals that had extensive quality improvement programs in place. Those hospitals clearly used their data to improve the quality of care. One-star hospitals had less data and fewer reporting processes, and when you look at the results, it's clear that the one-star hospitals clearly did not improve some key areas of care.

Heart surgery was a good example of differences in care outcomes between the five-star hospitals that have formal data based quality assurance programs in place and the one-star hospitals that rely primarily on good will and good intentions to make better care happen.

The hospitals that only had one-star ratings had one out of every 20 coronary artery bypass surgery patients die.

By contrast, the five-star hospitals in the Health Grades report has less than one out of 100 of their patients with that exact same surgery dying.

Earlier studies of mortality levels for that heart bypass surgery have shown that the death rate for the worst hospitals in America who do that particular heart procedure has actually ranged closer to one in ten of their surgery patients dying from that surgery.

So if you need that particular heart surgery and if you go to a high quality, data supported five-star hospital, and have the surgery, your likelihood of death is only one in a hundred. If you go to a one-star hospital, your chance of dying jumps to one in twenty. And if you go to an even lower performing hospital -- if you go to a worst care performers for that particular surgery -- your chance of dying from the same exact surgery jumps to roughly one in ten. One in ten is a very different risk level for a patient than one in a hundred.

Heart attacks also result in very different outcomes when you compare one and five-star hospitals.

The difference in death rates between the one-star hospitals and the five-star hospitals for basic heart attacks is also worth knowing. Look at the chart below. Over ten percent of the heart attack patients die in the one-star hospitals. Less than five percent of those some patients die in the five-star hospitals.

Figure 2.5

Differences in Risk of Mortality: 5-stars Hospital vs. 1-star Hospital

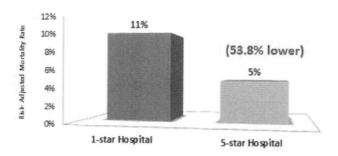

Heart Attack Death Rate

Source: 2012 Health Grades Report

Our current business model for care makes no differences in the way we buy care for any of those fairly dramatic differences in care outcomes. We don't change the cash flow for care in any way based on these very difference care outcomes. That is obviously a flaw in the way we buy care today.

As we build our business model for care, we definitely should -- at a bare minimum -- insist that any of the patients who will be undergoing those surgeries should know clearly what those relative mortality risk levels are for each site before having the surgery. Likewise, we need a business model for care that creates an information flow so that patients who have heart attacks can easily know that their personal death risk doubles if they go to a hospital that only gets one star for its safety programs and its care processes instead of earning five stars.

Ideally, we should pay hospitals less for a bad mortality rate and more for a good mortality rate. The chapter of this book on how employers should establish performance specifications addresses those issues in more detail. At this point, we just need to keep in mind that the business model we use to buy care should probably be set up to encourage data supported care because the hospitals included in the star rating system who had the best results were the hospitals with the most intense care data.

Sepsis Death Rates Vary As Well

The patterns of sepsis care -- not surprisingly -- look very familiar for the hospitals included in the star rating system.

The wide variation in performance that exists now relative to mortality levels for patients with sepsis in American hospitals and the many opportunities we have for care improvement for sepsis patients have both already been discussed in this book. The National Health Grades report looked at sepsis care, as well, and their data confirms the points made by this book. Their outcomes numbers directly reinforced the point that was made earlier about the benefits of systematic care improvement for sepsis care patients.

The next chart shows the impact of systematic care improvement in hospital settings for sepsis patients. The 12 percent mortality rate for sepsis they report for the top performing five-star hospitals that were included in their study is clearly a great success story. That 12 percent number is a bit higher than the best hospital performance results in the other care system that was mentioned earlier in this chapter -- but their five-star hospitals mortality level for sepsis is clearly a lot better than the 23 percent mortality number that is the average death rate the National Health Grades organization uncovered in their one-star hospitals. In some hospital settings, the death rate reaches 30 percent of sepsis patients.

The chart shows the sepsis mortality rates for the one and five-star hospitals rated by Health Grades.

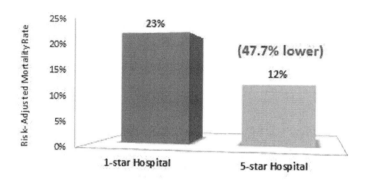

Figure 2.6

**Differences in Risk of Mortality:
5-stars Hospital vs. 1-star Hospital**

Sepsis Death Rate

Source: 2012 Health Grades Report

Not surprisingly, the same relative performance paths existed for pneumonia data in the Health Grade study. Those differences were fascinating, as well. Pneumonia is one of the hospital acquired infections that happen most often to patients in this country. The success level variation for treating that disease is huge. As you can see from these charts, the best "five-star" hospitals only lose about two percent of those patients. The one-star hospitals, however, lose over seven percent of the pneumonia patients. Being more than three times more likely to die is a very important difference in the survival rate if you personally are a pneumonia patient.

Again -- the business model we use today to buy care does not differentiate in any way between those differences in care outcome. If anything, the way we buy care today rewards the hospitals with the worst death rates because the pneumonia patients in those less effective hospitals tend to have their pneumonia longer than the cases in the best hospitals and they spend more time in the very expensive intensive care units.

We clearly need a business model for care that insists on making that kind of comparative mortality rate information available to patients who need those levels and categories of care. We also need a business model for care that pays hospitals more for higher survival rates and pays hospitals less for higher rates of death.

Figure 2.7

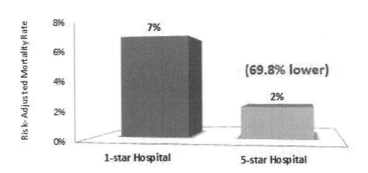

Differences in Risk of Mortality: 5-stars Hospital vs. 1-star Hospital

Pneumonia Death Rate

Source: 2012 Health Grades Report

We Need Care Delivery Innovation

We also need a business model for care that incents providers of care to be much more innovative in developing alternative care delivery tools and support systems.

As one example -- one important care delivery improvement that patients tend to appreciate and use is to give patients e-connections with their caregivers. E-visits can actually replace face-to-face visits for multiple levels of care. When people deliver care by the package, e-visits are easily included in the package. But when care is sold only by the piece, e-visits are rare and they are sometimes not available at all.

That makes economic sense for the caregivers because the current piecework payment model for care doesn't usually pay for e-visit, and that lack of payment penalizes any fee-based care sites that use e-visits and telephone connectivity as an efficient tool for delivering care. It penalizes those sites and those care teams because those electronic connections, information flows, and remote venues of care delivery are not paid for by the typical insurer or medical fee schedule.

That rigidity in payment decisions for those electronically connected levels of care is unfortunate because we need to design and implement care innovation approaches that use those new tools. It is a flaw in the business model we use now to buy care to not pay for improved connectivity. We obviously need a business model that supports reengineering the delivery of care to make it more affordable and more accessible using any and all of the new connectivity tools available to us.

We need to use the available sets of new connectivity tools to achieve a more flexible connectivity goal. Enhancing connectivity should be a very conscious goal. We need to fully and creatively use the new connectivity tool kit that is increasingly available to us through all of the new smartphones and internet connectivity devices so that we can deliver care in highly patient-focused ways in multiple care settings and deliver care that is both less expensive and much more patient friendly from a logistical perspective.

The Cusp of a Golden Age for Care Support Tools

We are actually on the cusp of a golden age for health care support tools. If we take full advantage of the new tool kit that is being made available to us, we will be able to deliver better care with major improvement in the access to care and achieve a significant reduction for the overall cost of care in the process. These are exciting times for health care support tools. We are on the cutting edge of a connectivity revolution for health care. The new computerized connectivity revolution and an explosion in data purchasing capabilities and operational functionality has already transformed many work flows and has fundamentally changed many basic customer/vendor interactions and transactions in multiple other areas of the economy. That new connectivity capability is now reaching health care and if we use the new tools well, that connectivity revolution will change care as well. If we know what we are doing, we will change care significantly for the better.

Hospital Care Will Also Have Better Tools

The new tools will make care better at all of the various sites we use to deliver care. The next generation of care delivery will have hospitals that are supported with great technology and with databases that will give hospital caregivers all of the information about each patient and their care needs.

Hospital care will get better with the new tool kit and it will become safer and more effective when hospitals adapt both continuous improvement approaches and data based core tracking as care competencies.

Hospitals are much more likely to do that work and use those tools well if the business model for care buys team care instead of piecework care and if the hospitals are allied as team members with appropriate caregivers for each patient.

So hospitals will still be a primary site of care. Hospitals will not disappear. If we design the entire process well, hospitals will be increasingly embedded into a care team approach rather than simply continuing to be free-standing functionally unconnected care business units that deal with patients in the pure context of the patients' situational care needs.

Clinics Will Also Have Much Better Tools

The second site of care that will survive and thrive going into the future will be the clinics and doctors' offices where people have a direct face-to-face encounter with licensed caregiver who will provide needed elements of care.

Those clinic-based sites of care will also continue to be needed for the foreseeable future. Those doctors' offices will also have much better technology and they should be supported with electronic information about each of the patients they serve if we put the right linkage in place. In many settings, the electronic data will come from an electronic medical record that are installed and operated at the clinical care site. In other settings, the electronic data will be available from patient focused electronic care registries and the data may be independent of any care sites. The goal for both approaches needs to be to have all of the needed data for each patient available at the point of care.

The patient-focused medical homes and the Accountable Care Organizations that are described in Chapter Four of this book will both be a very powerful source of patient supported registry functionality. The medical homes and ACOs will need systems that anchor that data for care settings that do not have a full electronic medical record in place.

There will be variations relative to the patient data connectivity tools -- but we should be headed very deliberately for a functional future where all face-to-face care sites will have either EMRs or an electronic patient registry of some kind to support care.

The physician's office part of the care delivery system is clearly also destined to survive as a key element of future care delivery. There will be a growing level of variability in site size, site scope, site scale and functionality for those medical offices. At one end of the continuum, we will see face-to-face care delivered at microsites -- tiny care kiosks -- where licensed caregivers will see patients face-to-face in very small care settings.

Some of those settings will even be mobile. A number of care vans exist already and are being used to bring face-to-face care more conveniently to patient locations.

As we go forward to create team care and accessible care, even the micro care kiosks should be well supported with electronic medical records and extensive levels of patient information.

At the other end of the physician's office care continuum from the micro clinics will be a growing number of medical macro clinics. In a number of settings, care delivery organizations are building full service, full capability macro care sites -- mega care hubs. The care hub model has the potential as a medical group to provide almost all of the care needs of their patients in one very large care sites sometimes available to provide multiple levels of care in one visit.

Those care hubs will also be heavily supported by the new electronic tool kit. The care hubs will also be supported by extensive levels of connectivity tools that will allow for video links, team consults, and care connectivity levels that will allow key levels of care expertise to flow electronically to the patient rather than having the patient moving from one physical site to another.

The ability of really well designed care hubs to do that work well is already being proven. One of the large multispecialty care settings is already using video consults so well that over 20 percent of their dermatology visits are now being done by video from the office of the patient's primary care doctor.[105]

The ability to redesign work flows and to build care delivery around the patient can be enhanced significantly by the use of those tools in a multi-specialty team care context and setting.

In any case, the doctors' offices will continue to be a major site of care -- in multiple sizes and permutations -- and those physician anchored sites will also have all of the information about each patient available electronically in real time.

For some elements of care -- like drawing blood, removing a cyst, setting a broken bone, or getting a tissue sample for diagnostic analysis -- sheer logistical realities will require physical medical office sites to continue to exist.

The Home Will Become the Third Site of Care

One obvious problem with delivering care in either a hospital or a clinical care site is that the patient who is receiving care has to actually physically travel to those care sites. Travel can be inconvenient and sometimes difficult for patients. Any time a patient can receive appropriate care without having to travel to a care site to get that care, that approach to care delivery has the potential to make life easier for the patient.

If we really want to build care delivery around the patients and not around the business units of care delivery, the ability to receive basic care without travelling to a care site has obvious value and merit.

That fact –- combined with the fact that most of the care dollars spent in this country are spent on patients with chronic disease who generally benefit physically from consistent care monitoring and care support –- have caused quite a few caregiver organizations to conclude that the third primary site of care in the future should be and will be the home.

The new tool kit for care monitoring and care connectivity is already allowing the home to be the primary site of care for a growing number of patients. A whole array of in-home care support tools can already track key elements of a patient's physical status. In-home EKGs are now possible. Basic function monitoring can be now done relatively inexpensively from the home for an increasing number of patients.

Caregiver contact with the patient in the home can be very often video-linked and tied to a blend of phone connections and email connectivity. That in-home care package already can replace many of the patient doctor encounters that have always required the patients to go in person to a clinic or a hospital for care.

In-home care can be far more convenient, significantly less expensive, and –- for many patients –- faster, more consistent and better care.

That in-home care support model works best in the context of accountable care and a care team. It's hard to do isolated pieces of care in a home. But team care makes sense for home care. The use of patient-centered medical home team care approaches can create an easy to manage context for care delivery where in-home care is part of a total care package and a total care agenda for a patient instead of being an incidental, siloed, unconnected array of services that can be individually provided in the home as a site of care. Preventable care can also often be done remotely.

The best accountable care teams will also look at in-home care tools as a key and easy way to react quickly to patient needs when patient need quick interventions. The ability of care teams to monitor physical statuses of patient in their homes will be at a level that is far superior for many patients to the traditional monitoring that has happened in person when the patients have a monthly or even weekly appointment for a face-to-face care at a medical office.

The home could be the primary site of care for quite a few people -- and that will be most effective in the context of team care being delivered to those in-home patients.

The Internet Will Be the Fourth Site of Care

In addition to those three increasingly well supported physical sites of care, we are on the cusp of seeing care delivery evolve very quickly to an entirely new care concept -- care everywhere.

Internet supported care can happen whenever an internet connection exists.

Care everywhere is clearly going to happen. There are thousands of computerized care opportunities already available on the internet that can do some levels of care diagnosis, care monitoring, and various kinds of care consultations. Second opinions on the web are becoming easy to do. So are initial diagnoses for some conditions.

Health care apps already abound. Many elements of care that once required a face-to-face doctor's office visit can now be achieved on the internet. The new monitoring tools that exist on the web today can give patients the ability to track their activity levels, their food intake levels, and even their relative levels of heart activity or emotional status. Electronic tools to help monitor patients who are suffering from depression exist now. Monitoring for congestive heart failure patients is also available as a web tools. There are a number of tools now and more are being developed.

Group therapy session and individual counseling are even available electronically.

The new tool kit of care is exploding -- and it will transform care delivery.

We Need To Avoid New Electronic Siloes

That could be wonderful. It could also be -- for some patients -- dysfunctional and even dangerous. That new tool kit could also create entirely new data silos. It would be more than a little ironic if one consequence of using the internet as a care support tool would be to replace paper data silos with new electronic data silos that are equally segregated and equally dysfunctional.

As we look at the business models we need to use to buy care in the future, we need to make sure that those new business models embrace and support the best elements of this new world of care delivery rather than rejecting, derailing, defusing, or ignoring it.

Again -- building a level of accountability for the care of each patient can be a key thing to build into the new tool kit. If Accountable Care Organizations actually become accountable and are functionally responsible for the total care needs of a patient, we will need those ACOs to embrace team care, connected care and continuously improving care.

E-visits, done well, can replace some face-to-face office visits for the new care organizations and can both improve care and reduce costs. As noted earlier, quite a few existing care sites that could do various kinds of e-visits well do not do them at all today because the piecework business model we use to buy care pays well for a face-to-face visit and doesn't pay at all for an e-visit.

Patients Love E-visits

Again, that perspective is not theoretical or hypothetical; that set of assumptions about what is possible when providers of care sell care by the package and not by the piece is based on direct observation of patient behavior and care delivery in settings where that model is used.

Kaiser Permanente is currently paid a lump sum today for all care as a care system. KP is not paid by the piece for care -- so Kaiser Permanente has already built electronic patient connectivity tools and uses e-visits today for many patients. Last year, there were over 13,000,000 e-visits in that particular care setting that would or could have been face-to-face visits in other care sites.[106] Over 30,000,000 Kaiser Permanente lab results were delivered electronically to Kaiser Permanente patients -- with several million of those lab results going directly to people's smart phones.[107] In the past -- and in other care settings -- patients would need to visit their clinic to see their doctor in person to get those lab results.

Patients love that that electronic connectivity for e-visits and lab results. It doesn't happen in too many other care sites today because those electronic connections tend to replace a face-to-face billable event and any care redesign that eliminates a billable event is frowned on by people who rely on that cash flow for their livelihood.

We don't need care delivery built around entirely those kinds of billable events when other and better alternatives exist for meeting patient needs.

What does that tell us?

It tells us that the business model we use to buy care should very intentionally and effectively support the evolving delivery opportunities in care. The new ACO's and Medical Homes that are being worked to sell and deliver packages of care are highly likely to use that same set of tools and use them well.

Before describing what that new business model for buying care should look like, it makes sense to look at one more key issue that has a huge impact on health care costs in America. The next chapter focuses on that key issue -- the prices we spend for care. Any solution to health care costs that doesn't look at prices as part of the strategy to reduce costs is overlooking a major opportunity. So read the information in the next Chapter about the reality of prices in this country today and then look at various ways how we might change the way we buy care.

CHAPTER THREE

PRICES ARE HIGHER HERE

Prices matter a lot.

When you look closely at health care costs for this country, the one point that stands out as the biggest single difference between us and everyone else in the world is prices.

We almost never talk about prices. Until very recently, prices have not been a significant part of the public debate in this country. Medicare has recently triggered some public discussion of actual prices changed in some hospitals by releasing some Medicare data, and a couple of news media outlets have done some very interesting pricing stories -- but that information has only triggered media attention, and it hasn't triggered policy focus in any settings.

Almost no part of the current official health care reform agenda deals with prices or even mentions prices. But when you look at the U.S. health care spending levels and when you compare us to the rest of the world, the single most glaringly obvious thing that stands out as the overwhelming difference between us and everyone else on the planet is the unit prices we pay for care.

If we took the exact same prices that the single payer system in Canada uses to buy each piece of care in Canada and if we directly substituted their prices for the prices we pay today for each piece of care that we buy in the U.S., the truth is we could deliver every single piece of care we deliver today -- changing nothing about the volume of care received by our patients and changing nothing about the type and scope of care delivered today to our patients -- and we could provide all of that care for about forty percent less money. We would spend about the same percentage of our GDP on care as Canada spends on care if we just paid the same prices for each piece of care that the government pays for each piece of care in Canada.

Prices are -- when you look at real numbers -- the overwhelming difference between us and them.

Insurance premiums are based on the average cost of care for insured people. Insurance premiums paid in this country could drop hugely if we used the Canadian fee schedules to pay for care here. If American insurers suddenly paid Canadian prices for each piece of care, the insurance premiums charged in this country would drop by that same 40 percent, and it would happen instantly. That isn't a speculation or a guess or a hope. It's the law.

The new health care reform law would require that premium reduction to happen if the prices we spend for care went down to those levels, because the new law specifies that insurance premiums have to be based on a percentage of the money that insurers use to buy care. Loss-ratio lows have already caused some insurers to pay rebates to their customers. Using Canadian prices to buy care would increase those rebates hugely.

All Other Countries Have Lower Prices

Prices really are the major financial difference between us and them.

That means that prices are an incredibly important health care cost factor that we need to understand and address as we look at how much money we spend for care and as we try to figure out how to spend less money on care.

This chapter of this book is intended to put the whole picture about the price situation in this country on the table so that everyone who reads this book can clearly understand this fundamental financial reality and can work to help figure out how to factor prices into the goal of making care more affordable. We need to start by looking at real numbers that show how much we actually pay. The price charts that are included in this chapter show how much we Americans pay for several key pieces of care compared to the amount that is paid in other industrialized counties for those same exact pieces of care.

It isn't just Canada who pays less than we do for each piece of care. Every other industrialized pays less to buy each piece of care. The charts in this chapter show the prices that are paid for care in several other industrialized countries.

The comparative prices for pieces of care in this book come from countries that use the same basic care delivery models and the same basic care delivery equipment and the same basic procedures that we use in our country to deliver care. CT scans are a universal commodity. Scans are scans. We all use the same equipment from the same manufacturers and we all basically do the same scans. The price comparisons for scans in this chapter are, as the saying goes, apples to apples. The data shows that prices for those identical CT scans vary hugely from country to country. We pay two to ten times more for our scans than other countries pay for their scans.[108] Prices for surgeries also differ by a significant amount -- and the prices paid for a day in the hospital vary by an amazing amount from country to country. Even drug prices for the exact same drugs made by the exact same drug companies differ quite a bit from country to country. We need to understand what those price differences are and we need to understand why those differences exist if we want to make care more affordable in this country.

Our Prices Are Often Double or Triple the Prices Paid in Other Countries

So what are the actual price differences between us and the rest of the world? Let's start with appendectomies.

Figure 3.1

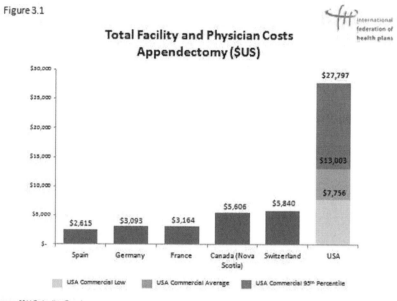

Total Facility and Physician Costs Appendectomy ($US)

Source: 2011 Federation Report

Appendectomies are a good example of price variations that happen between countries. Look at the price chart above. The total cost for an appendectomy in Spain in 2011 was $2,615. The cost for that same procedure in Germany was $3,093. France was slightly higher -- at $3,164. Canada actually had higher prices than any of those counties -- running $5,606 per appendectomy, and the Swiss paid $5,408 for each appendectomy patient.[109]

How much did those surgeries cost here? The average price for an appendectomy in the U.S. was $13,003.[110]

That is the exact same procedure being done in each and every country.

Appendectomy techniques are about the same from country to country. The human body is the same in each country. The quality of care is pretty consistent, site to site. We definitely do not get higher quality appendectomies for our higher prices. Other countries have appendectomy success rates that are as good as or better than ours, and patients in some of our hospitals are actually more likely to get post-surgical infections and be damaged then hospital patients in other countries. People don't fly to our country from Europe or Canada to have their appendix removed. An appendectomy is an appendectomy everywhere. But the prices paid for appendectomies are far higher in the U.S. than in any other country.

We Don't Pay Just One Price in the U.S.

It's useful to take a close look at each of the bars on that appendectomy price chart. There truly is a lot to learn from that array of data. The variation of prices for that surgery that is shown on the U.S. data bar is a particularly good data point for us all to study and understand.

The U.S. prices shown on that chart are actually a wide range of prices. That is important to know. We don't pay just one price in the U.S. for that procedure. We pay a wide range of prices. Every care site in the country sets its own prices -- and those prices vary a lot. Prices vary from site to site and prices in this country can even vary significantly from patient to patient at the exact same care site.

Other countries tend to have a single price for most procedures. That same standard price for each procedure is usually paid at every care site in each geography in those countries and that same exact price is typically charged by each caregiver to every payer in that geography. Many other countries achieve that level of multisite and multi-payer price uniformity by literally mandating prices. The pricing mandate that they use in other countries can be pretty rigid. A doctor in Canada can actually lose their license to be paid for care by their national health service for any of their government paid patients if the doctor charges any patient even one dollar more than the government approved fee for any of the services on their approved fee list.[111]

So prices for pieces of care are very rigid in that lovely part of the world that sits just north of our borders.

Prices Vary a Lot in the U.S.

By contrast, prices in the U.S. vary. A lot.

In the U.S., the $13,003 price mentioned above was the average fee that was actually paid in the U.S. in 2011by health plans or health insurers for an appendectomy.[112] There was actually a very wide range of fees charged that year for that procedure in this country, however. The American bar on that appendectomy chart shows the range of fees that were used in the U.S. for that surgery.

Twenty-five percent of the time, U.S. care sites that year charged less than $7,756 for the procedure. Five percent of the time, U.S. care sites charged more than $27,797.[113] Those are huge price differences. It is particularly important and useful to know, understand and remember that those major price differences that are charged in our country don't just vary between care sites. Some people who have heard that caregiver prices vary in this country think -- in error -- that the price variations that exist in U.S. are actually based on price and cost differences that occur between different sites of care. That seems logical -- but it is actually is a wrong belief. Prices charged to patients often vary hugely in this country for the exact same procedure done at the exact same site of care -- with the care delivered at that site by the exact same caregiver. Because of the business model we use to buy care, any given American care site might actually have dozens of different prices for each specific procedure. What causes the fees to vary from patient to patient? The answer to that question also surprises some people. The actual fee that is used by each American care site to deliver a particular service to any single patient usually depends directly and entirely on who the official payer is for each patient receiving care. The fees charged for each patient are based on the patient's health plan. Each health plan payer in this country tends to negotiate their own fee schedule with individual providers of care. Because of those negotiations, the fee that is charged in this country to any given patient usually is based on whoever the actual specific insurer or payer is for that patient. A care site that has contracts with a dozen local insurers could charge a dozen different fees for the same procedure for insured people.

Medicare and Medicaid Have Their Own Fee Schedules

To complicate the situation a bit more, each care site is also very likely to have a separate Medicare fee and a separate Medicaid fee for that same procedure.

And for the patients who do not have Medicaid coverage, Medicare coverage, or private insurance coverage of any kind, the providers tend to use a master fee schedule often called a "chargemaster." That chargemaster fee schedule basically sets the fees that are charged to uninsured patients.

The chargemaster fees tend to be the very highest fees of all. Those fees are high, in part, because the care sites often negotiate their contracted payment levels with health plans using a payment formula that is based on a fixed percentage of discounts from the provider's chargemaster. A health plan might negotiate a 30 percent discount off the chargemaster fees for a care site, for example.

Obviously, the care providers who use that negotiation approach to set their fees are strongly incented to have the highest possible chargemaster fee levels. It is better for the care site to have a high fee when the chargemasters serve that mathematical purpose as the key determiner of the actual revenue they receive from their contracted and discount paying health insurers.

The actual chargemaster fees can be so high as to be almost unbelievable. Several are listed later in this chapter. The prices on these charts, however, are based on the actual fees that were paid in 2011 by the health insurers.

Are Any Prices Inherently Legitimate?

So what does that wide variation in fees paid in this country tell us about the inherent legitimacy and appropriateness of any given fee?

People who receive care often believe that there must be an inherent legitimacy of some kind to each price that is being charged to them by their caregiver for their personal care. People who get care and then receive bills from their caregivers often believe that the pure price on the bill that is being charged to them by their care site must be "right" in some important way or it wouldn't be used by a caregiver they trust as the fee that is being charged to them as a patient for that piece of care.

That sense that there is actually a "right" price for any given piece of care is clearly not an accurate way of thinking about prices. There really is no such thing as a "right" price for pieces of care in this country. In the real world of health care cash flow, all prices tend to be functionally situational and all prices tend to be linked to payment mechanisms and tied to negotiated price levels. To the extent that the price variations happen at the care sites, those variations are not patient based, functionality based, or resource based in any way. That is an important reality to understand. Variation happens. The business model we use to buy care has created an amazing range and array of prices for most pieces of care and every provider who sells care in this country lives with that pricing reality every day.

Angioplasties Fees Are a Lot Higher Here

The U.S. price ranges for each procedure are fascinating. As noted earlier, all American health insurers tend to negotiate fees with their care sites -- and most of the negotiated fees are discounts of one kind of another from the full "chargemaster" fee schedule that is set up by each care site. Some of the negotiated fees are actually based on the Medicare fee schedule -- with insurers using Medicare fees as the base and then negotiating a private insurer fee that might be, for example, 120 percent of Medicare.

But even with both sets of those negotiated discounts -- either basing discounts on the chargemaster or basing payments on percentages of the Medicare base fee for that service -- we clearly pay a lot for each piece of care in this country than any other country in the world.

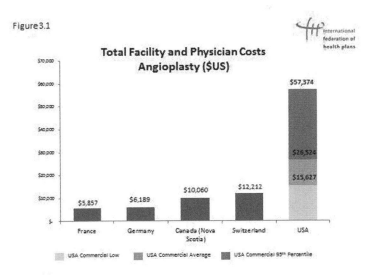

Figure 3.1

Source: 2011 Federation Report

The next chart shows the angioplasty cost in the same countries that were cited above. Again, the U.S. clearly pays more for that care. Various payers in the U.S. range from paying under $15,000 for that procedure to paying more than $57,000 to have an angioplasty done. The average cost here is $26,000. No other country spends more than $12,000 for that procedure. You can buy a very nice angioplasty in Paris for $5,857.[114]

All of those price charts in this book with the data from the other countries were compiled by the International Federation of Health Plans. The Federation is an interesting confederation of roughly 100 private health plans from 25 countries.[115] The prices on these charts from those other countries were usually the amount that was paid by the private health plans in those countries to buy each piece of care. The Canadian prices came from a government fee schedule. The prices on this set of charts for the United States were calculated from a massive American claims payment database that included actual payment data for over 100 million covered people.

As noted earlier, the U.S. price ranges shown on these charts were based on the actual amounts that were paid by U.S. payers…and do not include or show the inflated chargemaster prices that have been set up at the care sites. The numbers on those charts are what we actually paid in this country to buy that care. The prices are real.

In some cases, the prices are also stunning.

We Spend Ten Times As Much To Deliver a Baby

Delivering a baby is another area where the U.S. has a clear lead on prices. Look at the next chart. A doctor in Germany gets paid $226 to deliver a baby. A doctor in Canada gets paid $460. The average price paid in the U.S. to deliver a baby is $3,390. The lower end of the baby delivery price range in the U.S. runs down to $2,326. At the top of the range, 5 percent of babies delivered in this country triggered a fee in excess of $7,222.[116] Some care sites in this country now charge $15,000 to $20,000 to deliver a baby.[117]

Again -- when anyone wonders why Germany spends 11.6 percent of their GDP on health care[118] when the U.S. spends nearly 18 percent, [119] -- a quick look at the fees charged to buy care in Germany and the prices used to buy that same care the U.S. makes the explanation of that GDP percentage difference pretty simple.

Medicare and Medicaid Prices Tend To Be Lower

Most of the charts in this chapter do not include the amounts that are paid by either Medicare or Medicaid to buy each piece of care. The prices paid by those programs are discussed below. Both Medicare and Medicaid tend to spend significantly less money than the private payers in this country to buy pieces of care. Why do the Medicare and Medicaid programs pay less for care? They pay less because they can. Both of those government programs have the legal right to simply impose prices rather than having to negotiate prices with various providers of care. As a result of that authority, both of those programs tend to pay prices that are significantly below the average price levels shown on those charts for private payers.

Medicaid generally is the lowest payer for any piece of care in the U.S. The amount paid by Medicaid in California to deliver a baby for example, is $544.[120] That number looks very similar to European prices for delivering a baby and it is far below the private market prices that are paid in this country for doing that same procedure. Those relatively low Medicaid price levels obviously help to explain why it has been increasingly difficult to get many U.S. doctors to accept high numbers of Medicaid patients in significant areas of the country.

Figure 3.2

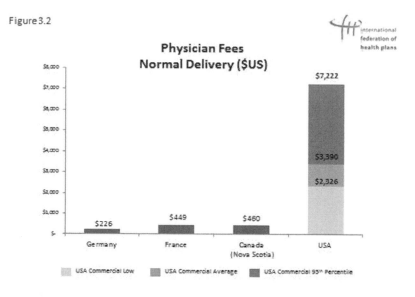

Source: 2011 Federation Report

Delivering a baby tends to be fairly similar from country to country. Cultural differences do exist relative to the way people approach giving birth, but those cultural differences should not be sufficient enough to cause a procedure that costs under $500 in France or Canada to generate an average fee of $3,390 in the U.S.

Heart Surgery Prices Vary a Lot

Heart surgery follows that same pricing pattern.

One of the more common heart procedures that is done here and elsewhere is coronary artery bypass surgery. That is a lovely surgical procedure. It saves and prolongs lives. It can be transformational for patients' lives. It is very much a high value procedure.

It is also a high cost procedure. Every country charges significant amounts of money to do that procedure. In France and

Germany, as you can see in the upcoming chart, that surgery costs over $16,000 per heart. That is a lot of money. In Switzerland, doing that same procedure costs the payer $25,486 per heart.[121]

Canada is even more expensive -- currently averaging about $40,954 per heart.[122] That is even more money than Switzerland.

What about the U.S.?

We win again. The average price paid in this country to do that basic heart surgery procedure was $67,583 per heart in 2011.[123]

Twenty-five percent of the fees to do those by-pass surgeries in the U.S. actually ran below $42,951...very near the Canadian numbers. At the other extreme, five percent of the fees in this country to do that bypass surgery exceeded $138,050[124]... with no improvement in safety levels and no guarantee of better outcomes for the higher priced surgery sites.

People Have the Illusion That Prices Reflect Quality

As the first two chapters of this book pointed out clearly, there is actually no mechanism linking high fees to higher quality care in this country. Many people do have the illusion that prices must reflect quality in some way, but the heart surgery sites that are charging over $100,000 to do those surgeries can actually have much worse outcomes and higher death rates than the care sites that are charging $20,000 or $40,000 for that same procedure. In fact, a number of studies have shown that the care can be less safe and less consistent in some of the higher priced care sites.[125]

So for that very basic heart procedure, we currently have care sites in the U.S. charging ten times as much as the average fee in Germany or France.[126] The outcomes in Germany and France are generally the same or better than the outcomes in U.S. care sites that charge a lot more.

Figure 3.3

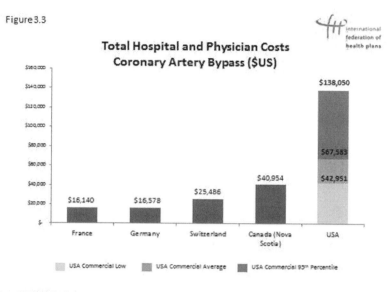

Source: 2011 Federation Report

This is actually a surgery where some of the best care in the world now is coming from some extremely low-cost surgery sites in the Middle East and India.

In a couple of developing countries, a few hospitals have recently built world-class heart surgery care sites that do that particular procedure with great effectiveness and skill. The very best sites in India have better outcomes and lower infection rates than the typical American hospital. The American hospitals do that work for an average piece of $67,000 -- and those very best Indian surgery sites now charge between $3,000 and $10,000 per heart for the same procedure.[127] The Indian prices and the surgical results in those Indian hospitals prove again that prices and quality have no inherent linkage in health care delivery. Best care is not inherently more expensive and the worst care sites sometimes have the highest price tags.

The Highest Cost Sepsis Sites Had the Highest Death Rate

One fascinating recent study of sepsis patients showed that the hospitals who charged the most for sepsis care actually also had some of the highest death rates from sepsis.[128] That inverse relationship between cost and quality can shock people who think that paying more for care means that higher priced care is better. For the sepsis patients in the hospitals that were included in that study, the higher prices meant bad care was happening. Those higher prices actually resulted from the bad care to a significant degree. Significantly more patients died of sepsis in the higher cost hospitals that were involved in that study.

That fact -- about prices and quality not being somehow linked for care delivery -- really does confuse a lot of people. The confusion is understandable. That linkage is how things usually work. Prices and quality are usually linked in other areas of the economy. "Spend more; get more," is the economic norm. We tend to believe that a $20,000 car is better than a $10,000 car -- and we tend to believe that a five thousand dollar computer will be better than a one thousand dollar computer. We have come to expect and believe in that direct relationship between value and price in many other things that we buy. So it is hard for people to understand that the current business model we use to buy care in this country does not have that linkage built into either the purchase process or the pricing process for care. Value does not drive prices in our business model for care delivery. Prices are created and driven by each business unit's financial goals, by each business unit's revenue strategies and by the various circumstances and historical charge patterns that exist at each care site.

Medicaid Tends To Be The Lowest Payer Everywhere

There is some pricing pattern consistency for some parts of the health care ecosystem. As noted earlier, our government programs do tend to have some price consistency for the care they buy. The government creates that pricing consistency for Medicare and Medicaid by imposing prices rather than by negotiating prices for Medicare and Medicaid patients. Those government imposed prices are usually not very high...relative to the "retail" prices charged to other payers.

Medicaid, in fact, tends to be the lowest payer everywhere in the country. Hardly anyone in any care setting in this country pays providers less than the local state-imposed Medicaid fee schedule. Many care providers argue that the Medicaid prices are so low that almost all caregivers lose money on every Medicaid patient and most caregivers have to make up for those losses by charging more money to their non-government patients. Some caregivers state that their Medicare prices are also below their cost of actually providing care -- and they often say that they make up for Medicare losses as well by shifting the care costs to their insured patients through higher fees for those patients. Some care sites argue that the "cost shift" from their Medicare and Medicaid patients actually are a "hidden tax" -- and argue that their fees are higher in large part because of that "hidden tax" and "cost shift" to other payers.

Is that a true set of assumptions? It probably is true for some care sites -- particularly the sites who serve a lot of Medicaid patients. The cost shift argument is probably less true for the care sites that have both very high fees and very few Medicaid patients. The cost shift argument is often not supported with any volume numbers that justify the high prices being charged in a number of care sites. That situation is very care site-specific in its relevance.

Medicare Pays More Than Medicaid but Less Than Everyone Else

In any case, Medicare clearly also imposes a fee schedule on care-givers that runs significantly below the usual amounts that are paid to buy care for insured people. Anytime we use taxpayer money to buy care, the government tends to set the prices that are paid for each piece of care. Medicare simply sets fees that are fixed, non-negotiable, and significantly lower than the usual private market fees for the same procedure. Some Medicare payment levels are shown below.

The next chart includes the U.S. average fee and the Californian Medicare and Californian Medicaid fees for the three procedures that were outlined earlier in this chapter -- appendectomies, delivering a baby and coronary artery bypass surgery.

As you can see, the payments made by those two major government programs fall well below the average payment for private health plans for each of the procedures.

Figure 3.4

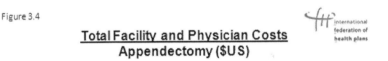

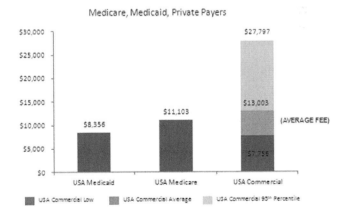

Source: 2011 Federation Report. Medicare and Medicaid estimate was compiled by Deloitte Consulting LLP on behalf of Kaiser Permanente Health Plan.

Figure 3.5

Total Hospital and Physician Costs
Coronary Artery Bypass ($US)

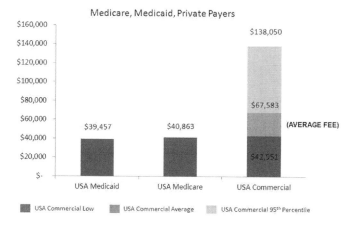

Medicare, Medicaid, Private Payers

$138,050

$67,583

$39,457 $40,863   (AVERAGE FEE)

$42,951

USA Medicaid   USA Medicare   USA Commercial

■ USA Commercial Low   ■ USA Commercial Average   ■ USA Commercial 95th Percentile

Source: 2011 Federation Report. Medicare and Medicaid estimate was compiled by Deloitte Consulting LLP on behalf of Kaiser Permanente Health Plan

Figure 3.6

Total Hospital and Physician Costs
Normal Delivery ($US)

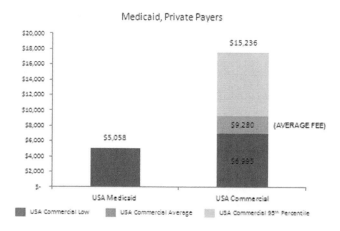

Medicaid, Private Payers

$15,236

$9,280   (AVERAGE FEE)

$5,058

$6,995

USA Medicaid   USA Commercial

■ USA Commercial Low   ■ USA Commercial Average   ■ USA Commercial 95th Percentile

Source: 2011 Federation Report. Medicaid estimate was compiled by Deloitte Consulting LLP on behalf of Kaiser Permanente Health Plan.

What we can see from each of those charts is that both Medicare and Medicaid pay significantly less than the commercial average payment. It is also true that some patients in the U.S. who have commercial insurance are charged fees that resemble the Medicare and Medicaid fee schedules.

The patients who are not shown on these payment charts are not the people who are the most damaged and abused by the overall spectrum of fee levels used in this country.

The Uninsured May Pay the Most for Each Piece of Care

As noted earlier, the prices shown on those charts basically represent either negotiated fees or mandated fees. People who have Medicare or Medicaid coverage or who have private insurance all have someone either negotiating fee on their behalf or imposing fees on their behalf. The uninsured people in this country, however, have no one helping mitigate the fees charged to them for care. They tend to have the pure top level chargemaster retail fees imposed on them when they seek care.

So the people who are charged the most for each piece of care in this country are almost always the uninsured people who are paying for their own care. Those uninsured people, unfortunately, not only do not have either a health plan negotiating their prices or a government agency mandating prices on their behalf.

They also have no legal protection today against abusive fees. There are no laws that limit the chargemaster top fees or address their use for low income people. There are no laws that limit these fees to a level that might, for example, be a multiple of Medicare fees -- or an average of all negotiated fees in that care setting, plus 10 percent -- or some other formula-based regulatorily-defined fee cap.

As a result, the chargemaster prices that are used to create bills for the uninsured consumers who get care in this country can run quite high.

A recent article in Time Magazine looked at a number of those charges that are being used today as the fees that are charged to uninsured people. Time Magazine showed chargemaster fees for an emergency room visit by an uninsured person for $21,000 and Time showed a stress test that was billed to the uninsured person by the care site at a chargemaster fee of $7,997. Then the Time article showed that Medicare would have paid $554 for the same stress test and less for the emergency room use. The Time article also showed chargemaster fees to an uninsured patient of $157.61 for a CBC (complete blood count). That was the fee when that service was billed to an uninsured person. Medicare, Time pointed out, would have paid the doctor $11.02 for that same exact CBC test in Connecticut if it had been done for a Medicare patient.[129]

The Chicago Tribune wrote an article about the chargemaster fees based on the Medicare data report. The Tribune article showed a variation on local fees for a major hip replacement ranging from $36,141 at one care site to $117,102 at another care site -- for the same exact procedure.[130]

Medicare payments for that procedure were $21,072, according to the Tribune.[131]

The Los Angeles Times wrote a similar article showing price variations based on the Medicare report. The Times reported that the price range for an artificial joint replacement varied from a top price of $220,881, to a low price of $35,524.[132]

That same Los Angeles Times article cited prices for the treatment of simple pneumonia that varied from $19,852 at the bottom of the range, to $54,400 at the top of the price range.[133]

The Denver Post wrote an article on that same set of issues showing price variation for joint replacement, ranging from $32,000 at the bottom of the local price list, to $84,000 at the top.[134]

Medicare pays $13,000 to $20,000 for that procedure in that geographic area according to The Post.[135]

So the patterns are widespread. Price variation in those chargemaster prices is massive and has no relationship to care quality or even care availability.

There is clearly no rational expense-based reason or resource-linked reason that can be used to justify either of those horrific chargemaster fee levels being charged for those services. The truth is, of course, that many of the uninsured people end up being charged those very high fees by the care sites simply don't pay those very high fees. Many uninsured people have very little money and absolutely cannot afford to pay those extraordinary fees. So they often don't pay them.

Those people can be damaged twice in the process. Look back to the Time magazine article cited above.

The impact on an uninsured person for not paying that $7,997 fee for what was actually a $500 stress test[136] is that the credit status of that uninsured patient can be impaired or ruined. The future debt capacity of that uninsured person can be destroyed by having that particular bad debt. And -- to add insult to injury -- the hospitals that created those exorbitant and entirely artificial fees might actually get to write off the unpaid fees by the low income patients as "bad debt" for their tax-related issues.

Many hospitals and medical care sites do not fully enforce those kinds of abusive pricing approaches and consequences for their patients. Many care sites also do not wreck the credit rating of the lower income uninsured people who cannot pay their medical bill. But too many care sites do manage to bankrupt patients with those kinds of financially abusive bills -- or ruin the patient's credit ratings -- and then get public credit for charity care in the process.

Many people work very hard to pay off the debts incurred by those high bills. Look back again at the Los Angeles Times article. It is painful to think of the basic injustice of a minimum wage worker having to take $50 out of every paycheck for years to pay off an incident-based health care bill -- shelling out cash every month for two years to pay for a care service that would have generated that particular care site only a single $50 paid-in-full fee if Medicare had been the payer. Too many uninsured people have been ruined financially and even bankrupted by those prices.

Low Income Uninsured People Will Still Face Abusive Prices

The new health care reform legislation will significantly reduce the number of uninsured people in America. It is a good thing that our very-low-income people in this country will now qualify for Medicaid coverage. These kinds of pricing dilemmas will no longer be relevant for those very low income people who join Medicaid next year because Medicaid will now buy their care.

Other low income people who are currently uninsured will now also be able to buy subsidized coverage though the new insurance exchanges. These horrendous and crippling chargemaster prices will be completely irrelevant to all of those people once they have insurance coverage of some kind and they have either insurers or the government mitigating prices on their behalf.

So those abusive prices will damage fewer people a year from now.

But even after many people move to Medicaid and even after millions of others move to subsidized private coverage, we will still have over ten million uninsured people in this country.[137] Those ten million people with no insurance will all still be at the mercy of the abusive chargemaster prices that will continue to be charged to uninsured people.

Those high chargemaster fees, of course, are often charged to an uninsured person at the worst possible time in a person's need for care -- an emergency situation. The next chart shows emergency room activation fees at several Californian hospitals. Some of the prices charged by some care sites are reasonable, and some can only be labeled as abusive.

Again -- the variation in fees from site to site is almost mind-boggling. The fee that is paid by Medicare for that service is shown at the bottom of the chart. Health plans pay more than Medicare and more than Medicaid, but less than full chargemaster prices.

Figure 3.7 — FOR ILLUSTRATIVE PURPOSES ONLY

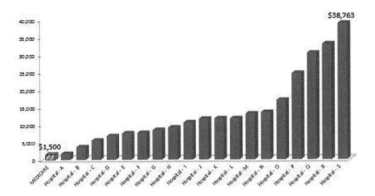

Fees for Trauma Unit "Activation"

Source: Trauma Activation Fees in the State of California 2011 as prepared by Deloitte. Medicare number obtained from Office of Statewide Health Planning and Development (OSHPD) 2009: http://www.oshpd.ca.gov.

Prescription Drug Prices Are Also Higher Here

Overall -- when you look at the average amount we spend for each piece of care -- our prices are the highest in the word.

We pay more for just about everything. We see very significant price differences between us and other countries for medical technology and for prescription drugs. Medical technology prices in other countries tend to be significantly lower for the same exact pieces of equipment. Implants also definitely cost a lot more here. Prosthetics cost more here. We pay a lot more in this country for most pieces of medical technology.

Drug prices also tend to be much higher in the U.S. Nexium, for example, costs $23 in France. That same drug costs $36 in Canada and the price jumps to $56 for Germany.[138]

In the U.S., the average price paid for Nexium is $193 -- and five percent of American patients pay more than $357 for the drug.[139]

The following chart shows the Nexium prices.

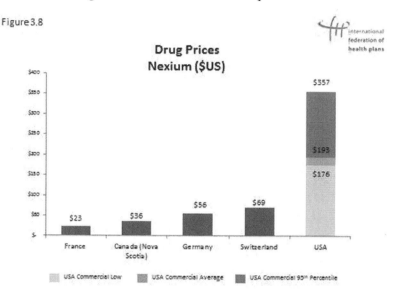

Figure 3.8

Source: 2011 Federation Report

Likewise, Plavix prices run from $49 in France to $74 in Canada and those prices run way up to $109 in Germany.[140]

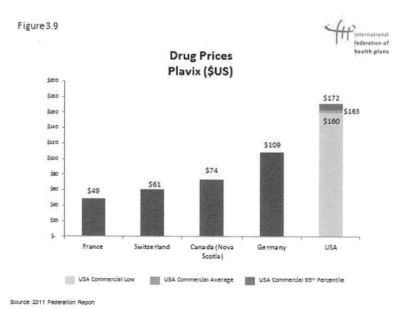

Figure 3.9

Source: 2011 Federation Report

The U.S., of course, beats Germany. We pay an average price of $163 for that drug.[141] Is that a fair price for us? That question has been asked many times. It isn't easy to answer. What exactly constitutes a fair price for a prescription drug? That really is an interesting and important question. Other countries clearly pay less. We can safely assume that the drug companies are not taking financial losses for each sale they voluntarily make in each of those other countries.

We know from sheer common sense that the costs of providing those drugs must be below the prices they currently charge to sell those drugs to patients in those other industrialized countries.

Our prices are higher -- but higher for no functional, operational, or logistical reason. There is no higher cost factor here for drugs that is created by some expense-related issue that is unique in the U.S. What we can obviously conclude from the evidence in front of us is that all of the prices shown on those charts for all of those drugs in each country are simply invented by those drug companies for each market.

Drug prices here and in those other countries clearly have no inherent unit price relationship in any country that ties each price directly to the actual cost of producing those drugs, storing those drugs, or delivering those drugs in those countries. The prices are obviously set in each case and in each country based on what each local market will pay. The U.S. clearly will pay a lot. So prices here are very high.

An example of countries paying what the markets allow to be paid is the price range for the breast cancer drug, Herceptin. Herceptin extends life for some breast cancer patients.[142] It doesn't technically save lives but it clearly extends some lives. It is a very expensive drug.

One of the recent ongoing debates in the health policy world in this country has focused on whether insurance companies in this country should pay for Herceptin. An ancillary debate that has also occurred in this country has focused on whether the insured patients who have cancer who want that drug should pay a larger share of the Herceptin price. It is a very expensive drug. Herceptin currently costs about a $100,000 per patient in the U.S.[143] A hundred thousand dollars per patient is a significant amount of money. That price makes it extremely expensive for any people who need to use their own money to pay for that drug. That high price also increases the premiums that are charged by health plans when that drug is a covered benefit and the health plans pay for the drug. That payment for that drug by health plans arithmetically increases the average cost of care for all of the insured people in each health plan that pays for the drug.

So how do actual U.S. prices paid for that drug compare to the prices paid for that same drug in other countries? The answer, of course, is the same one we saw for other fees. We pay more. That same exact drug with the same exact dose runs about $40,000 per patient in Great Britain.[144] We pay $100,000. British patients pay less than half that amount.

Much of the ethical debate, the political debate, and economic concern about whether any level of constraint or limitation on the use of that drug is needed or appropriate in the U.S. could be ended fairly immediately if the drug company that is selling that drug simply stopped charging American patients two or three times as much for that drug in the U.S. as that same company charges breast cancer patients for that same drug in other countries. The ethical debate would not be needed if the economic reality was that our patients were charged the same prices charged to patients in other countries.

The Drug Has Been Assigned an Unaffordable Price

This is a basic truth we ought to understand. That drug is only unaffordable in the United States because it has been assigned an unaffordable price in the United States. That debate about rationing that particular drug is a little like having a debate about rationing food in a setting where the only baker in town is charging a thousand dollars per loaf for bread and people are starving because they can't afford bread. The debate in that town about how to respond to that thousand dollar loaf of bread should not be about how many people should starve. The debate in that town should be about repricing bread.

Insurance premiums could clearly be lower in the U.S. if this country paid British or Canadian prices for that drug and then also paid the same prices that those other countries pay for all other prescription drugs as well.

Paying Canadian Drug Prices Could Cut Insurance Premiums by 7 Percent

At a more macro level, we need to understand the basic economic fact that prescription drugs currently consume about 14 percent of the average premium costs for U.S. health insurance companies.[145] The basic economic reality is that 14 percent of the premiums collected by the insurers are used by the insurers in this country to buy prescription drugs. If American patients -- and American insurers -- could suddenly buy all drugs at Canadian prices, the total premium levels that are charged to their customers by American health insurers could drop by 7 percent over night just to reflect the lower prices that would be paid for drugs.

Seven percent is real money.

We Have Never Had the Political Courage To Address Those Issues

We have never had either the political courage or the political momentum in this country to address those issues. We don't ever link those prices for pieces of care to the premiums we charge.

We have never publically looked at how much less our insurance premiums would be in this country if we paid either Dutch or Swiss or Canadian prices for our prescription drugs.

The new loss ratio laws in the Affordable Care Act now very clearly mandate that the premium levels that can be charged by each health insurer must be based directly on the actual cost of care that is paid by each insurer. It's probably time to have a meaningful discussion about the impact of prescription drug prices on insurance premiums because the relationship is pretty clear at this point.

The Extreme Price Variation for a CT Scan Has To Be Seen To Be Believed

Drug manufacturers are actually not the worst unit-pricing offenders. Scans win that award.

Perhaps the most extreme level of price variation in American health care currently relates to CT scans and MRIs. CT scans and MRIs are wonderful technology. Done well, those scans can unveil important information about patients that can save lives, improve diagnosis and then help guide and monitor care plans for individual patients in very important ways. No one doubts the value and the benefits of those lovely scanning technologies.

What is a little less clear as a value and a benefit is the relative array of prices that are being paid today for those particular imaging procedures and the number of times that those scans are done. This book does not address or discuss the scan frequency appropriateness issues. Work done at the Virginia Mason Medical Center in Seattle can shed huge light on that topic.[146] That care team did some excellent quality redesign work relative to the need for scans. They have published their results. Take a look at what they have concluded. It is a well-done study. We do more scans, overall, than we need to do. We do more scans than any other country -- other than Japan -- by a wide margin -- so we win on both volume and price when it comes to scans.

We pay more per scan than anyone in the world.

The next chart shows the price range for a CT scan of the abdomen. In Canada, the price paid for that scan is $122. France pays a price of $141. Germany and Switzerland pay much higher amounts, with the Germans paying $354 per scan and the Swiss paying $425 per scan.[147]

In the U.S., the average scan price was $584 -- nearly five times higher than the prices paid in Canada or Spain. The range of prices paid in the U.S. was amazing -- with five percent of the scans in this country running over $1,657 and a number of scans running under $200.[148] The Medicare prices for those scans is now $316.[149] In California, the Medicaid price paid for those scans is $311.[150]

Some care sites have charged nearly $10,000 for a scan.[151] Other care sites in the U.S. have publically advertised the availability of $49 scans.[152] That is an amazing range of prices. What is even more amazing is the fact that it is actually possible to charge $40 for a scan and not lose money.

How can that be true?

Once a piece of scanning equipment is in place and once it has been paid for by other customers, the incremental real cost of doing the very next scan is close to zero. The production cost of doing an additional CT scan is actually less than the cost of doing an additional traditional x-ray, because doing a traditional x-ray involves the care site having to buy a piece of actual film and then use a mixture of expensive chemicals to process the film. Film based X-rays create real incremental costs and they create both supply and purchasing expenses that do not exist when you do a purely electronic scan. A CT scan may have the radiation exposure for each patient of a thousand low-dose x-rays[153], but that scan can cost less than a single x-ray in pure per scan production costs.

The variation on scan prices is huge.

Figure 3.10

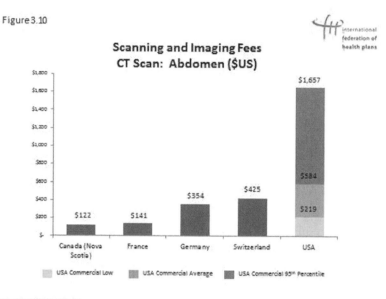

Scanning and Imaging Fees
CT Scan: Abdomen ($US)

Source: 2011 Federation Report

So a market-based purchasing model of some kind that is focused on bringing scan prices down in this country obviously has a high likelihood of success. There is already a range of more than ten to one for American care site scan prices. When we are trying to keep health care costs flat in this country, it's clear that if we simply -- on average -- brought our scans a little further down the existing price continuum for scans in this country, we could meet and exceed a very aggressive cost reduction goal for scanning costs and we could achieve those savings within the range of prices that already exist today in this country for scans. Take a good look at the chart. We pay more than the other countries and we have an amazing range of prices here.

We Also Have the Highest Hospital Costs in the World

When you look at prices charged in this country for pieces of care, some of the most interesting information relates to hospital prices. Hospital prices in this country -- not surprisingly -- tend to be the highest in the world by a large margin. The following chart shows that every single country in Europe spent less than a thousand dollars per day for hospital care in 2011. Our average cost per day in this country exceeded three thousand dollars in 2011.[154] We spend a lot more money for each day in the hospital than any country in the world by a wide margin. Our daily hospital costs usually run three to five times higher than the daily hospitalized costs in other industrialized countries. We pay more per day and we pay more stay.

Figure 3.11

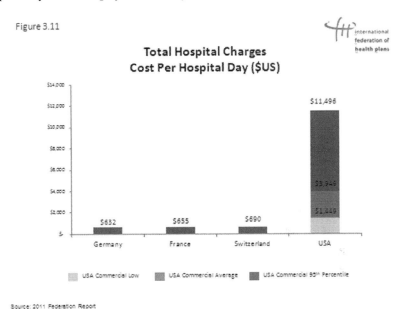

Source: 2011 Federation Report

The next chart shows average cost per stay in the hospital. We clearly win on both charts. The average cost per stay in Germany -- the second highest priced country -- is $5,000. We spend on average, more than $15,000 per stay -- and five percent of our hospital stays exceed $50,000.[155]

Figure 3.12

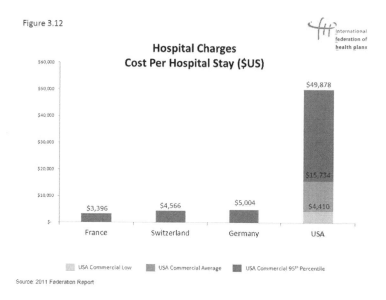

Hospital Charges
Cost Per Hospital Stay ($US)

Legend: USA Commercial Low | USA Commercial Average | USA Commercial 95th Percentile

Source: 2011 Federation Report

Why Isn't Our GDP Percentage Triple Other Countries?

So when we look at hospital care, medical care, many tests, scans, medical equipment and prescription drugs, we see prices in this country for each piece of care that tends to be two to five times higher than any other country. Those extreme ratios raise a very interesting and important question.

If our unit prices for all of those pieces of care are also that much higher than the European prices and if our prices are so much higher than the Canadian hospital, medical, procedural and pharmaceutical unit prices, why aren't we spending even more of our GDP on care compared to their percentages? We spend roughly 18 percent of our GDP on care. Those other countries now spend nine to twelve percent of their GDP on care.[156] If our unit prices are more than triple their prices, why isn't our total GDP percentage difference also triple their GDP percentage? Why are the GDP amounts spent for care in each of those European countries actually running at about half of our percentage instead of running at a third of our expense? That is actually an important question that we need to answer in order to understand the reality of our health care delivery expenses.

People in Other Countries Get More Care Than We Do

Why aren't we spending three times as much money in total for care in this country instead of spending -- in total -- roughly twice as much?

The answer to that question surprises most Americans. Some people who have read this book chapter were shocked. It is a very important point to examine, understand and discuss. The truth is, by most measurements of care delivery, the people in those other industrialized countries actually get more care than we do. We spend more money -- but we get less care. The urban legend that we hear very often in American health care debates is that all of those countries in Europe spend less money than we do on care because they ration care. Again -- facts can often be useful when dealing with health care policy thinking. That particular urban legend is not true. Look at the numbers. In just about every major category of care delivery, the Europeans have both higher volumes of care and faster access to care.

Let's start by looking at hospital days. A popular urban legend in this country is that we, Americans, have too many hospital beds and that we, in fact, significantly over use hospital care compared to all other countries in the industrialized world.

That is not true.

We Have Nearly the Lowest Hospital Use in the Industrialized World

We Americans actually have among the lowest hospital admission rates of any country. Our hospital admission rates are lower than almost every other country in the industrialized world.[157] The next chart shows the relative number of hospital admissions per capita in half a dozen countries. We clearly admit patients to our hospitals far less often than those countries admit patients to their hospitals. We Americans are, in fact, significantly less likely to be admitted to the hospital for care than folks from almost every other industrialized country.

Figure 3.13

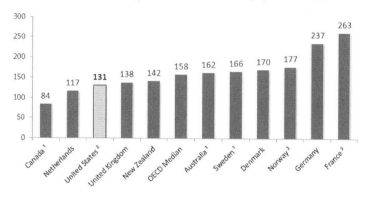

Utilization of Hospitals OECD Countries

Hospital Discharges All causes, Per 1000 population, 2009

Note: OECD 2008 numbers for Canada, United States, New Zealand, Australia.
1. Excludes discharges of healthy babies born in hospital (between 3-6% of all discharges).
2. Includes same-day separations.

Source: OECD Health Data 2011, WHO-Europe for Russian Federation and national sources for other non-OECD countries.

Only Canada and the Netherlands have lower hospital admission rates then we do. The average length of stay for delivering a baby in the Netherlands is less than two days.[158] It is very low because the Dutch prefer to deliver babies at home. Just about every other industrialized country is much more likely to admit a patient to a hospital than we are. Germany and France are roughly twice as likely as our country to admit patients for hospital care. Admitting patients to hospital care twice as often as we do clearly isn't hospital care rationing by those other countries. That urban legend is wrong. Even Great Britain is slightly more likely to hospitalize a patient then we are.

They Also Have Longer Lengths of Stay

So if we admit fewer patients to the hospitals, do the people we admit to the hospital stay there longer than the people in those other countries who admit more patients?

Again -- the answer is no. Look at the next chart.

We also have one of the shortest lengths of stay in hospitals of any industrialized country.[159] The following chart show the actual numbers. Only the Scandinavian countries that use government hospitals and tend to employ their own physicians tend to have their patients leave the hospital faster than we do.

Figure 3.14

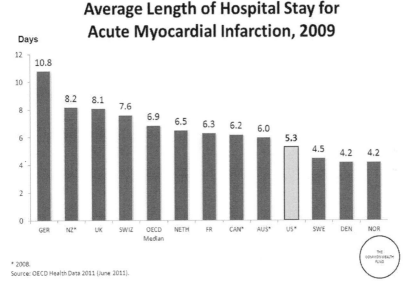

Average Length of Hospital Stay for Acute Myocardial Infarction, 2009

* 2008.
Source: OECD Health Data 2011 (June 2011).

Other countries -- as you can see from these charts -- currently keep their patients in the hospital for significantly longer lengths of stays than our average stay in this country. This next chart shows the length of stays for a basic heart attack. The average length of stay in hospitals for a heart attack in Germany is almost eight days. In Great Britain, the patients who have heart attacks stay in the hospital for over seven days. Our average length of stay in this country for a heart attack is slightly over five days.[160]

So the urban legend about our care costs being so much higher than European care costs because we have too many hospital beds and because we use our hospitals a lot more than Europeans use their hospitals is simply not true.

Do Other Countries Ration Medical Care?

What about medical care? If these countries don't ration hospital care, do they ration medical care? Another commonly held belief in this country is that our overall health care costs are so much higher because we Americans have much better access to physician care. Many people in our country believe that urban legend that those other countries who spend less money overall on care spend less money and keep their costs down primarily by rationing access to physician care. The urban legend is that we Americans use medical care far more extensively than people in those other industrialized countries use medical care. Is that belief about higher levels of physician care for patients in this country true?

No. That belief is also wrong. Again -- looking at real data on a given issue is often useful in figuring out what is true about that topic. Look at the actual numbers. We Americans actually see our doctors less often than the people in most other industrialized countries see their doctors.[161]

We Americans see our doctors -- on average --slightly less than four times a year. Canadians, in contrast, see their doctors five point five times a year. The French see their doctors almost seven times a year.

The Germans and the Japanese see their doctors the most -- with Germans going to the doctor over eight times a year and the Japanese seeing their doctors -- on average -- an amazingly high level of 13 doctor visits per year. Our four visits per year are significantly lower than their 13 visits. So the basic data about how often we see our doctors tells us that those countries are not rationing access to their doctors.

Anyone who believes that we see doctors more often and that is the reason why we spend more money on care should look carefully at the next chart.

Figure 3.15

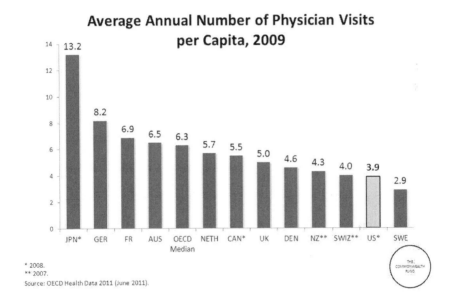

The other countries on this physician visit chart are clearly not rationing access to medical care. Again, only the Swedish -- with their government owned and government-operated care system -- see their doctors less often than we Americans see our doctors.

So if we look at the actual data, we can see that patients in other industrialized countries see their doctors more often than we see our doctors. They are also more likely to be hospitalized than Americans and when they are actually hospitalized, the patients in those countries tend to spend more time in the hospital.

So where do we Americans get real value for all of that additional money that we spend on health care? Do we at least get faster access to our doctors when we need faster access to our doctors?

The answer to that question is the same answer.

No.

We also do not get faster access to basic medical care than the other industrialized countries.

Other Countries Get Better Same Day Access

Several other countries that spend half as much money as we spend on care actually tend to have significantly better access than we do to same day care. Again -- look at the numbers on the next chart. Our numbers are over on the right hand side of the chart. The lower side. Just over half of American patients who want same day care can get it. By contrast, the Dutch patients currently have their same day care needs met almost 70 percent of the time. [162] We do get faster access to doctors than patients in Canada and Sweden. We lose to all the other industrialized countries on that basic measurement of care access. All of these countries have more doctors per capita than we do. We do tend to have more nurses per capita than those other countries, but we have fewer physicians.

When you measure how long people actually waited in each country for primary care, we were in the middle range -- with 16 percent of Americans waiting 6 days or more for basic care. The French had half as many people waiting 6 days for care — with only 8 percent of the French population not getting that level of care within a week.

Figure 3.16

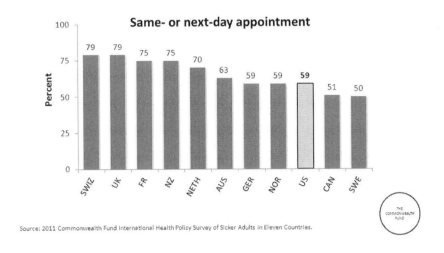

Access to Doctor or Nurse Last Time Sick or Needed Care

Source: 2011 Commonwealth Fund International Health Policy Survey of Sicker Adults in Eleven Countries.

Figure 3.17

Waited six days or more for a doctor visit

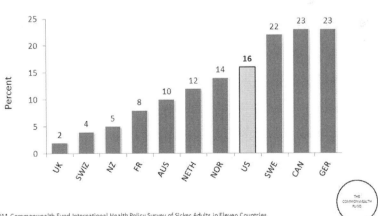

Source: 2011 Commonwealth Fund International Health Policy Survey of Sicker Adults in Eleven Countries.

The clear winners on getting fast access to primary care doctors are the British. They use a different care financing model. They don't buy care by the piece. They buy care as a package -- with primary care doctors paid a lump sum each month to meet the total primary care needs of their patients. People in Great Britain chose a primary care doctor and each doctor is then paid a flat amount per month per patient. Every primary care doctor has a known panel of patients. That approach somewhat resembles the patient-centered medical home model we are learning to use in the United States. Using their primary care model -- where their doctors sell packages of care rather than pieces of care -- the British only had two percent of their people who were not seen by their doctor within six days. Our16 percent six-day access to care performance was not the worst in the world but our performance was far from the best.

Figure 3.18

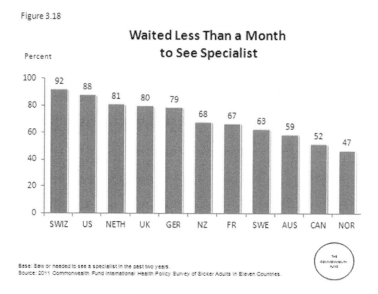

Waited Less Than a Month to See Specialist

Percent

Base: Saw or needed to see a specialist in the past two years
Source: 2011 Commonwealth Fund International Health Policy Survey of Sicker Adults in Eleven Countries

Access to Specialty Care

The one area where we are not at or near the bottom of the care access performance charts is in access to specialty care. On the specialty care access chart shown below, we do fairly well. We don't do as well on access to specialty care as the Swiss -- but we do slightly better than the Dutch and the Germans and we do quite a bit better than Canada, Sweden or Norway. We spend significantly more money on specialty care than any of those other countries. We spend over than twice as much money on specialty care compared to most other countries. Our access to specialty care numbers aren't twice as good -- but they are roughly tied with the best performance in Europe.

The Business Model Affects Availability

So what is the impact of all of those accesses to care performance levels for care delivery on our total health and on relative outcomes of our care?

The next chart shows life expectancy levels for people in each of the countries listed on these charts. We do not win on the scale of life expectancy. The U.S. currently rates 51st in life expectancy in the world.[163] On this next chart -- comparing just the industrialized countries -- we rank in last place. We pay the most money for care and we get less access to most categories of care. We rank dead last in our survival statistics. Primary care access seems to help prolong lives. Timely access to specialists doesn't seem to have the same life extension impact.

That is, of course, due in part to the simple biological fact that by the time you need a specialist, your health has probably already deteriorated. Having access to heart transplant surgeons twice as fast as another country is a good thing until you recognize that patients in those other countries are less than half as likely to actually need a transplant surgeon. As this book keeps saying -- we get what we pay for.

Figure 3.19

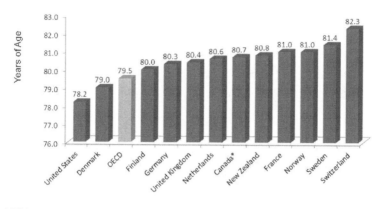

Life Expectancy at Birth, 2009

* 2007 data
Source: OECD Health Data 2011

Care Financing Sculpts Care Delivery

One of the interesting points to discuss is the fact that care delivery seems to be influenced quite a bit by the financing approaches used by each country.

There seems to be a fairly strong correlation across countries between easy or delayed access to specialty care and the type of business model that is used by each country to buy and sell care. Countries that use private insurance plans to pay for the care of their citizens tend to have faster access to specialty care than countries that use only government payers. Switzerland, The Netherlands and Germany all use both private health insurers and private care sites to deliver and finance care. Those countries do well on access to both specialists and primary care.

By contrast, the countries that deliver and fund their care entirely using either a single payer approach or a government-run and government-owned care system tend to have measurably slower access than other countries to specialty care and slightly slower access to primary care. Sweden, Norway and Canada all fit that model. It's an interesting and fairly obvious pattern and correlation. The care systems in the countries with the most government control over financing and care delivery operations clearly have the slowest access to specialty care.

Figure 3.20

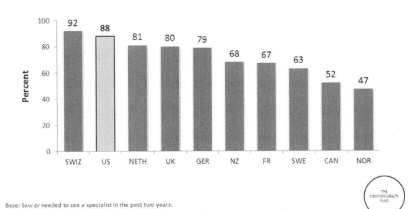

Waited Less Than a Month to See A Specialist

Base: Saw or needed to see a specialist in the past two years.
Source: 2011 Commonwealth Fund International Health Policy Survey of Sicker Adults in Eleven Countries.

We Pay Primary Care Doctors Half As Much Money

Most of the other industrialized countries place a very strong emphasis on primary care. Most other countries do not encourage as many of their doctors to be specialists. We do the exact opposite. We encourage specialty care. We generally pay our primary care doctors only about half as much as we pay most of our specialists. Lower paid primary care doctors in the U.S. can take a decade to repay medical school debts that higher paid specialists and subspecialists can repay in a couple of years -- sometimes a couple of months. Other countries tend to have their doctors graduate from medical school with little or no debt -- and usually only specialists in those countries end up with educational debt. We set up very different financial realities for our medical students.

Other countries tend, -- as a matter of policy -- to have two thirds or more of their doctors in the primary care specialties and a much lower percentage of their doctors in the specialty and sub-specialties care areas.[164] The people who do health planning in those countries believe that patients will get better care overall and will live longer if patients have quick and easy access to primary care. The charts above that show both relative access to care and the better life expectancy levels that exist in those countries might indicate that those could be good and valid theories and strategies. Their goal and their key strategies are to prevent medical disasters. Our model and care strategy is to let a large number of disasters happen and then throw large numbers of specialists and subspecialists into the intensive care units of our hospitals to provide an avalanche of purely reactive and very expensive care for those patients who are in dire need. Patients in other countries live longer than we do. Our specialists make a lot more money. Those are not unrelated facts.

Rationing Is Not the Winning Strategy

So what does all of this data about access to multiple levels of care tell us relative to the prices we spend to buy care? It tells us that other countries do not spend significantly less of their GDP on care delivery because they ration care. Switzerland spends a lot less money than we do on care. We know that to be true. It is also true that no one in Switzerland rations care. When we compare ourselves to other industrialized countries, the people in those countries actually tend to have more doctor visits, faster access to doctors, more hospital admissions and longer stays in the hospital than we do.

So why are overall care costs so much higher here? This chapter also answers that question. Prices are the key difference between us and them. We get less care but we spend a lot more for each piece of care. As the opening of this chapter stated very directly, prices for pieces of care are clearly the key cost driver that is the difference between us and them on the total cost of care in each of our countries.

How Did Prices Get So High Here?

Our world record prices for care obviously raise another key question that it is useful to answer. How did we manage to end up with all of those prices for pieces of care that are so much higher than the prices that are charged in all other countries?

The next two charts are fascinating. They outline an extremely important piece of data that we need to understand. The first chart shows the decrease in hospital lengths of stay and in hospital admissions that has occurred in the U.S. for the past couple of decades.

We obviously don't have our current very low levels of hospital use numbers by accident. We have been reducing both hospital admission rates and the length of stay for hospital patients in our country steadily over the entire timeframe shown on this chart. This chart shows that we now have the lowest hospital admission rates in the world. We made that happen. Those very low hospital utilization levels did not happen serendipitously. Market forces and the business model we use to buy hospital care created that hospital use outcome. We made important changes in the way we buy care and those changes helped point us irreversibly and irrevocably toward that overall reduced hospital use performance level.

Figure 3.21

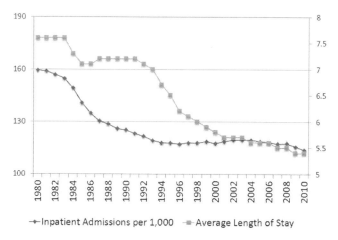

Inpatient Utilization
(American Hospitals)

→ Inpatient Admissions per 1,000   → Average Length of Stay

Sources: American Hospital Association, "AHA Trendwatch Chartbook 2011," 2011.

DRGs and HMOs Reduced Length of Stay

We changed the business model we used to buy hospital care roughly thirty years ago. Hospital use was going up. We were buying hospital care in those days entirely by the piece -- with every day in the hospital generating a new avalanche of fees. Medicare believed they were facing a hospital cost explosion and they had a mild panic attack. Medicare decided to change the way they bought hospital care to keep those costs from exploding. Medicare is a huge purchaser of care. When Medicare changes the way it buys care, care changes. So what did Medicare do?

Medicare decided to stop buying hospital care by the piece. Medicare decided to pay for hospital care using package prices for each patient. The new package prices were based on the hospital admission diagnosis for each patient. Medicare based their new payment approach on what they called "DRGs" -- Diagnosis Related Groups.

The DRGs had a huge impact on the business model and cash flow reality for the hospitals. It no longer made sense for a hospital to do an entry level, cost-generating X-ray for every patient because the new DRG-payment approach did not pay for each separate X-ray. Those hospital admission X-rays actually used to be done routinely for just about every hospital patient. They were done in the days when hospitals were paid by the piece and when those X-rays were a very profitable thing to do.

Then the payment approach changed. Hospitals could no longer send a separate bill to Medicare for each of those pre-admission X-rays. Hospitals looked very differently at the actual biological and medical need for that particular piece of film when the payment approach changed. That piece of film turned out not to be an important piece of medical data for new patients when those X-rays stopped generating revenue. That was just one example. DRGs changed the way hospitals thought about many areas of care. Many areas of care changed. Lengths of stay were high on the list of changes.

Then -- at about the same time Medical implemented DRGs -- "managed care" plans began growing in the private insurance market in this country. Employers who were unhappy with exploding insurance premiums turned away from the old simple insurance model and began hiring health plans to reduce their costs. The new health plans began replacing the old health insurance companies. The old pure health insurers had been simply functional conduits for cash. Those original health insurers generally made no attempt to influence the delivery of care in any significant way. They simply received a bill from a caregiver -- checked to see if the service on the bill was listed on the approved list of services -- and if it was on that list, they paid the bill. No questions asked. They didn't even negotiate the prices. Quite a few employers who were paying the premiums for those pure insurance plans found that the premium prices were increasing at unacceptable levels, so the employers began to move their purchasing decisions. The employers began using managed care plans -- HMOs -- instead of traditional health insurers instead to pay their claims.

The new health plans, by contrast with the old insurers, started looking at ways care could be made better and cheaper. The insurers who became health plans stopped functioning purely as a conduit for cash and began to try to manage the cash flow and care costs to reduce their premium levels.

The new health plan approach that began replacing the old insurance company conduit for cash approach began to functionally do a number of new things to actually "manage" care. The health plans decided to look for ways to eliminate wasteful and unnecessary care expenses. The new health plans immediately stopped paying for those preadmission X-rays on every patient. They also stopped paying for pieces of care like Friday hospital admissions for Monday surgery. Those Friday admissions actually were fairly common in some settings. Big bills were being incurred over the weekend for those Friday admissions but more often than not, there was no real care being delivered to those patients because the purpose of the admission was generally just for the patient to "rest." A hospital can be an expensive place to "rest" -- when there are no medical care needs for the patient to be in that bed.

Health plans found many opportunities of that sort to affect the costs of hospital care. Changing a number of elements of care delivery became a major goal of some plans. In the process, the new health plans started looking at lengths of stay for patients in the hospital, and they did that work initially by diagnosis. They worked to cut maternity stays, for example, from five days to three days and then to two days. Other lengths of stay were reduced as well. Health plans also started to figure out which inpatient surgeries could have been done just as well and much less expensively in an outpatient setting.

This book isn't a history book about those changes in care delivery that resulted from "managed care" -- other than to note that they happened...but it is important to recognize that some aspects of the business model for care changed in the process. Hospital days were affected.

When Medicare stopped buying hospital care by the piece and when the new health plans began to "manage" hospital care with one of their key goals being to reduce unnecessary hospital use whenever possible, then the number of days in the hospital went down at the levels shown on that last chart.

There was a lot of tension in some care settings as those health plan-triggered changes in practice and payments were implemented. Some of those changes were really needed and well done and some of the changes were clumsy, insensitive and more focused on cost reduction than care improvement. Revisiting all of that history in a lot of detail isn't particularly productive at this point in this book -- other than to say that the full scope of changes in the hospital business model that were triggered by both sets of payers clearly changed the delivery of hospital care in the U.S. You can clearly see the results on the hospital utilization chart above.

Changing some basic business realties for hospitals changed the way the hospital product in this country was both structured and produced. That chart tells a very powerful story about the impact of those changes over time.

If that chart is accurate and if that very impressive reduction in hospital use happened, why don't we now spend less money on hospital care than anyone in the world?

Again, the answer is simple.

Prices.

Hospital days went down. Unit prices went up.

The next chart shows the increase in hospital prices that happened over that same timeframe.

Figure 3.22

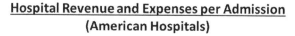

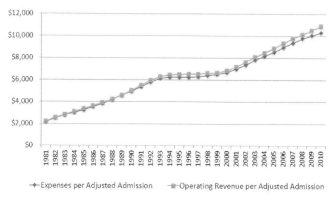

Clearly, hospital prices have gone up -- year after year. Operating revenue increased for the hospitals even when their utilization levels decreased.

Prices Offset Utilization Drops

The next chart blends the last two charts. The story of those two intercepting trends is pretty clear. Prices went up. A lot. Some of the price increases charged by the hospitals made obvious operational sense. The cost to produce a day of care should go up a bit when there are fewer people being hospitalized because the people who are still being hospitalized are -- on average -- sicker people, and sicker people do need more care. The Friday admissions for Monday surgery that were happening in 1982 and then eliminated -- and the final three days of a five-day maternity stay -- had not involved patients who actually needed a lot of care. Those patients were functionally resting in the hospital. Resting is a good thing, but those patients were not being actively treated in the hospital.

So some price increases for a day of hospital care made some sense when the hospital admissions went down and the length of stay diminished because the average intensity levels of the care for the patients in the hospital did increase.

The actual increase in prices, however, more than offset the reduction in hospital utilization and exceeded the increase in the care intensity levels. The net impact of all of those prices going up in hospitals has been to give America the highest per capita hospital costs in the world by a factor of two.

We now spend more than $15,000 per stay for hospital care. No other country in the western world spends more than $5,000 per stay.[165]

Figure 3.23

United States Utilization Drops and Price Increases

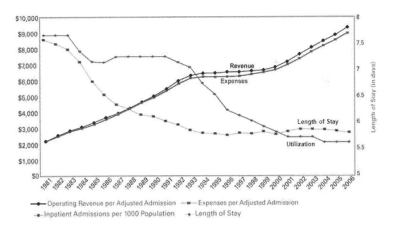

Sources: American Hospital Association, "AHA Trendwatch Chartbook 2011," 2011.

That is the economic reality about hospital costs we all need to understand.

Why Weren't Consumers Upset About Higher Hospital Prices?

Why weren't consumers outraged -- or at least upset and alarmed -- by all of those increases in hospital prices? Consumers were not upset because the increases were invisible. Consumers had absolutely no idea that those price increases were happening. Our insurance benefits very effectively hid those price increases from us as consumers. As those prices were increasing, we Americans either had full insurance coverage for our hospital care -- and that full coverage payment approach obviously concealed prices from patients really well -- or we had deductible plans with relatively low deductibles. The deductible plans showed us the deductible amount charged to each patient for care, but that deductible payment approach completely hid the full price that was being charged by each hospital for each patient and then paid by the insurers.

That's why consumers did not object to the price increases. They were invisible. Both types of insurance payment hospital benefit plans very effectively concealed all of those hospital price increases from all insured consumers. Those full coverage and low deductible benefit plans also concealed all of those hospital price increases year after year from our policy makers, our legislators, and our news media. The overall premium increases that were being charged by the health plans were sometimes somewhat visible to the public and the media. But the actual price increases that were created each year by American hospitals were totally invisible. Those prices increase were out of sight, out of mind. But they were obviously not out of the health care economy.

Why Didn't Health Insurers Blow the Whistle on Price Increases?

Health insurers, of course, knew exactly what was driving their premium increases. They paid the bills. They cut the checks.

So why didn't health insurers blow the whistle and expose all of those price increases to the rest of the world? Health insurers chose -- for years -- not to draw any attention to those prices. Health plans had business reasons not to make a fuss about those prices increases. Many health insurers did not want the public or the government drilling down into any of the specifics of their cost structures, so insurers generally kept their mouths shut about the hospital price increases. The insurers also did not highlight or spotlight all of the other fee increases that have been set up over time by the various medical practitioners, drug companies, or technology companies. Why were insurers generally silent about the prices that were causing their premiums to go up?

For starters, insurers often compete with each other based on their relative level of negotiated discounts. So perversely, if a provider price goes up by a lot but the insurer can say to their client, "We have a thirty percent discount on that fee," -- then the perceived value of the discount is greater when the prices are higher.

Insurers can also tell their employer clients -- "We have a 30 percent discount and the other insurers only have a 20 percent discount. Thirty is better than twenty."

Any public reaction that might have been triggered relative to the per unit price increases by included consumers or well-informed news media could have resulted in some kind of legislation that might have made that relatively comfortable competition that was based on relative price discounts irrelevant.

In that timeframe, insurers also were not particularly interested in having their entire financial infrastructure exposed to the public eye. Once people started looking at the role that unit price increase actually played in creating premium costs increases, that set of discussions might have opened the door to looking more closely at other pieces of the total premium cost package. Those numbers used to be invisible to the outside world. So the old business model worked just fine for most insurers and there was no reason for insurers to highlight all of the hospital price increases that created that particular chart. It was easier to pay the higher prices and pass the costs on to self-insured employers and in premium increases.

That meant that silence prevailed about prices from the best and most relevant source of knowledge in this country about prices.

Journalists and health care economists have also both been singularly uninterested in prices as a topic for either reporting or study. The public media has done many stories about care developments, medical science improvements, and treatment innovations and have written some highly informative pieces -- those stories almost never reflect, touch on, or even mention the price that will be charged for the new treatment. Those stories never mention or even hint at the inevitable impact of that new price and new service on insurance premiums. Most journalists actually do not know that linkage between costs and premiums exists -- and health insurers have not explained it to them.

In addition, health care economists seldom mention either prices or price increases in their own analysis of health care costs. Professor Uwe E. Reinhardt of Princeton did a brilliant piece two decades ago for the Journal of Health Affairs where he explained the issue clearly. The piece was called, "It's the Prices, Stupid." [166] The piece was clear, concise, well-reasoned, well-structured, and amazingly accurate, and it was basically ignored literally for decades. The primary reason that it was ignored is that the paper made the intellectual and the academic points brilliantly -- but the author did not include one single actual price number in the article. If any of the price charts that are included in this chapter of this book had been in that article by Dr. Reinhardt, it would have been game/set/match for the health policy world for the argument and debate about the impact of prices on overall costs of care in this country. Because there were no actual unit price numbers in the article, the argument was regarded as pure theory.

Influential people who very much did not want this country to look at pricing issues were able to categorize it as an interesting but unsubstantiated theory instead of having to treat it as a deadly accurate statement of facts and reality about the actual key issue for health care costs in America.

We probably would have taken health care purchasing in this country down some very innovative and productive paths had that article been accepted as absolute fact at the time it was published.

In any case, even the health insurers who know exactly what was driving their costs up every month were silent about the impact of prices on premiums. The public had no idea of that impact and most people had no clue that prices were going up or that those prices increases had any impact on insurance premiums.

That legacy of silence about the actual causes of premium increases has recently not been good for the overall creditability of insurance companies. Some insurers are now paying a significant credibility price for that particular transparency deficiency. The credibility issues exist for insurers because surveys show that most people in this country now believe that premium increases are driven almost entirely by the health plan profits and even by health plan greed.

That transparency level is in the process of changing. It isn't voluntary. Insurers today are far more likely to point out the impact of prices on their premiums because the Affordable Care Act has now mandated that premiums are to be created by care costs, and that is creating significant insurance company transparency relative to their cost factors in the new premium-setting process. Hiding the expense factors is no longer allowed by the new rating rules for insurance premiums. One result of that change is that an increasing number of insurers are now beginning to tell the unit price story, and some are even pointing out some price abuses. The public will be well served by that new flow of data from insurers to the world. No one has better data about prices than the organizations that pay those prices.

We Should Not Make That Mistake Again

In any case, the chart that shows us both sets of lines for hospitals utilization and hospital prices tells us a really important story.

We did not get the cost benefit from the utilization changes. We clearly made a mistake. We need to make very sure we don't make that same mistake again. It is actually possible for us to make that mistake again as we go forward with the approaches outlined in this book and as we make care better and more efficient.

As we create team care, and as we bring computer-supported, continuously improving care to levels where we can reduce in-hospital utilization in this country even more, we need to be very sure that we don't once again lose the financial benefits of all of our care improvements and have those gains in better care destroyed and erased by another generation of simple, per-unit price surges for hospital care. If we lose the next generation of that particular price war, we could make the next set of care delivery performance gains disappear entirely as financial wins for the country.

We need to achieve and hold price gains at this point in time and not simply face and pay for another round of price surges.

The Urban Myth of Fee Legitimacy

To deal with prices, we do need to have more people understand exactly how the price-setting approach usually works for care prices in this country. We need the public to better understand care prices.

One of the urban myths of American health care economics is that the prices that are being charged by a caregiver to any given patient somehow have a basic fundamental validity and an inherent legitimacy. People who get care generally feel like each fee that is charged to them by their care site or their caregiver must be legitimate or their caregiver would not make them pay that amount of money for their care. We tend to grant the prices that are charged in this country an amazing level of legitimacy, and we tend to assume in our future thinking that prices for care will always be either stable or perpetually increasing. That is a bad way to think. Instead, we obviously should be looking at price flexibility and price variability as a key and easy to use cost mitigation factor.

We have not traditionally looked at prices as being an opportunity to bring down costs. We don't think like that as individuals. Amazingly, even health care economists and policy "experts" who look long and hard at health care cost issues far too often don't think of prices as a possible tool for making care more affordable.

It's a bit easier to understand the public thinking on that issue than it is to understand why very intelligent health care economists and policy gurus think that way.

It is really fascinating that so many health care economists who are deeply immersed in the economic issues of care don't even look at price or think of price as a potential cost variable when they are doing future financial projections about health care costs.

Even very intelligent economists who should know better often assume in their own thinking that all current prices are somehow collectively "right" and inherently legitimate. Those economists who believe in the inherent rightness of overall prices then tend to base their own future cost projections and their strategic thinking for health care expenses on the aggregate set of today's prices, with the assumption that prices for all pieces of care will perpetually and inevitability rise -- like some kind of inexorable economic tide.

Economic projections and policy strategists both tend to be anchored for too often intellectually in the inevitability of perpetual price increases. That is a highly simplistic and singularly unproductive way to think about prices.

Prices Are All Invented

What is true is that the private market prices for each piece of care are all invented for the business purposes of the health care business units that are charging the prices. The business units generally set overall revenue goals for themselves, and they each then create an array of prices that will -- in the aggregate -- achieve those total revenue goals. In that context, the truth is that individual prices are extremely variable in multiple directions almost all of the time. We really should not assume that any of those prices for any piece of care ever has an inherent legitimacy on its own merit as being a pure and accurate and direct reflection of the actual cost of producing care for that particular service in that place and that time. Private market prices are all invented by the business units of care to meet their business goals. As noted earlier, government prices for each piece of care are simply set arbitrarily by the government and then those prices are imposed on each caregiver to meet the government's budget goals.

Those non-negotiated Medicare and Medicaid prices do not pretend to reflect the actual cost of care for care sites. Both of those government-run programs simply impose their prices on the caregivers. Those imposed prices reflect how much money the government is willing to pay for each piece of care for the people they insure.

As noted earlier, many other countries also use that government imposed price approach for their patients. Those government-mandated prices are also used to set payment levels for the patients who are covered by private health insurers in most counties. Some countries do allow some levels of market forces or competitive factors to be involved in setting some of their care prices. Others governments just mandate all prices that are paid for each piece of care.

All Other Countries Have Lower Prices Than We Do

Regardless of which approach each country uses, however, the other countries all end up paying a lot less than we do for each piece of care.

The appendectomy, angioplasty and coronary artery bypass surgery fee schedules examples that were shown above each gives us some sense of the price variation that exists between countries and also gives us some sense of the individual price variation that exists today within our U.S. health care ecosystem.

One Role of Health Plans Is To Negotiate Prices

As noted earlier, one of the major roles played by health plans and health insurers in this country has been to negotiate prices on behalf of the people who buy their insurance. The first Blue Cross plans began that tradition during the Great Depression.[167] To have an affordable premium level, those early Blue Cross plans all negotiated significant hospital discounts for the people who bought health insurance through the plan. Those price discount negotiations and volume-purchasing processes have always been a major role that health plans play for their customers.

Health plans in this country are allowed by law to negotiate the purchasing of care. Most plans use their purchasing volume and their market leverage to negotiate lower than list prices with most of their caregivers. Since insurance premiums that are incurred by any health insurer are always based on the average cost of care for any set of insured people, each of the negotiated discounts for those individual pieces of care helps to reduce the premium levels that are needed by the health plans to buy care for the people they insure.

Plans that have strong market leverage tend to negotiate prices based on the Medicare fee schedule -- with the actual payment being "Medicare, plus a defined percentage." Health plans that have less market power and who deal with local care businesses units that have some levels of local market control or market dominance tend to pay based on a discount from the care provider's chargemaster fee schedule that were described earlier in this chapter.

That is almost always weaker price leverage. Those prices that originate with the chargemaster fee tend to be higher than the ones that are based on the local Medicare fee level.

Other plans have their own payment level -- and negotiate a whole array of fees based on local market realities. Approaches vary from buyer to buyer.

Providers Don't Like Price Negotiations

For all of those approaches, providers often complain to media, patients, and politicians about those health plans' price negotiations. Many providers of care express both public and private unhappiness about the fee discounts or the pricing arrangements that result from their contracting process with health insurers.

One of the almost humorous ironies of the American health insurance marketplace and the health care policy world has been that some of the same consumers who have been most unhappy with the high premiums that are being charged to them by their insurers sometimes both publically and privately criticize those same health plans for negotiating any fee discounts with their caregivers. That actually does make emotional sense -- because patients everywhere tend to like their personal caregivers. Fee negotiations by health insurers can make providers of care unhappy and patients generally don't like it when their personal caregivers are unhappy. But the basic arithmetic of health care coverage and unit prices is pretty clear. Higher fees for prices of care that are charged by providers to insurers directly result in higher premiums for those insurers.

Price Transparency or Price Relevancy?

One of the strategies that some people have proposed to reduce health care spending levels in the U.S. is to require price transparency of some kind. Creating transparency relative to prices has been a goal and preferred strategy for some health care policy strategists and for some segments of the purchasing community. Some people believe strongly that if patients in this country somehow could come to know what the actual and relative prices are for various care sites and various care procedures, people who would have that transparent set of price data in hand about pieces of care would see the actual price differences between the various caregivers and between various sites of care and those patients would then move their own care to the lower cost care sites.

Price transparency, those people believe, will -- all by itself -- bring down prices and reduce health care spending levels. Is that true? Is pure transparency a good price reduction strategy?

Will we save money on the purchase of care if we somehow make all key care prices transparent to patients?

Probably not. Transparency is not enough.

Prices need to be both transparent and relevant before people will make decisions to use lower priced care sites.

Transparency Can Have Unintended Consequences

That hoped-for movement of patients to lower priced care sites when the actual prices of all relevant care sites become transparent to the patient tends not to happen unless the prices for individual pieces of care are both transparent and financially relevant to each patient. Relevant is the key word. Relevant is essential. Transparent is not enough. In fact, transparency, all by itself, can have serious unintended consequences.

When prices are merely transparent, the patient who chooses between a hospital that charges $2,000 to deliver a baby versus picking a hospital that charges for their care $8,000 to deliver a baby generally tends to believe that the $8,000 care site must somehow be better. Pure and naked transparency about the relative prices that are charged by caregivers can actually cause many patients who know both sets of prices to migrate to the higher cost site in the mistaken -- but entirely understandable -- belief that prices and quality are somehow linked.

That set of decisions by patients to pick the higher priced site instead of selecting the lower priced site is highly likely to happen when prices are transparent because the benefit design for insurance we generally use to buy care in the U.S. makes the price difference between those care sites financially irrelevant to the patient.

Our standard insurance benefit package designs very clearly make most caregiver prices differences for significant caregiver completely irrelevant to the patient.

Deductibles Hide Price Differences for High Cost Procedures

Deductibles create a real problem for that particular set of care site choices.

When the insurance benefit plan for a patient is a flat $1,000 annual deductible, then the consumer only pays -- at most -- the deductible cost of one thousand dollars -- regardless of the care site that the consumer chooses. The obvious arithmetic truth is that both the $2,000 fee charged by Hospital A and the $8,000 fee charged by Hospital B to deliver a baby both blow right past the flat $1,000 deductible. So the actual out-of-pocket cost difference that would be charged directly to the consumer for choosing and using either hospital is zero -- even though the pure price to deliver a baby charged by Hospital B is actually $6,000 higher than the fee charged by Hospital A.

In that cash flow reality, patients often decide to use the high priced care site in the simple, unsubstantiated but entirely understandable belief that the higher priced site must somehow offer better care because it charges a lot more. That's why pure stand-alone price transparency can actually sometimes be both dangerous and counterproductive.

When prices are simply transparent but when the price differences are not financially relevant to the individual patient, then the patients have a tendency to prefer the higher priced site in the belief it must be better or it wouldn't cost more. The standard insurance benefit designs that we use in this country make those price differences on most significant care purchases irrelevant to the patient.

Prices for pieces of care that happens before the deductible is met each year can be relevant -- but we know for a fact that 80 percent of the cost of care in this country actually comes from the patients who have exceeded their deductibles. A few people incur most care costs, and those people easily exceed their deductibles.

The French Model Makes Prices Visible and Relevant

Is there any other way to buy care? Yes.

The French, for example, use a very different payment model. The French model does make price differences between caregivers relevant to the patient. The French have made some very intelligent decisions about both benefit plans and prices. Instead of using a front-end deductible and then having the insurer pay all of the price differences between the care sites, the French set up a fixed fee for each procedure and they pay that predetermined fixed amount to the provider when that care is delivered to a patient.

The French also, however, allow each provider to charge the patient more for doing the procedure than that predetermined base-level fee. If the provider wants to change more than that base fee, the French require the consumer to pay the cash difference between the base government fees and the higher fee that is charged by the care sites. That two-tier payment approach makes prices both visible to the patient and directly relevant to both the patient and the caregiver.

If we used the French approach for the care decision example that was listed above -- where there is a choice between two maternity care sites with very different prices -- there would have been a very different consumer choice dynamic for the patient.

The French predetermined baseline fee for that service might be to have a $2,000 flat fee basic insurance benefit for maternity care. In that case, the patient who went to the care site that charged $2,000 for the care would pay nothing from their own pocket to have their baby delivered. Those patients would, functionally, have full coverage for that service. Their $2,000 base payment insurance benefit would pay the full $2,000 fee for the delivery.

Using the American price examples that were mentioned earlier -- if that same French patient decided to go to the eight thousand dollar site, however, and if the patient had her baby there, then the patient would have to pay the $6,000 difference between $2,000 flat insurance benefit payment level and the actual $8,000 provider fee. Just like caregiver prices in the U.S., the second French care site would still be allowed to charge $8,000 to deliver the baby. But that higher fee would not be invisible or irrelevant to the patient in France. That price difference between the two sites is made moot and irrelevant by the American deductible-based insurance plan payment approach -- but any higher prices are very relevant in France. Any care site in France that decides to charge a lot more money to deliver the baby than the baseline fee would need to convince the patient that their care was so good that the care at their site is worth the patient paying the extra money. Suddenly, with that payment approach, market forces actually became very relevant and very real. Prices in France are more than just transparent -- they are relevant. Prices become relevant decision factors both for patients and for caregivers when they occur.

That is a very different market reality. Price transparency helps keep prices down in that French model instead of price transparency driving costs up.

Market forces become very relevant when price-based decisions must be made by both patients and caregivers.

Interestingly, that approach and that base payment insurance plan benefit design also gives consumers in France the first dollar insurance coverage that consumers everywhere love. Consumers in France receive immediate benefits from their insurance coverage every time they need care -- rather than having to pay their full deductible first before getting any insurance benefits for the care they use.

The Choice of a More Expensive Care Site Doesn't Increase Insurance Premiums

Any time higher prices are charged in our country, someone has to be the source of cash for the higher prices.

In this country -- because insurance is the mechanism we usually use to allow each of us to pay for the costs of our care using other people's money -- the higher prices that are charged when we pick Hospital A instead of Hospital B are paid by the insurer. When an insured consumer chooses to use Hospital A, the higher expenses from hospital A are simply added to the average cost of care for that group of insured people. That choice to use higher priced Hospital A by any insured patient simply increases the premiums that are charged to all patients who have that same insurance plan. Premiums paid by all insured people in that risk pool pay for that high cost provider choice by any patient who chooses the higher cost site. In France, people use their own money to buy the higher priced care. That is a very different cash flow, a very different cost sharing reality and a very different market model.

Our cash flow model actually encourages, supports, enables, funds and rewards high prices. So we get what that model creates -- high prices that exceed the prices paid for prices of care anywhere else in the world.

Why Don't We Use the Approach Other Countries Use To Keep Prices Low?

So why don't we just change the way we pay for care and use one or more of the approaches that the other countries use who spend a lot less than we do on care? That question is worth answering. To do that, it makes sense to look quickly at the approaches that the other countries actually use.

The opening pages of this book pointed out that the high cost of care in America is both a blessing and a curse. Health care creates great jobs. It anchors a number of communities. Health care is a thriving part of our national and local economies. That's why we don't simply decide to use the Canadian approach or simply adopt Canadian fee schedules. Setting up mandatory price levels here and moving to the current Canadian fee schedule would cripple our care infrastructure. It would badly damage our local economies. That strategy of using Canadian fee levels in the U.S. would be dead on arrival as a political agenda -- for very good reasons. We clearly do not want to cripple the care industry and damage local economies in this country by paying Canadian fees.

The Canadian model does have its obvious charm as a much simpler way to buy care. Canada uses a single payer system, with one government payer for each province. Each province in

Canada sets all prices for all insured medical procedures that are done in that province.

Most Canadian Provinces Don't Cover Prescription Drugs

Canada also sets prices for all prescription drugs sold in each province. What a great many otherwise well informed people in this country do not know is that most provinces in Canada actually don't cover prescription drugs as an insured benefit in their government insurance plan. That coverage decision is a useful point to understand in a book chapter on care prices. Drugs are actually not a covered benefit for most of Canada for their single payer system. Patients in most Canadian provinces actually pay for their own drugs.

Why do Canadians accept that benefit plan gap? Prices help. Canadians pay prices for each of those prescription drugs that have been set by their local government. The provinces that don't cover drugs simply set the actual drug prices that are paid by consumers in the province to buy drugs.

The basic benefit design strategy is to set those prices low enough for each drug so that people in Canada who use prescription drugs for their care can afford to buy their own drugs. In other words, they use mandated drug prices -- not mandated drug benefits -- in most provinces of Canada to create consumer and patient affordability for drugs.

The number of health care policy people or political leaders in this country who know that six of eight Canadian provinces actually do not cover prescription drugs for their own citizens is tiny. The Canadians very cleverly use prices as a major tool to help people with their drug expenses instead of using government insurance and tax money to buy these drugs for people. Those Canadian provinces have chosen mandating low drug prices over offering prescription drug coverage in their tax-funded single payer system as their basic drug strategy. They have successfully kept that drug purchase expense away from the single payer tax-payer funded part of health care costs in Canada by simply having each patient in those six Canadian provinces buy their own drugs.

They do allow people who want to buy private health insurance to pay for their drugs to buy that insurance. Some people do buy that insurance.

Several Countries Set Prices

The Canadian government also sets very specific prices for every other piece of care delivered in Canada.

In Canada, the government is the single payer. The government, as the single payer, simply sets the prices for each and every piece of care. Most people believe that all countries in Europe use that Canadian model for their coverage. That isn't true. European countries actually do not use the Canadian single payer model. No country in Europe uses the Canadian approach.

In most European countries, private health plans are the preferred insurance approach. Most people actually have private insurance -- not Canadian-style government insurance -- in Europe. The government is absolutely neither the primary payer nor the insurance administrator in most European countries. The Netherlands, Switzerland and Germany all use competing health insurance plans to provide coverage to their populations.

There are both for-profit insurers and not-for-profit health insurers in those countries. The private insurers in those countries compete in multiple ways for customers. They tend to have very competitive private insurer markets in those countries -- with competition and television ads that look a lot like the private insurers' plans and ads in the U.S.

But the private insurance plans in those countries generally all use the same exact local fee schedule that has been set up, created and mandated by the government when those insurers buy care from the caregivers in those countries for their insured people. Those countries use private insurers, private doctors, mostly private hospitals and they all complete for patients and customers -- but they all tend to pay the same amount for each piece of care in each geographic area.

As noted earlier, the French government also sets a basic fee schedule for each piece of care as well. The French model is different than the Swiss or Dutch models because the French government allows caregivers in France to charge more than the government set amount if the providers want to charge more. That model was explained earlier in this chapter. Quite a few French patients currently buy private insurance plans to pay for the difference between the government set fee and the actual price charged by the care sites.

We are not very likely as a country to transplant the approach used by any of those countries to the U.S. because we are highly unlikely to allow the government in our country to set all fees for all American caregivers.

They Don't Use Fees in Sweden and Norway

We are even less likely to use the payment approach they use in the Scandinavian countries. The Scandinavian countries technically do not provide health insurance to their citizens. They provide care -- not insurance -- to their citizens.

The Scandinavian countries actually don't regulate fees for their caregivers because they actually do not use fees in any way for pay for most care. They do not buy care by the piece in the Nordic countries. They don't use fees in other care settings because they deliver almost all of their health care in those countries from care sites that are owned by the government.

People in each of those countries are legally entitled to have care from those care sites, not insurance coverage. The

Scandinavians only have insurance-like "coverage" with actual insurance functionality if they leave their country and then need to buy care elsewhere. In that case, their national system will accept the bill and pay for that foreign care. Inside each country, fee schedules are completely irrelevant to the functional cash flow of care delivery.

Physicians in those Scandinavian countries tend to work for the local health authorities. The doctors in those countries are paid by the month -- not by the piece. So formal government budgets directly control the total costs of care in those countries and controlling specific fee levels is not relevant for most care in Scandinavian countries. Even though the Scandinavian approach has its obvious merits, the likelihood of converting all of American health care to a model of integrated hospitals and salaried physicians -- with no fees used to pay for any care -- is so challenging that the problems of full system to that model conversion are fundamentally insurmountable.

Great Britain Skips Fees By Using Capitation

They use a different model in Great Britain.

Great Britain, as noted earlier, has its own unique model where all of the primary care doctors have an enrolled list of patients and each doctor receives a flat lump sum payment per month for every patient on their panel. The doctors receive that monthly fee from the National Health Service.

The British in effect, "capitate" their primary care doctors. Each doctor's revenue is based on the size of each doctor's patient pool -- or "panel." As in the Scandinavian model, there are no fees charged, paid or recorded for any care that is delivered by those doctors to their own panel of patients. The cash flow for those doctors is a little more complicated than just the flat fee.

The British National Health Service has actually also set up a few performance-based bonus plans for their primary care doctors. The bonus plan payments are based on the doctors achieving some process-based performance goals -- with a focus on their patient who have chronic conditions. So some bonuses are paid to those doctors but there are no actual fees collected by or for any patients by those NHS-reimbursed doctors.

Most hospitals in Great Britain are owned by the government. The government-owned hospitals in Great Britain tend to operate very much like the Scandinavian hospitals, the government-covered Canadian hospitals and the Veterans Administration hospitals in the U.S. -- with annual macro budgets set by the government for each hospital and no individual fees for pieces of care inside the hospital. The budgets for the hospitals are usually modified somewhat based on volumes of patients -- but not in a way that creates any fees for any explicit services.

The British are constantly experimenting with their payment approaches for specialist care. Each new government in Great Britain tends to have its own variation on specialty care management. These efforts seem to be a perpetual work in progress everywhere.

So those are the basic ways that the other countries that are shown on the price charts in this chapter fund the delivery of care. Would any of those approaches that are used in Europe or Canada work in the U.S.? Probably not very well.

It Would Be Hard for Us To Use Any of Those Payment Models Here

We are not likely to transplant any of those care delivery or care financing approaches in their current form into the U.S.

It's pretty hard to imagine the U.S. turning all American hospitals over to the government. It's also pretty hard to imagine our government directly hiring all of the doctors in the country. Having the government own our entire care delivery infrastructure isn't likely to happen. Our government does own some care sites now –– so we Americans will probably continue to get our care from a mixture of both private- and government-owned care sites for the foreseeable future.

The truth is we are highly unlikely to disrupt our current infrastructure of care and business model for care to move to an entirely government-owned care system for either hospital care or medical care.

We Probably Will Not Set Up Primary Care Panels for All Patients

We are also highly unlikely to set our primary care doctors up with panels of patients and then pay the doctors a flat sum of money every month for every patient. That model works well for primary care in Great Britain, and it creates the fastest access to primary care in the industrialized world, but the potential and the sheer logistical complexity of transplanting that approach here as the way we pay our physicians is unfathomable.

Moving to that model would be extraordinarily disruptive. It is also unnecessary. We will, however, as the next chapter of this book points out, probably get some of the key care coordination benefits that are achieved by that British model as we begin to move some patients in this country to receiving some basic levels of care from well-designed patient-centered medical homes and Accountable Care Organizations. The team care that can result from that patient-centered medical home care delivery approach can achieve some of the care coordination and care access successes of British primary care. But we are highly unlikely to assign all people to patient-centered medical homes in this country. We are far more likely to incent our patients and our caregivers to use team-based care than we are to mandate the use of team-based care or move to anything resembling a primary care capitation model for our patients.

So we are not likely to convert as a nation to any of the care delivery or financing model used by any other country. We will not bring down the prices for care by moving to a different funding model for our overall care.

Growing Interest In Simply Dictating Fees

A growing number of people who look at all of our cost and price issues are beginning to believe that we should and probably will evolve over time more to a system where we will control key costs by mandating fees. An increasing number of people are beginning to suggest that we Americans should follow the lead of many other countries and begin to pay for all care using some level of standardized fees -- with the government setting the exact prices and determining the fee levels that are charged here for each piece of care. It's easy to see why that strategy has its fans.

The Germans, Swiss, and Dutch all use that model. We actually do know how to do that payment model here. We already do exactly that now for both Medicaid and Medicare fees. The infrastructure to use a mandated set of fees to buy all care is in place in this country today.

So why not have our government follow the Canadian or Dutch model and control care costs by simply setting fees for every single piece of care?

Fee Schedules Cripple Care Improvement

The most fundamental problem with simply using a government-imposed fee schedule to pay for all care for this country is that fee schedules are a really bad way to buy care. The last two chapters of this book have tried to make that point. The next couple of chapters will make that same point again -- with some vigor and several examples. Fee schedules are very limiting. Buying care by the piece is flawed at multiple levels. Fee schedules cripple innovation. Fee schedules cripple process redesign. Fee schedules and buying care entirely by the piece dictate particular approaches to care delivery and then lock those dictated care approaches firmly in place.

We very much need care in this country to continuously improve. Continuous improvement should be our top strategic care priority for the country. Fee schedules as a business model stifle continuous improvement. Fee schedules are both rigid and limiting by their very nature. When the only care that is paid for in a health care delivery infrastructure is just the specific pieces of care that are explicitly included on the list of approved care procedures that is embedded in an authorized fee schedule, then that all-powerful fee schedule literally defines and dictates the delivery of care.

When you buy care entirely by the piece and when you then try to reengineer any care processes, that reengineering process has a high potential to streamline care delivery, but it will not be done if it reduces cash flow for the caregiver for any pieces of care.

Streamlining care delivery can eliminate -- for example -- duplicate processes. Duplicate tests exist. They add no value for care delivery. Duplicate tests are a source of revenue, however, that is now rewarded totally and well by the piecework purchase model of care. Those duplications are rarely eliminated in any care setting as long as care in that setting is paid for by each billable piece. That piecework payment model really does dictate care. Care redesign and care innovations are almost impossible to do when the cash flow for care is defined, channelled, and controlled by an authorized and regulatory enforced piecework-based fee schedule.

We Need Care To Continuously Improve

Why is that a problem? The next two chapters of this book explain why that is a problem. We need care to continuously improve. When care continuously improves, care will be higher quality, safer, and more affordable. Continuous improvement -- as a culture, a skill set, and an operational reality -- will give us much better care outcomes than status quo care. We need a business model for care that triggers and rewards continuous improvement -- not a business model and cash flow approach that stifles improvement. That's why pure discounts are bad. That's why a government fee schedule is not a good thing to do. Using government-imposed fee levels as our cost control tool would simply reinforce and solidify the fee-based approach to care delivery. The fee-based payment model restricts care innovation and strongly worse incents higher volume of pieces instead of helping use figure out optimal care. There is not viable fee-based path to optimal care.

Continuously Improving Care Cut the HIV Death Rate by Half

Instead of buying care by the piece, we need to buy care by the package. Fees become financially and functionally irrelevant when care is purchased as a package. The fees for those old preadmission S-rays for all patients become entirely irrelevant immediately when Medicare started using DRGs to buy hospital care and stopped paying for pieces of hospital care. No fee control was needed for those X-rays because X-rays were included in the overall purchase package for hospital care. Once that X-rays status happened, only the patients who needed those X-rays continued to get them.

Buying a full set of care for a fixed packaged price instead of paying for each item of care by the piece is very empowering for the people who delivery care because the care site can eliminate that unnecessary X-ray without losing needed revenue generated by that piece of film.

Selling and buying full packages of care is a much better payment approach that can improve care and bring down the costs of care. That approach is very familiar to the author of this book for obvious reasons. Kaiser Permanente -- the author's employer -- sells care by the package...not by the piece. Kaiser Permanente receives a fixed payment per month for each patient -- not a revenue stream based on each piece of billable care.

Kaiser Permanente has cut the death rate for HIV patients to half of the national average.[168]

How did that happen and why is that relevant to a chapter on fees and prices? Care at Kaiser Permanente has been reengineered around those HIV patients. Care in other care settings for those patients would be based entirely on the fees authorized by payers like Medicare, Medicaid, and insurance companies for specific services delivered to those patients. Only services with an authorized CPT code would create revenue under that model.

Those successes in dropping the death rate for HIV patients hugely have happened because the Kaiser Permanente care teams are not bound to only doing pieces of care that are defined by that pay schedule of fees. Kaiser Permanente sells packages of care. Kaiser Permanente also engineers entire packages of care. Kaiser Permanente is paid a lump sum every month for all care needed by each patient, and that lump sum for each patient buys a full package of care for each patient. Kaiser Permanente is not paid piecework fees -- so Kaiser Permanente is not limited by any list of authorized services or by any insurance-based fee schedule to define its care.

Why is that freedom from services defined on an "approved" fee schedule relevant to price issues? Fourteen of the things that are done now to cut the HIV death rate to half of the national average at Kaiser Permanente do not show up on a Medicare, Medicaid or typical Blue Cross fee schedule.[169] If care in the Kaiser Permanente care settings was limited to doing only the pieces of care included on those fee schedules, twice as many HIV patients would be dead.

Likewise, Kaiser Permanente had cut the number of broken bones in the oldest seniors by over a third.[170] Nine things are done to achieve those success levels. Six of those nine things that are done to achieve that care success do not show up on a Medicare fee schedule.[171] So again, if the only care delivered to those high risk patients relative to broken bones was the approved and authorized pieces of care that are listed on the current Medicare fee schedule, fifty percent more very elderly seniors at Kaiser Permanente would have broken bones.

Likewise, the number of stroke deaths has been dropped by forty percent at Kaiser Permanente.[172] Those successes were achieved by doing multiple proactive things that don't show up on a fee schedule. The number of highly convenient e-visits between doctors and patients at Kaiser Permanente now exceeds 12,000,000 visits a year.[173] Those millions of e-visits between patients and doctors happen because Kaiser Permanente is pre-paid and doesn't need to collect a separate fee for every visit with a patient in order to survive financially.

Pressure ulcers were mentioned earlier in this book. Most hospitals have seven to ten percent of their patients with pres-sure ulcers.[174] Many of those pressure ulcer patients are dam-aged for life. Kaiser Permanente has less than one percent of their patients with pressure ulcers.[175] Some Kaiser Permanente hospitals have not had one single pressure ulcer for more than a year.

Why is that data point relevant to a chapter on prices and to the issue of selling care by the package and not selling care by the piece? It takes incredible nursing care that is focused on every single patient to get the pressure ulcers that occur in a hospital down to zero. Some patients have to be turned every hour to avoid those ulcers. There is no fee on a standard approved standard piecework fee schedule that would pay Kaiser Permanente to turn those patients every hour. There is also no fee to have the highest risk patients in beds that have special liners. There is no fee for monitoring the care results continuously at each micro care site to deliver that great care for those patients.

So great care that saves lives actually generates literally no money in coded fees from a standard fee schedule. But if that great care was not there, if the care for those patients failed and if pressure ulcers rebounded, those ulcers would each generate an abundance of fees.

If the Kaiser Permanente hospitals were paid by the piece instead of being prepaid for all hospital care, those patients would generate significant revenue when ulcers happened. The average revenue increase that would happen for each pressure ulcer payment is literally over $40,000 per patient.[176]

In the rest of the country -- where hospitals are paid by the piece -- seven percent of patents get those ulcers.[177] Those piecework-paid hospitals average over $43,000[178] in piecework fees for each damaged patient. Other hospitals who are not prepaid do not usually have those care success levels for pressure ulcers -- and if they did, the revenue for those piecework paid hospitals would drop significantly.

Which set of care outcomes do we want? Fee schedules can never reward zero ulcers. Fee schedules do, however, create care settings all over this country where 10 percent or more of the patients have those horrible wounds[179]...each triggering a rich flood of fees for the piecework care site.

So the point here is that the right answer to prices for pressure ulcers is not to negotiate steeper discounts on fees charged for pressure ulcer care. The answer is not to pay lower or discounted fees for each piece of that care. The answer is to transform care. The answer is to transform care so those levels of care are not needed. Care transformation solves the unit price problem much more effectively than using a Canadian fee schedule.

We Need Care To Be Continuously Improving

The point made earlier is that we need care in this country to get continuously better. Continuous improvement should be a goal.

The pressure ulcer work at Kaiser Permanente has gotten continuously better. The care model of being paid by the package rewards continuous improvement. With that payment model, the ulcer level has dropped from 3 percent to 2 percent of patients and now it averages less than 1 percent. Very smart people did things in systematic data supported ways to continuously improve that care.

We need all care in this country to continuously improve. We should be obsessively focused as a country throughout our infrastructure of care by the goal of continuous improvement. We need to set targets for care outcomes -- like having less than 1 percent of your patients with pressure ulcers or less than ten percent of sepsis patients dying of sepsis -- and then we need to engineer and reengineer care to achieve those goals everywhere in a context of continuous improvement.

You really can't redesign care well in a piecework payment business model where care delivery is made entirely rigid by a fee schedule.

We very much need care in this country to be continuously improving. We need care delivery models to be redesigned and continuously reengineered to be more patient-focused and more affordable. That work will not happen while the cash flow for care in this country is generated by a piecework payment model and restricted to doing the things that are listed on an approved fee schedule.

That's why following the lead of those other countries who set fees and then simply setting up a discounted government fee schedule for all care in this country that arbitrarily pays a lower amount for each piece of care could obviously reduce the immediate cost of care for America -- but that pure fee-based approach would impair the ultimate care improvement we need for the future. We can't achieve optimal care while we are paid for care by the piece. We need great care. We can't get great care in the context of a piecework payment model. We really do want care in this country to get continuously better -- not just get temporarily cheaper.

Paying entirely by the piece for care also creates a wide range of opportunistic gamesmanship and levels of fraud and abuse relative to defining and reporting the pieces of care. The growing and painfully expensive issues of Medicare and Medicaid fraud are largely driven by the fact that both of those programs buy care by the piece and that piecework payment approach is highly vulnerable to fraudulent billing. It is very hard for a care team to achieve fraudulent billing when you sell a package of care. It is very easy for a care team to achieve fraudulent billing when you sell care by the piece.

We Need To Sell Care by the Package and Not by the Piece

We clearly need to bring down the cost of care and we need to make both care and coverage affordable. We need to make unit prices either meaningfully relevant to the patients or we need to make those prices irrelevant to the caregiver because the caregiver is selling care by the package and not by the piece. If we sell care by the piece, we need to stop paying a lot of money for care that damages patients and undermines patient safety and health.

If we do need to pay for care by the piece, then using some version of the French model is a far better way to introduce real market forces and price relevance to the purchase of care...with prices probably going down for many pieces of care when they become relevant to the business model in a better way.

The next chapter deals with those purchasing and cash flow issues very directly. The next chapter talks about business models that can help refocus care on better outcomes, continuous improvement and lower costs...buying packages of care rather than just pieces of care. The next two chapters discuss various ways caregivers and health plans can connect and collaborate to create better and more affordable care.

If We Can't Reengineer Care, We May Need To Reprice Care

We need to take all of those issues on as a country and we need to make market-based payment reform very real.

The truth is, however, that if we can't achieve those repackaging and reengineering goals, and if we can't create affordable care with those approaches, then we may need to surrender to that cold reality and we may very need to simply set macro fees for all care. Repricing care is clearly a better model to use than borrowing money to pay for care and transferring the debt created by the overpriced care being received by us today to our children and our grandchildren. Repricing is also clearly a much better path going forward than rationing. Rationing is a very bad cost-containment strategy. The pure repricing model -- if it is ultimately needed --- actually works better than either rationing care or deferring care costs to our kids. As this chapter has shown, other countries who deliver more care than we do for their citizens at multiple levels have lower costs because they clearly understand their local care pricing model, and they use it to keep costs lower than their costs would be if they didn't use that approach.

Let's not go down either the path of rationing or the path of borrowing if we can use reengineering, refocusing and process redesigning to make care better and more affordable instead.

The next chapter deals with those issues.

Chapter Four

CARE DELIVERY IS A BUSINESS

Cash flow has an incredibly powerful impact on the delivery of care. The specific ways that we channel the flow of cash to caregivers in this country dictates almost all of the care that is delivered by those caregivers. If we want to change the care that is being delivered in this country, we will need to identify the care we want to buy, and then we need to change that flow of cash so that the money we spend to buy care will buy the care we want to buy.

Before we change the flow of cash in any meaningful way, we need to collectively recognize and address three very basic realities about health care in this country.

1) Care Is a Business

Reality one is that care delivery is a business. We need to think of care delivery as a business and understand care delivery to be a business. It is a huge, well connected, cash-flow rich business that consumes roughly 18 percent of our total economy.[180] The people who deliver care are all paid money to deliver care -- and the care industry functions as a business in a very functional way -- with the care that is delivered to patients based very directly on the specific business model we use today to pay for that care.

2) Care Is a Politically Powerful Business

Reality two is that health care is a politically powerful business. We will need to solve our massive cost problems and achieve both our cost reduction and our care improvement goals and targets in the political and economic context that is created by the massive and well-connected care delivery infrastructure of this country. That infrastructure of care delivery business units currently consumes nearly three trillion dollars a year in revenue.[181] The infrastructure has great collective political power. As one result of that power, that entire infrastructure has almost no quality or performance oversight. It has very effectively managed to put in place and protect the highest prices for pieces of care that are paid to caregivers anywhere in the world. That massive and extremely well-financed infrastructure of care business units has -- for obvious reasons -- great political leverage and huge and very powerful regulatory influence.

So the truth is that any solutions that we would like to use for our cost and quality problems will have to be created, designed and implemented with that political reality in mind. The answers we will be able to use to address the cost of care crisis in this country will need to be acceptable to major elements of that very powerful infrastructure. As we design solutions to our cost challenges, we need to know that the answers we use will need to provide benefit to major portions of the infrastructure of care. We need to recognize that the proposed solutions to care cannot just somehow simply deprive that very powerful infrastructure of any significant amount of its revenue. Major portions of the care infrastructure of this country will need to receive positive financial benefits from any new business model. If that does not happen, well organized and very powerful provider resistance to any new approach will be fatal to just about any proposed new approach.

3) We Get What We Pay For

Reality three is that we get what we pay for. We get exactly what we pay for. This is also an important reality to understand. We need to recognize clearly that the massive infrastructure of care delivery that exists in this country today is based on and built very specifically around the exact business model we use now to buy care. We get exactly what we pay for and we will keep getting exactly what we get today from the American infrastructure of care until we change the way we currently buy care.

In order to get a better set of products and services from the infrastructure of care, we will need to first define those better products and services. Then we will need to put in place functioning cash flow mechanisms that will actually and explicitly buy those better products and services. Cash flow will continue to very clearly and directly both determine and define care. To change care, we will need to rechannel some aspects of the flow of cash that actually buys care. That is a very simple but incredibly powerful truth.

We Now Sell, Produce and Buy Care by the Piece -- And Pieces Rule

So -- how do we buy care now?

The key point to understand about the way we buy care now is that we almost always buy care by the piece. We have a piece-work business reality in this country for care. Because we buy care by the piece, we sell care by the piece, and we produce care by the piece. Pieces rule. We have almost a purely piecework based economy for most of the care that is delivered in this country. It is a very simple cash flow model. We buy care by the piece and cash flows are based on direct payment for each piece of care.

There are some very important restrictions in place that define which pieces of care we pay for. That set of restrictions is another very important fact about the business model we use to buy care that we need to recognize and understand. Restrictions exist. We need to understand what those restrictions are and we need to know why they exist. Those clearly defined restrictions on which specific pieces of care will trigger payment for our caregivers often create their own challenges to care flexibility and their own very powerful array of barriers to care improvement and care affordability.

Those restrictions on the pieces of care that will be paid for in this country have been created by the two major sources of cash for caregivers. Those restrictions on the reimbursable pieces of care have been defined and determined by the government and they have been defined and determined by the health insurers who pay for most care in this country. That is also an extremely important point to understand. The exact pieces of care that we buy and pay for today are not defined by the patient, or by the caregiver. They are not defined by the market. They are not created by any market process or by any care engineering approaches that continuously create a set of patient-focused care services. Cash flow for the pieces of care that are delivered by caregivers is restricted to paying only for a defined set of services and our major payers have defined those "allowable" services based on their own determination of what pieces of care they want to buy.

Care That Isn't on the Approved List Generates No Revenue

Those lists are very powerful. People do not appreciate the power of those lists to both dictate care processes and restrict how we deliver care in this country. Care that is not on those lists generally generates no revenue for any caregivers from the major payers. Care is -- as this chapter pointed out at the very beginning -- a business. Businesses inherently pay attention to revenue. Caregivers usually do nothing that doesn't generate revenue. So any care item that is not listed on the approved insurer, Medicare or Medicaid payment list generally does not happen.

That payment process is clearly defined, and it is very tightly and skillfully administered by each payer. Claims examiners for each of the payers look carefully at every bill that is submitted by each caregiver to see if the bill represents a piece of care that is on the approved list.

Each business unit in this country that sells care by the piece understands that model well. Each business unit that sells care by the piece builds its operations, structure, work flow, functionality, service capability, and products around that specific piece-work cash flow. Care is defined by those lists.

The Care Infrastructure Only Delivers Care Defined by the Fee Schedule

The power of that defined and approved procedure list to sculpt care should not be underestimated.

The care delivery infrastructure very rarely performs any services or does any pieces of work for patients that are not specifically listed on and included in the standard insurance–process blessed piecework fee schedule. Having a nurse call an asthma patient to make sure that the patient has refilled their prescription is a very good thing to do. Having asthma patients refill their prescriptions helps reduce the number of asthma attacks. That particular service is not, however, usually included on any of the approved fee lists. So those very useful and high value calls from nurses to asthma patients rarely happen in most care settings.

At the other extreme -- having an emergency room treating an asthma patient who is in crisis and is actually having an actual asthma attack triggers a set of services that are very much on the approved payer fee list. So treating an asthma patient who is horribly and painfully in crisis creates a flood of approved cash that flows freely to the various care sites that see and treat that patient in the context of that crisis.

Because that crisis care is paid for, the emergency rooms are set up to handle those patients and those crises. Because we do not pay for those nurse calls, most care sites have not been set up to have nurses do that array of work. The nurses, therefore, who work in the doctors' offices where the asthma patients get their primary care seldom make those unbillable phone calls to see if the asthma patient has had their prescription filled for use in an asthma crisis.

We get exactly what we pay for.

That process of defining functional care delivery for each patient through the approval process screen of an insurance company or a government program approved fee list creates a sometimes crippling and often highly dysfunctional rigidity in care delivery. Innovation is usually crippled and entirely legitimate care process enhancements are sometimes actually criminalized by the rigor of that piecework payment model. Criminalized is a relevant word to use to describe the enforcement power of those payment rules for government payers. Billing a government payer for a nurse making a phone call to check on an asthma patient can actually be considered billing fraud by the government because that is not an authorized bill for a nurse to send to Medicare or Medicaid. The bill for the nurse's service is considered fraudulent if it is sent in. Fraud is considered a category of criminal behavior. The payer defined lists tend to be very inflexible -- both for the sets of services that can be provided and for the type of caregiver who is allowed to perform them.

The list of approved services that exists today in the fee schedules reflects a rigid model of thinking about what constitutes reimbursable care. The lists of services that we use today to approve claims payments tend to be a snapshot of specific individual care services that have traditionally been done by particular subsets of licensed caregivers in the context of our historic, completely piecework approach to producing and buying care in this country.

That payment model and cash flow rigidity clearly creates some real problems if our goal is to continuously improve care.

Optimal Asthma Care Should Be a Package –- Not an Avalanche of Pieces

Asthma care is a very useful example of how the rules set by those approved billing lists can create inferior care.

Chapter two made this same point.

If we really wanted to provide optimal care for asthma patients, we would actually structure the care around each asthma patient. We would build a plan for each asthma patient to both prevent asthma crisis for that patient and to intervene quickly when crises do occur for that patient. An overall patient-focused model that looks at the full scope of asthma care -- done well -- can reduce asthma crises by half or more.[182] That would be the approach that providers would create if asthma care was sold as a package of care for asthma patients. That's not the approach we use. We just buy defined pieces of asthma care. When we buy asthma care only by the piece and use the approved procedure list to define the pieces -- there is no payment for that nurse doing that care delivery preventative patient-focused intervention work. There is not only a lack of payment for those proactive prevention services –- there is actually a lack of needed tools to perform those services. Chapter one talked about our data deficits and our tool deficits. There sadly are no tools today in most care settings to link multiple caregivers for an asthma patient because there is currently no fee that will be paid to any of the caregivers for using those tools or doing that linkage work when payment is determined by today's standard fee schedules. We waste a lot of money on asthma patients and we get bad and unnecessary asthma care in the process because of that clearly inferior and entirely reactive way of dealing with asthma care that is dictated by that fee schedule.

The current piecework payment model we use to buy asthma care does create a lot of money for caregivers, however. It is not without irony that the piecework approach we use to pay for care actually generates huge revenue for caregivers when an actual, full -blown asthma crisis happens for a patient. Hospitals, emergency rooms, and doctors' offices can each bill for a lot of pieces of care when asthma attacks happen. By contrast, those very same piecework reimbursed caregivers can completely lose their revenue when their well-done prevention efforts work well for a patient and when those horrendous asthma attacks do not happen for that patient. As this chapter clearly pointed out at the beginning, health care is a business, and we get what we pay for. So what do we get? We pay for crises.

We get a lot of crises. We have twice as many asthma attacks as we would have and should have in this country if we were delivering optimal care and buying asthma care by the package and not by the piece.[183]

This isn't simple speculation or academic theory. There currently are a few prepaid health plans and care teams in some settings who now basically do sell care by the package instead of just selling care by the piece. Those plans that are paid for a full package of asthma care tend to look carefully at the whole patient relative to asthma care because they know that they reduce their expenses when they reduce asthma attacks. The care sites that sell a complete package of care can benefit financially when asthma attacks do not happen. By contrast, there is no reward or financial advantage given to any fee-based care site of any kind who might be equally successful in preventing an asthma attack.

We Have Twice As Many Asthma Crises As We Need To Have

The result of that perversely designed payment approach is that we have twice as many asthma crises as we need to have in this country and we spend a lot of money unnecessarily on overall asthma care.

One very inflexible piece of that typical payment rule set is that doctors must directly deliver all pieces of care in order for care to be paid for. The fee schedules usually mandate that only doctors can do the billable units of care.

The infrastructure that we have set up to provide the care pieces for asthma care are therefore usually organized so that each allowable and billable piece of care will be delivered by a physician rather than done by any other member of their care team. So we have physicians doing services that really do not need to be done by a fully trained physician. That exclusive mandate that physicians must deliver many services happens in this country today because the approved fee schedule that defines allowable care for a piece of care is usually only activated for payment if an actual physician provides those pieces of care to a patient. Having a nurse do some key points of that work may make great logistical, practical, operational, functional, programmatic, and medical sense -- but that level of nursing care usually doesn't happen in most care settings because the standard third-party payer fee schedule doesn't pay nurses when they do that work.

Asthma care is, of course, absolutely not alone in having the business model we use to buy care cause the current infrastructure of care delivery to perform in sometimes perverse and frequently suboptimal ways. This chapter describes asthma care as an easy illustration of the perversity and dysfunctional aspects care delivery that result from the way we buy care, but those same dysfunctionality issues extend across almost the entire spectrum of piecework-reimbursed care in this country.

The Cash Flow for Care Rewards Crisis and Bad Outcomes

The truth is, as Chapter Two pointed out, the current business model we use to buy care very directly rewards both medical crises and bad care outcomes for just about all medical conditions. The pattern is pretty clear. As noted earlier in this book, the current way we buy care richly rewards heart attacks and it very much underfunds heart attack prevention. The current way we buy care pays way too much money for hospital infections and it does little or nothing to reward or even fund hospitals for preventing or minimizing those infections. The very best care sites have less than one percent of their patients who get pressure ulcers.[184] Average hospitals have seven percent of their patients with those ulcers.[185] How does our payment model deal with those very different consequences of care? The current fee schedule we use to buy care doesn't pay a dime to have all of the highly skilled patient-focused and extremely competent nurses in the best hospitals checking all of the high-risk patients in those hospitals hourly for those infections. Those hospitals get no fee schedule "credit," and they get no cash for the amazing amounts of work that are done in those hospitals by those nurses on behalf of those patients. But the fee schedule we use to buy care actually will easily pay each of those hospitals -- on average -- more than $40,000 per patient when those nasty and dangerous ulcers do happen. That is a lot of money paid for failure and no money paid to achieve success.

Buying Care by the Piece Discourages Care Reengineering

Those perverse payment approaches are actually not the absolute worst consequence of buying care entirely by the piece. An even more negative consequence for both care quality and care affordability is that the current piecework model of buying care also discourages and even penalizes many aspects of basic care process reengineering. That particular point was also made a couple of times earlier in this book. It is important to be understood. That piecework approach we use to buy care keeps continuous improvement approaches from becoming a major aspect of the way we deliver care in far too many care settings. The impact of cash flow considerations literally financially crippling and penalizing any significant reengineering efforts most of the time is a major flaw of that piecework payment approach.

Buying care by the piece usually financially penalizes clearer, simpler, and better processes that are designed by care sites. It financially penalizing the care sites if any of the process redesign work that is done by the care site eliminates a billable piece of the original care process. Far too often, implementing very reengineered beneficial changes in care approaches will directly and immediately reduce the revenue flow for the care site that does the reengineering. The amazingly effective work process redesign work that was used to get pressure ulcers for hospitalized patients in the best hospitals to less than one percent of patients is not currently reimbursed by any fee schedule. The sad reality is that when fee-based hospitals actually do that wonderful prevention work, they lose an average of $40,000 in piecework revenue per patient when that work succeeds and the patients are not damaged.

That is obviously a very dysfunctional and perverse way to buy care. The financial consequences of reengineering key pieces of care are often fiscally dire for the hospital who reengineers. The medical consequences of not reengineering that care are, of course, dire for the patient. Cash flow wins. Very few hospitals do the work needed to achieve those highly improved levels of care.

There Are Many Opportunities for Care Process Redesign

There are actually a great many opportunities that result for care process redesign in the delivery of care in this country. Many of those opportunities are strongly obvious to just about everyone who delivers care. There is a lot of "low-hanging fruit" available and waiting for some basic care process redesign -- but that process redesign very rarely happens in real care settings because the piecework model of payment reduces cash flow to any fee-paid care sites that actually redesign and improve processes.

Remember the points that were made at the beginning of this chapter. Care delivery is a business. We get exactly what we pay for -- and we don't get what we don't pay for.

The perverse economic equation that exists can be hard for patients, the news media, and policy makers to believe, but every care site in this country that is paid by the piece knows it to be true.

That crippling of process redesign innovation work may be the single most damaging impact for this country that results from buying care by the piece. That piecework payment model literally cripples both process improvement and reengineering processes for many important areas of care.

Process Reengineering That Improves Care Can Cut Revenue

People often ask why health care hasn't taken advantage of the process reengineering approaches that have transformed so many other industries. The answer to that question is actually pretty easy and very basic.

Process reengineering rarely happens in health care delivery settings in this country today simply because any care process engineering improvement approaches that actually streamline the processes of care tend to also reduce the number of currently billable care steps that now generate real cash for the care business unit that does that redesign. Reengineered processes and innovative new care approaches that deliberately eliminate redundant, unnecessary and duplicative tests for a hospital admission, for example, almost never happen in the real world of care delivery.

Those obvious and easy to do reengineering steps to eliminate unnecessary pieces of care do not happen in the real world of health care very often because each of those care improvement changes will clearly cut off at least some of the existing revenue stream and reduce the current cash flow that has been created for that particular piece of the business infrastructure of care by running those unnecessary, duplicative -- but very billable and highly profitable -- tests.

No Industry Ever Reengineers Again Its Own Self-Interest

We obviously need to improve those aspects of the business model of care if we want to get rid of even obviously unnecessary tests and procedures.

As this book points out in several places, no industry ever reengineers against its own self-interest. Wal-Mart has done some spectacular and brilliant work relative to the processes involved in distributing their products. They have done brilliant interactive work with their vendors. Their just-in-time inventory control is legendary.[186] The truth is -- if the consequences to Wal-Mart of doing that wonderful just-in-time inventory reengineering would have been for Wal-Mart to lose twenty percent of their customers and to lose thirty percent of their net revenue for those specific products, then the likelihood of Wal-Mart going down that particular reengineering path would have obviously been significantly diminished. If the old way of getting supplies on the shelf in the Wal-Mart stores would have generated thirty percent higher profits, the old way would probably have prevailed. Wal-Mart brilliantly reengineered key processes. Why? Wal-Mart benefited directly from the redesigned process. Wal-Mart made more money as a result of that new process -- not less money. Any redesign work in any industry that impairs profits instead of improves profits is a lot less likely to happen in any business setting. That is true in any industry and it is very much true in health care.

That's another reason why we need to change the business model we use to buy care. We need to put a business model in place that rewards reengineering and rewards patient-focused process improvement work. The current way we buy care badly flawed when it comes to incenting reengineering.

We also need a business model that rewards price competition. Every other industry tends to have some level of price competition. Health care has almost none.

Price Competition Is Not Rewarded by Market Forces in Care

The business model we use to buy care today clearly does not reward caregivers for making care more affordable. That is another question people often ask. Why don't caregivers figure out how to reduce prices? The odd but very real truth is that caregivers do not benefit in most settings as businesses by being able to reduce prices. That is sad but it is sadly very true. That economic reality usually isn't true in other industries. In other industries, price cuts can often improve profits because lower prices can very often increase the sales volume for whoever cuts their prices. Basic price cuts often don't damage businesses in other industries because sales generally go up when prices go down for most products in most industries.

That specific cycle of achieving financial rewards as a business based on reducing costs and prices does not happen very often in health care. The price chapter of this book made that point clearly. Price competition is almost non-existent for caregiver business units in this country. In the business model we use today to buy care, cutting the prices for any piece of care usually just reduces the caregiver's total income without increasing the caregiver's volume or without improving the bottom line of caregiver organizations.

Health care providers are all very intelligent people. Anyone smart enough to get into medical school or into a health care administration program is more than smart enough to understand that basic financial reality. Doing things that damage their own business interests isn't something that intelligent people who run businesses usually do.

We Will See a Golden Age of Care Process Redesign When Care Is Purchased by the Package

That means we need to change the way we buy care to make reengineering of key processes to reduce prices an approach that directly and clearly benefits caregiver business units rather than an approach that directly penalizes and economically damages caregiver business units. This is another very basic point to understand. We clearly need to make reengineering to create lower prices something that benefits care sites -- not damages them financially. When that happens, reengineering in health care will flourish.

Many Caregivers Are Ready for a New Market Model

When the business model changes, we will see an explosion of creativity -- a golden age of care process redesign.

Caregivers are -- in many settings -- ready for that change to happen. There are brilliant caregivers who will improve processes in amazing ways once those process improvements create a financial reward for the care sites instead of creating a financial penalty.

So how can we create those rewards? A key next step will be to buy more care in packages in a way that changes the cash flow for caregivers and moves the flow of cash away from a total dependence on selling care entirely by the piece. The piecework approach to buying care incents volumes of inappropriate care and it clearly limits our ability to strategically and functionally reengineer care. We need a business model that allows us to buy packages of care -- not just pieces of care -- so we can liberate the care redesign thinking in health care and see care become more efficient, more effective, and more affordable.

Providers Can Do Wonderful Reengineering When Care Is Sold as a Package

Providers of care can and will do really smart things -- both alone and collectively -- when care is purchased in packages.

Buying packages of care empowers and enables caregivers to reengineer both the pieces and the processes of care in very positive ways that can meet both the business needs of the caregivers as well as the cost needs of the people paying for care.

There is ample evidence showing that to be true. Many people who do health care policy work know some of those examples. But a couple of those examples need to be described more heavily in this chapter of this book. The examples that are described below show significant successes for both care delivery costs and care quality that have actually resulted from buying packages of care -- instead of pieces of care -- in real world American health care settings. The first two examples listed below are two specific procedures -- eye surgery and heart transplant surgery. In both cases, care was reengineered and transformed when the business model moved away from buying that care by the piece to buying it as a package. The third example of positive care engineering described below came from a care site that actually guaranteed the success of their key surgeries and agreed not to charge for any needed "redos." The care site that guaranteed their surgical results reengineered both their processes and their services and their patients ended up with better care at less cost.

Perhaps the most powerful example described below shows the great care that can result from buying all care as a total package from a team of caregivers for an entire population of patients for a fixed monthly price. That particular example is one that the author is very familiar with, because it is an example from his own workplace. All four of those very real business model examples make the case that care can be reengineered in very effective ways when the cash flow model that is used to buy that care changes.

In each of those settings, real world caregivers in this country have used the cash available from a package payment to reengineer real care. Each example is worth understanding at a level that is less superficial than just describing the impact at a vague and macro level.

Eye Surgery Sold as a Package Worked Well

Let's start with eyes.

One very good example of real-world experience and care delivery changes that can happen when we buy care by the package has been Lasik eye surgery. People who look at selling packages of care often use Lasik eye surgery as a really good example of what can happen when you start buying and selling care by the package instead of by the piece.

The basic elements that resulted from that change in the business model for that particular surgery are also pretty clear and worth understanding.

Lasik eye surgery improves people's vision. It is a very useful surgery.

When Lasik eye surgery was first introduced to the market, the total surgery cost almost $2,000 per eye[187] and that fee didn't always involve all of the ancillary charges that are generally incurred for all of the related care sites and connected procedures. Three thousand dollars is a significant amount of money to spend for a procedure that basically functionally replaces eyeglasses.

That procedure and that price is relevant to this chapter of this book because the market model we used in this country to buy care for that surgery didn't simply follow our usual purchasing approach for basic surgeries. Instead of selling all of the individual service that related to that eye surgery as a pile of billable pieces, the economic model that is now used to pay for that surgery now includes all aspects of that surgery as a package of services -- with one price for the surgery and the entire set of related services.

Why did this country use a different business model to pay for those particular surgeries?

Insurance companies made a very important decision about that eye surgery very soon after it was made available.

They did not make it an insured benefit.

Insurance companies and health plans decided not to cover and pay for that specific procedure when it was invented. The insurers called that eye surgery "cosmetic" rather than therapeutic. Cosmetic procedures are usually not covered by insurance. Those particular surgical procedures for eyes did not, therefore, go on the approved payment list for insurance coverage. You may disagree with that definition and with that decision by the insurance companies relative to the approved benefit status for that particular eye surgery -- but the consequence of that payment exclusion decision by the health insurers was fascinating. The impact of that payment decision on provider behaviors and provider practices relative to that surgery is definitely worth understanding and discussing.

If the Services Had Been Insured, the Initial High Price Would Have Been Permanent

If the insurers had decided to simply include that new eye surgery procedure as another covered benefit in everyone's insurance plan, then the care improvement story and the affordability issues for that particularly surgery would both have been ended by that decision by insurers to simply pay for the procedure. If the insurers had routinely added that eye surgery benefit to their list of approved services as a standard covered procedure, then insurance companies would have simply paid that initial designated price for each surgery. The future prices that would have been charged for that particular eye surgery would have stayed at the initial $2,000 per surgery price total cost level. That's how pricing usually works for pieces of insured care in this country.

Some insurers would inevitably have negotiated some volume discounts with various eye surgeons who did that service, but those price discounts would probably not have steered very many patients in any particular direction to any care site because -- as we know -- insured patients usually only pay the flat deductible amount for any service. That flat amount of deductible expense would have made any insurance plan negotiated discounts and price differences for that procedure invisible to the patient and therefore irrelevant for any actual patient decision making about that surgery.

That's how we buy most care in America. That point was discussed earlier in the chapter on prices. Our most current widely used insurance benefit plan design -- the deductible -- tends to hide both prices and price differences from consumers once the deductible is met. Deductibles tend to make prices invisible and irrelevant for every piece of care that costs more than the deductible. That would also have been true for that particular eye surgery if the surgery had been insured and then paid for by the deductible benefit package insurance plans.

Insured Premiums Are Based on the Average Cost of Care

Insurance premiums are always based on the average cost of care for each population of people who are insured. So if the Lasik eye surgery had been a covered benefit, then each health insurer for each patient who had that surgery would have paid those full fees to each eye care surgery site on behalf of each patient. Those additional payments that were made by insurers to buy that new surgery would then have caused insurance premiums to go up. Each payment made by each insurer for each patient for that new benefit would have simply and directly increased the average cost of care for their entire set of insured people. That higher total care expense would have triggered higher premium levels -- and the insurers would have used that premium money collected from all of their customers to pay for the Lasik surgery for the customers who choose to have the surgery done.

We Use Other People's Money To Pay for Our Care

That is actually a very important fourth financial reality we all should understand about the delivery and financing of care in this country.

In this country, we almost always use other people's money to pay for our care. If we are in a government program, we use taxpayer money to buy our care. If we have a private insurance plan, we use the actual money that comes from all of the other people who also pay premiums each month to our insurance plan to pay for our care.

Getting access to other people's money is the primary purpose and the function of insurance premiums. The next chapter of this book discusses that business model in more detail.

In the case of the eye surgery -- if the health insurance companies had simply decided immediately to make the Lasik surgery a covered benefit -- then the consumers who choose to have the surgery done would each have paid only the deductible amount, and the rest of the fee schedule for each surgery would have been paid by each insurer -- using other people's money collected in premium as the source of that cash.

Insurance Premiums Is a Good Way To Collect Other People's Money To Pay for Our Care

New benefits always have that impact on insurance premium. New benefits always increase the average cost of care. So new benefits always increase premium. The math is pretty simple and pretty direct.

In this case, however, that particular fundamental cycle of premium calculation mathematics -- with new benefits creating premium increases -- is entirely irrelevant. You don't need to raise the premiums if the insurers don't need money to pay for the care.

That decision by the insurers not to insure that service changed the business model for both caregivers and patients for that piece of care. Consumers who wanted that service now were forced to use their own money to buy that care instead of just paying a flat deductible and then using other people's money to pay for the care. That new financial reality and that new cash flow very directly changed the functional and economic model of care for those eye surgery caregivers.

Direct Payment by Consumers Created a Different Business Model

Fees for that surgery were suddenly highly relevant to both the patients and the caregivers. Fees were actually highly visible to each customer instead of being quietly buried behind the obscuring financial fog of an insured deductible benefit plan.

So what happened next? Adam Smith would have recognized and probably saluted the process.

The market worked. Market forces became relevant for that surgery. Those market forces changed both the way that surgery was done and the way that surgery was priced.

Market Forces Became Relevant

What market forces were activated?

Price competition happened very quickly. That makes sense. When people had to pay for that surgery out of their own pocket, prices for that surgery become extremely relevant. Price competition very quickly developed and that competition structured the marketplace for that particular surgery. When the actual prices for the surgery became highly relevant to customers, care sites started competing for customers by both lowering prices for the surgery and by aggressively advertising their lower prices. Patients made their choices of caregivers and patients also made their personal care delivery purchase decisions based to a large degree on the highly visible price levels that were set by each competing care site. Competition worked. Sales volume followed prices. Lower prices created significant sales increases for the lower priced care sites. Prices for the surgery dropped from that initial $2,000. The prices actually dropped incrementally for several years. Some surgery sites dropped their prices below $1,000, and a few sites ultimately sold the procedure for roughly $300 per eye.[188] A thriving market developed for that surgery. It is very important to note that doing the surgery was actually profitable the entire time for the care sites that were competing for that business even though their prices for doing that surgery had dropped significantly.

Reengineering Became a Relevant Skill Set

How did those care sites manage to make money and be profitable doing a highly skilled surgical procedure at those very low prices?

The answer is simple. Every other industry knows both the answer and the approach that was used by those surgeons. They reengineered. They very directly improved processes. Reengineering was suddenly relevant to the care teams who did the surgery.

The business units who did that surgery very skillfully reengineered care. When prices became relevant and when providers were rewarded financially for dropping prices, the care teams changed the operational processes that were needed to support the surgery in order to bring down the actual functional operating costs for doing the procedure.

Those eye surgery care sites created new work flow for their care teams. They did very smart things about functionality. Efficiency became relevant, so efficiency happened. They reengineered their surgical lasers to allow the machines to move easily from patient to patient. They changed the recovery space and they changed the recovery staffing and they changed the recovery process. They even changed the record keeping for the surgery. They changed the anesthetic to a simpler process. The eye surgery units and care teams took a hard and clear look at each piece of the care process for that surgery. Care actually got a lot better. They computerized and improved the pre-surgery exam process. They actually improved the outcomes for that surgery in the process and they reengineered almost all of the steps involved in doing the surgery. They did that work and they did it well because the provider business units that were selling the surgery for a package price wanted to reduce the operating costs to each provider site that were being incurred for each patient by doing that surgery.

Health Care Is Not Immune To Reengineering

Reengineering works. It can be done. Health care is obviously not immune to reengineering. Providers of care just need to have a business reason to do that work. If the insurance companies had decided at the very beginning when the surgery was invented to simply cover that eye surgery -- and if the insurers had decided to simply charge each insured patient who received the surgery only their standard flat insurance benefit deductible -- there would have been absolutely no value to any provider to ever reengineer any part of that specific care process because there would have been no financial reason to do that reengineering work. That surgery had been profitable at the original price of $2,000. There would have been no reason for any surgery site to drop that price if the service had been insured and if the insurers were all paying that $2,000 price, no questions asked.

This point was made earlier.

No industry ever reengineers against its own self-interest. But when there is a business reason both to engineer and to reengineer, then very smart things can be done in health care to achieve really important process improvement goals and to bring down the cost of care.

Heart Transplant Surgery Followed a Similar Path

Eye surgery isn't the only example of the business model of care changing for some aspect of care and then having care delivery reengineer itself to respond to the new business reality. As noted in the chapter on prices, when Medicare stopped buying hospital care by the piece and instead decided to use a new Diagnosis Related Group (DRG) payment approach that used a partial package payment for most Medicare-funded hospital care, hospitals in this country reengineered care immediately and well. That reengineering was done so well as a result of that change in the payment model that we Americans now have the shortest hospital stays in the industrialized world. Remember chart 3.13. The basic business model that was used by Medicare to buy hospital care changed. The care delivery infrastructure for hospital care followed that change in the cash flow so well that we are now the world leader in low levels of hospital care -- with one of the lowest number of hospital days used per patient and the shortest lengths of stay in the industrialized world.[189]

Heart Transplant Surgery Followed a Similar Path

Heart transplant surgery followed a path that was similar in several ways to the path that was followed for the Lasik surgery. The business model that was used to buy that care also changed for heart transplants a number of years ago.

How and why did the business model change for heart transplants? The approach that was used to change the business model to buy that particular transplant was elegantly simple. Major buyers who paid a lot of money for heart transplant simply put heart transplants out to bid and those payers asked the caregivers for a packaged price.

When several major players in this country started to use that very different business model to buy heart transplants a couple of decades ago, the care sites that did those complex heart surgeries went through a change in their care delivery approach. Those changes very much resembled the work that was done for the eye surgery. The transplant centers applied processes and skills sets that paralleled the steps used in the eye surgery reengineering successes. Focused reengineering that was done by several of our very best great care teams made heart transplants both less expensive and more successful in a relatively short time. Reengineering worked again. The new package price business model that was used for buying that care trigged a whole array of care delivery process enhancements. Reengineering happened for those transplants. Reengineering happened because the providers who sold the transplants at a package price benefited from doing that reengineering work rather than being penalized for doing that work.

The patterns of thinking and reengineering that happened for heart transplants strongly resembled the reengineering approaches that happened for the Lasik eye surgery. As with the eye surgery redesign, the new heart transplant process made those surgeries both better and a lot less expensive.

Initial heart transplants were highly expensive. Quality of care for the transplants was inconsistent and prices were very high and going up. Spending more than a quarter of a million dollars to do a single heart transplant was not rare roughly twenty years ago.[190] Costs of those surgeries were very high at that time and both the costs and the volumes of the surgery were increasing steadily. Heart transplants -- like the eye surgeries -- can be wonders of medical science. Patients benefit significantly from both procedures. So an increasing number of heart transplants were being done -- and all of the health insurers and the government programs who covered that procedure were simply paying the constantly increasing bundles of fees that were being charged by each care site to do those complex and expensive procedures.

As was noted earlier, we always use other people's money in this country to pay for our care -- so health insurance premiums were being increased for all insured people to give the insurers enough money to pay for those transplants.

All insured patients were paying through their increased premiums for the growing costs of doing those lovely, life-enhancing transplants for the people who clearly needed them.

At that point -- as was noted earlier -- a few key buyers decided to simply put those surgeries out to bid. Those high volume buyers asked the very best care sites to give them a package price for that procedure.

That request, of course, changed the market model for those transplants. The insurers didn't just ask for a percentage discount of some kind from the typical avalanche of transplant-related fees. They asked for a single flat fee to do the entire procedure. The insurers who went down that path very wisely made the decision to only use the very best care sites with the best care outcomes and the best success levels to do the transplants and then they asked those best care sites to give them a package price for the whole procedure.

Packaged Prices Created the Opportunity To Reengineer

The buyers didn't simply try to negotiate steeper discounts. They also did not go to low quality vendors in order to get a low price. They very deliberately used the best care sites. The insurers knew that there were a number of great care sites around the country that did very good heart transplants. They believed that the best sites for that transplant were likely to get continuously better. Winners win. That's not always true, but it is generally a good way to bet. The insurers also knew that heart transplants were a medical procedure where the practical logistics of care for the procedure allowed a patient to travel safely to a care site -- so the care site for a heart transplant did not need to be in the same city or country as the patient's home. The willingness of patients to travel to get great transplant care was clearly enhanced by the fact that the care sites chosen by the insurers were care sites with great brands and wonderful reputations.

The insurers used several of the right "R" words in the process. The health insurers did not ration transplants. They repriced transplants. They also rewarded the reengineering of transplants. They repackaged transplants. Repricing, reengineering, repackaging and then rewarding caregivers are all good "R" words to use.

The Surgery Care Teams Looked At Prices Improvement Opportunities

Some of the transplant centers were initially not happy with that change in the market model for heart transplants. But then the care teams and the leadership teams at the various transplant centers looked at the proposed package cash flow approach and at the reality of a package price, and they realized how liberating that cash flow approach can be relative to empowering care reengineering and directly rewarding creating process improvements for care. It was clearly very empowering for the care sites to be paid a package price for each heart instead of having to sell their transplant care services patient by patient and piece by piece. The great heart care centers each took a careful look at their heart transplant process and then they simply reengineered multiple steps in the process to make the process both better and more affordable.

They often started by eliminating unnecessary duplication in the tests that were ordered for each patient.

They Reduced Test Duplications

Those unneeded and duplicative tests all used to be direct revenue for the care sites when they were paid entirely by the piece. When the new revenue stream became a single package-based fee, those unneeded tests stopped creating revenue and they simply became excess expense generators. Those tests were useless for care purposes so they become irrelevant to the revenue stream. So the people designing the flow of care inside those packaged price care teams usually very quickly reduced the number of duplicated and unneeded tests. They also changed some sites of care. Some transplant centers began to have some of their heart patients who were not at immediate medical risk sleep in hotel rooms next to the hospital for some days prior to surgery rather than having those same patients sleeping for those pre-surgery nights in very expensive -- and relatively uncomfortable -- hospital beds. Having a pre-surgery patient sleeping comfortably for a night or two in a very nice $200 to $300 per night hotel room rather than sleeping uncomfortably in a $3,000- $4,000 per night hospital bed makes a lot of sense when you are selling care by the package and not selling care by the piece.

When you are paid by the piece in a piecework cash flow model, however, having your pre-transplant patient stay in your $4,000 a night hospital bed to simply rest for a couple of days is very profitable for the care site. In a package price model, that use of an expensive hospital bed to be a pure resting site created an expense for each transplant patient that was clearly not a medical necessity. The actual medical needs of the patient were met as well or better by resting in a nearby hotel.

They Also Improved Recovery Time and Sites

The transplant centers also worked out better and faster post-surgery recovery agendas and sites. They did some serious process improvement work and the surgery centers created actual significant internal operating efficiencies around each piece of care.

That change in the business model for that element of care worked. The change was good for the patient and it was good for the caregivers. Outcomes were better. Processes were standardized. Survival rates went up. And the whole pile of pieces and procedures that had been billed under the old piecework payment model to add up to total fees in excess of $200,000 per heart were soon being done at some of the best hospitals in the world for roughly $100,000 to $150,000 per heart. Two decades later, basic transplant prices are still below where they were when the business model for heart transplants changed. Costs are down, prices are down, and the success rates from that surgery are much higher. Care got better and costs went down when the cash flow and operational thinking was centered on a package of care and not on pieces of care.

Guaranteeing Successful Results Also Triggered Reengineering

Care teams can and will do very smart things when the business model rewards doing smart things.

As noted earlier, one famous East Coast care site changed its business model a couple of years ago to guarantee the results from several of their key surgeries.[191] Making those very clear guarantees of surgical success was a very different business model for that surgical care. That care site basically said to patients -- if this surgery fails, we will do the surgery again and we will fix it for nothing. There will be no charge for the redo.

That care site started as one of the best surgery sites in the U.S. They already had fewer surgical redos than other care sites in the area. When they guaranteed results, and changed their surgery business model to not charge patient or insurers for redos, they got even better. As a business unit of care delivery that was now making actual guarantees of surgical success, they knew that a failed surgery would no longer simply result in them making twice as much money for that patient because they would simply be doing the surgery again and charging the patient double for the redo. That care team never ever did anything at any time in the old business model to cause any surgical redo to happen -- but that care team also was not as focused on making sure that the redos did not ever happen before they put their guarantees in place.

The People Who Guaranteed Success Studied Each Failed Surgery Very Closely

Again -- just like the heart transplant sites and the Lasik eye surgery sites -- the care sites that were involved in making that surgery outcome guarantee did careful process design and redesign work. Data became a key tool. They expanded their use of care related data. They studied each failed surgery --going back for multiple prior years to look at old failures. They carefully studied each current failure. They looked very closely and candidly to see what had caused each failure to happen. And then they made a few very well designed process reengineering changes to reduce the likelihood of those specific problems reoccurring for their patients.

What was the result of that work? It was exactly what you would expect.

Process Improved -- Care Got Even Better

Processes improved. Data gathering became increasingly sophisticated and effective. Surgeries got better. The numbers of surgical redos were very low for that particular surgical center to begin with and they went down even further. That care team started with really good care and the quality of care in those centers went up when the business model changed. The total cost of care went down because outcomes were better and redos dropped significantly. The operating costs of the care sites were also reduced when the processes were reengineered and improved.

So how was that particular decision to guarantee success for surgeries rewarded by our current business model for care? Not very well. That surgery unit initially lost some volume - because they had fewer redos -- and they, therefore, lost some revenue because their good care got even better. In this particular case, however, there was some offsetting volume-based market rewards for that care site because more people in the geographic area wanted to get their care from the surgery sites that guaranteed results.

At a macro level, that care site benefited economically from better care because their public aura and their credibility as a high quality care team that guaranteed results was good for their overall volume of patients and good for their brand. For obvious reasons, it was great for their local and their national reputation to be the care team that actually guaranteed their surgical results. That care organization made a gutsy call as a business to guarantee those surgical results, but the overall impact of making that guarantee turned out very well at several levels.

The caregivers on that care team took great pride in continuously improving their care. When care sites anywhere develop cultures of excellence and build cultures of continuous improvement, those cultures result in better care. Those cultures also tend to be good for the morale of the caregivers and those cultures of continuous improvement tend to be self-reinforcing at very useful and important levels.

The key point for us to learn about that surgery-results guarantee example is this -- care design and redesign can be done in almost any care setting -- and the results of the redesign can be excellent. Redesign work can actually be done in a very functional context for many key areas of care. Real opportunities to improve care processes do exist and those opportunities will only be very real and relevant in American care sites when the business model for our care sites makes those opportunities relevant and real.

Selling a Package of Care Reduced Broken Bones by a Third

In each of the examples listed above -- selling eye surgery and heart surgery by the package, selling hospital care through DRG payment model, and selling packages of surgery with a guarantee of success –- the business model for the caregivers involved changed and the caregivers responded by coming up with care process redesign efforts that created financial successes under the new model. Cash flow changed for care for those purchases. As a result, care changed to respond to the cash flow.

Buying All Care for A Package Price Is Even More Liberating

We need to expand that purchasing model to make it more comprehensive to give caregivers even more flexibility in figuring out the right processes of care.

A number of health care policy experts are now recommending that we move as a country away from buying care by the piece and that we should begin buying care more by the package. The next chapter of this book deals with variations on that approach –- looking at how caregivers can create better team using new tools like patient centered medical home care settings and can create better coordinated care though the new Accountable Care Organizations –- or ACOs. The ACO proponents are advocating that physician and hospitals should come together to accept accountability for the total care of patients in settings where the cash flow can be blended in ways that create flexibility among the caregivers relative to use of the money. One major goal of the new ACO agenda is to have caregivers collectively accountable for the care of a population of people rather than just dealing with care for people one incident at a time. As the next chapter explains, that new ACO model isn't entirely defined or refined yet, but it obviously has a lot to offer in many respects. There is a very good reason to believe that the concept of accountable and the commitment to organized care is a good path for us to be on as a country. We know from real experience that the Accountable and Organized model can work.

There are some Accountable Care Organizations in existence and that have been in place for a relatively long time. Some care sites and some care teams actually sell all of the care needed by a population of patients for a fixed price as a total package today. There are existing multispecialty care teams now who are paid a single monthly payment for all care and who actually have no fee-for-service billing now for major pieces of that care. That is a very different payment model than buying care entirely by the piece. The care priorities and the care delivery approaches that result from that flat payment approach for a package of care can be very different than the priorities that are a fact of life for a fee-based piecework payment business unit.

Kaiser Permanente is one of those prepaid care teams that sells care by the package and not by the piece. With three dozen hospitals, 550 medical care sites, 180,000 caregivers, and 9 million members, Kaiser Permanente is paid a flat fee every month for each of the 9 million members, and uses that money to provide the care needed by the 9 million people.[192]

Less than 5 percent of the Kaiser Permanente revenue comes from fees.[193] Internally, there is no mechanism to transfer money in any way based on fees. Like the care systems in Sweden and Norway, the care delivery is based on the needs of the patients and not on the need to code a bill for a service that will generate piecework cash payment for each piece of care.

Being freed from the tyranny and structure of a piecework cash model allows the care teams to focus on the patients.

One example of how care can be different on that approach relates to broken bones.

The Kaiser Permanente care team looked at broken bones very differently than the way that the standard piecework, payment-focused care sites looked at broken bones. Most piece-work-paid care sites actually make a lot of money when bones break. By contrast, the Kaiser Permanente care team incurred only additional cost and generated absolutely no revenue when bones broke for their patients. Broken bones are an expense to that care team -- not a revenue source, so it made sense for those caregivers to figure out how to reduce the number of broken bones.

The care team worked systematically to prevent bones from breaking rather than just waiting for bones to break and then providing crisis care to those damaged patients. The number of broken bones for the more senior patients in that care system was actually reduced by an amazing degree. The care teams reengineered their care with a particular focus on high-risk seniors. The care teams introduced individual care plans for their senior patients and they targeted effective preventative services for their patients who were at high risk of breaking bones. Prevention worked. The care team in that system actually reduced the number of broken bones for their senior patients by more than a third.[194]

The basic economic reality is that Kaiser Permanente does not make money when bones break. Kaiser Permanente also does not make revenue when strokes happen or when patients have heart attacks or when asthma crises happen. Kaiser Permanente also doesn't make money when patients have pressure ulcers or any other kinds of hospital infections. As this book has pointed out several times, other hospitals generally have 5 percent to 10 percent of their patients with pressure ulcers.

Kaiser Permanente has less than 1 percent, overall, of patients with those ulcers. And some hospitals have not had a single ulcer in over a year.[195]

KP revenue is not based on chasing down and billing separate fees for each piece of care as their foundational source of cash. Fees actually don't exist for internal cost factors inside of the Kaiser Permanente care infrastructure.

As the introduction to this book noted, the author of this book worked for Kaiser Permanente for 12 years. The author knows the business model of Kaiser Permanente very directly and fairly well. It is a very effective business model. Because Kaiser Permanente is prepaid and doesn't have to base its business model on protecting units of piecework cash flow, Kaiser Permanente actually has significant flexibility in figuring out the best ways of delivering care.

There are some benefit plans sold to members that require Kaiser Permanente patients to pay some fees, but the total cash flow from all of those fees is less than 5 percent of the total revenue of Kaiser Permanente.

This book has stated several times that care design can be much more flexible when it is liberated from a piecework cash flow. That statement about liberation from the fee schedule isn't based on guesses, theory, conception, or speculation. The author knows from direct experience that the prepaid cash flow approach can be very empowering and highly enabling relative to designing care delivery approaches and processes. Being prepaid -- and not having to collect piecework fees to generate basic revenue -- changes the economic incentive and business model entirely relative to both designing and delivering care.

Functional Preventive Interventions Are Needed

As noted above, selling care by the package gives the Kaiser Permanente care organization a strong and direct financial incentive not to incur the cost of repairing broken bones. Functional prevention interventions are an important focus for creative thinking about the tools needed for optimal patient care. Those exact same incentives to prevent problems rather than waiting for crises and then treating problems also apply to Kaiser Permanente patients not having strokes, asthma crisis or heart attacks. Those same incentives encourage the care team at Kaiser Permanente to have cancer detected at very early stages, and to have many fewer patients damaged for life or killed by pressure ulcers or sepsis.

Kaiser Permanente has some of the highest levels of blood pressure control of any care system in America -- and that high level of control helps with multiple levels of chronic care improved care outcomes.[196]

Package Prices Can Reduce Overall Costs

That reduction in hospital use for all of those categories of patients has allowed overall Kaiser Permanente premiums to be lower because less hospital care was needed for these patients. Some insurance-linked processes that compare health plans with one another can become completely confused about how to evaluate those kinds of successful results.

Some process analysts know the piecework payment model well but they do not understand packages of care. These analysts sometimes weigh and compare health plans based on the relative discount levels that plans have negotiated for their fees. The plans with the biggest discount levels get the highest ratings on some consultants' comparative measurement scales. Those comparisons sometimes have trouble understanding or relating to Kaiser Permanente care performance levels. The analyst formulas can compare and weigh a discounted fee. They can't weigh the absence of a fee. Done well, the fee does not need to exist. Care improvement is the best measure of value in that setting.

Stroke Deaths Are Down 40 Percent -- Cancer Deaths Are Down 20 Percent

As noted earlier, Kaiser Permanente has also used team care and care reengineering processes to reduce stroke deaths by 40 percent.[197] Kaiser Permanente has colon cancer mortality rates that are about 10-15 percent lower than other care sites.[198] Kaiser Permanente also has used proactive and coordinated team care to achieve an HIV death rate that is half the national average.[199]

A major key to success for the Kaiser Permanente care team in those areas is simply to be liberated from the fee schedules that rigidly define the menu of care approaches that are used in other piecework-reimbursed care settings. To cut the HIV death rate to half of the national average – with some of the best care results in the world -- Kaiser Permanente does many things that do not show up on a Medicare or standard insurance company fee schedule.[200] Likewise, for the broken bones successes, Kaiser Permanente did six things that do not show up on a Medicare fee schedule.[201]

Care Processes Don't Need To Protect Billable Events

Those successes are relevant to the rest of American health care today, because both buyers and care organizations are trying to move away from fee-based payment models. The people who are proponents of the ACO model of providing packages of care to a population of people as a better way of buying care should be highly encouraged by the Kaiser Permanente examples and successes. Kaiser Permanente is functionally a prototype full service ACO -- with all of the essential ACO component parts -- and the model works well.

Because Kaiser Permanente is paid by the package and not by the piece, care in the KP care settings can be designed around the patients. That is also the goal of the new ACO's. Process engineering thinking at Kaiser Permanente doesn't have to be focused on protecting piecework cash flow and maintaining high volumes of billable events from a fee schedule create by someone else. That is also a major goal for the new ACO'S. Care at Kaiser Permanente is not limited to delivering pieces of care that are included on a specific list of fees that function to define the cash flow and determine the economic survival for most fee-based care sites in this country.

A major goal of the ACO's is not to be limited by that schedule of fees. So the successes at Kaiser Permanente should be encouraging both to the medical homes and to the ACO's that are described on the next chapter in this book. Both the Kaiser Permanente approach and the KP tool kits and data sets are relevant to these effects.

Eye Surgery Packages or Total Prepaid Care

Kaiser Permanente also has created high levels of electronic connectivity between its caregivers and with the KP patients. Care information is sent directly to patients over the internet. Electronically reported lab results and even electronic doctor visits are popular with patients in those care settings.

Over 13 million e-visits between doctors and patients happened electronically last year at Kaiser Permanente.[202] Patients loved them. Those e-visits don't happen in most piecework-based care settings in this country because the caregivers in those piecework settings need to see their patients face-to-face in order for the insurance companies or Medicare or Medicaid to pay them for their work. That is unfortunate. E-visits can transform some pieces of care. A prepaid system -- and a patient-centered medical home -- can do e-visits with no loss of revenue.

So millions of these visits happen now at Kaiser Permanente. Piecework care settings can't afford to do them. So very few of these visits happen in those other care settings.

Organizations that deliver packages of care for a fixed price have a much higher ability to bring the processes and skill sets of reengineering and all of the new connectivity tools and care support apps to bear in health care to improve outcomes and to reduce costs and prices.

Buying care by the package made a major difference for Lasik eye surgery and for heart transplants. It sets up an extremely new set up opportunities for caregivers who aspire to function in teams. The key will be to create cash flows that allow the caregivers to function in teams and thrive.

Someone Has To Change the Purchasing Model or It Will Not Change

How can care purchasing be done by the package far more often in our country than it is done today? And how can we create cash flow approaches that will encourage team care, care reengineering and patient-focused care approaches?

The truth is that changing the way we buy care will not happen spontaneously or serendipitously. It has to be intentional. Someone needs to make that market reality happen. Buying care by the package cannot happen until someone with real money buys care by the package.

The truth is that someone embedded at the key points in the total cash flow of health care in this country need to set up the mechanisms that can create those kinds of purchasing arrangements and those kinds of care delivery approaches or those mechanisms and those approaches will not happen. The fee-based caregivers of this country clearly will not spontaneously reorganize into entities that will begin to sell care in packages.

The current infrastructure of care that is now absorbing all of that money will not spontaneously do a better job of integrating care at the levels that are so badly needed by the patients who need integrated and coordinated care. The rest of health care has had 50 years to spontaneously evolve into being Kaiser Permanente or into being the functional equivalent at Kaiser Permanente. That evolution has not happened -- for a number of reasons. We can count the number of reasons. There are 2.8 trillion of them. The rest of health care generates $2.8 trillion in cash flow from the current way we buy care. The infrastructure of care that is absorbing all of that money and doing very well financially will not evolve on its own to deliver the kinds of care that were discussed in chapter two or even to creating care that is sold in packages rather than pieces.

A Spontaneous Integration Into Teams Will Not Happen

The cash flow model for care delivery in this country clearly can only be changed by one or more of the parties who are right now upstream in the actual flow of cash in this country. One or more of those parties needs to change the way they buy care. That is the topic and the agenda for the next chapter of this book. Who can actually change the cash flow for care? How should that cash flow be charged?

CHAPTER FIVE

SOMEONE NEEDS TO BE ACCOUNTABLE FOR IMPLEMENTING THE NEW BUSINESS MODEL FOR CARE OR IT WILL NOT HAPPEN

Cash flow is king. The last two chapters of this book have described how the cash flow we use to buy care sculpts the way care is delivered in this country.

If we really want to change the business model we use to buy care in this country. We need to change that flow of cash. To change the flow of cash, we need someone who generates some significant portion of that cash making real changes in the way we buy care. Real money needs to be involved. Changes in the business model we use for purchasing care in this country can and will only happen if those changes are made by someone who is functionally upstream now in the actual flow of cash that we use today to buy care.

So who actually is upstream in the flow of cash in this country today?

Who in the current massive flow of the $2.8 trillion dollars[203] that is used to buy care, has the sufficient leverage, motivation, capabilities, and functional abilities to actually make changes that can effectively rechannel enough of that cash flow to achieve any or all of the goals that we need to achieve to improve care?

We need to figure out who has the leverage to change the flow of cash and we need to have clear sense of how that flow can and should be changed. This chapter is intended to help answer both of the questions.

For starters, we obviously have four very clear sources for the money that is used to buy most of the care in this country today.

The Patients, the Employers, the Health Insurers and the Taxpayers Are the Key Sources of Cash

The four significant parties who are actually upstream in the flow of cash in this country today are: the patients, themselves, the employers -- who provide health coverage and health benefits to their employees, our health plans and health insurers, and the government.

Those are the four basic sources of the actual cash that is used to buy care in this country today. If we are going to change that flow of cash, and if we want to use any of that money to buy better and more affordable care, then we will need one or more of those upstream cash sources to make significant functional changes in the way they buy care.

How can that be done?

Who among those four sources of cash actually has the leverage, the expertise, the motivation and the tool kits that are needed to modify and enhance the way we buy care and -- in the process -- to change the business model of care delivery for at least some caregivers? It's a good idea to look at the strengths, weaknesses, and relative flexibility of each of the four sources of cash to figure out what might be our best strategy for using cash flow changes to achieve our care improvement goals.

Consumers Have Very Limited Leverage Today

Consumers cannot do that job. Caregivers are not going to be the cash flow change agents we need to transform either care or the business model we use to buy care.

It would be nice at several levels if the consumers of care in this country could be the change agents who improve the way we buy care. That is not at all likely to happen, however.

The truth is -- with the exception of some selective individual care purchasing decisions and some personal health-related behavioral decisions -- the individual patients in this country basically have no significant economic power and no relevant individual purchasing leverage that can be used to change the current business model of care.

The sad truth is -- at this point in time -- consumers have very little market power in health care.

Consumers have too little individual impact on provider business unit cash flow, and consumers have too little information about key issues related to care to function as either collective or individual agents of change. That is a shame. We clearly could benefit from involving consumers more in making informed choices about both caregivers and care. We definitely should put a business model in place that can allow meaningful consumer impacts on care delivery to happen to a much greater degree in the future.

If we set the new business model of care up well, the consumers in this country could ultimately have a rich array of informed choices. If we design the health care market model well, we could put in place a model where informed consumer decisions could, would, and should steer the actual delivery of care. But today, at this point in time, individual patients simply do not have enough individual purchasing power to either change the model of care delivery or to cause their caregivers to change the way they produce, provide, deliver and coordinate care.

Consumers can make a few meaningful choices today about both care and health today.

Consumers can and should actually make individual choices to become healthier. And -- in some market settings -- consumers can actually make some choices between competing health plans and between competing care systems.

In an increasing number of settings, consumers who have very high deductible health plans also have health insurers who are beginning to give the consumers information about the prices changed by each available provider for a given set of services.

When a consumer has a $2,000 deductible plan and has to pay for the first $2,000 in care each year, then the difference between two care sites that change very different fees for their office visits can be relevant to the consumer.

If one site charges $75 for a basic visit and another site charges $125 for that same visit, -- if the consumers have tools to know what those price differences are -- that knowledge can drive some choices, and it has the potential to create price competition for some areas of care that cost less than the deductible amount.

As noted earlier, once the deductible amount is paid, prices become irrelevant to the consumer. But as deductibles get higher -- moving from $500, as it did a few years ago to $2,000 or more in many care sites today -- that can make predeductible prices relevant to some consumers.

In some settings, consumers get to choose between competing health plans. That can be an important and highly influential choice.

The opportunity for consumers to make choices between competing care systems doesn't happen as often as it should in this country today -- but it does happen in some settings, and those consumers choices can improve local care when they happen and when consumers can make informed choices based on good and relevant data about the comparative performance of plans.

Medicare has set up a very robust set of choices with their Medicare Advantage plans. In any given market, consumers can choose between several plans. Prices vary and care service levels and quality vary. Medicare makes quality and service data available -- and consumer choices for those products do influence care delivery and local markets for care.

High levels of voluntary enrollment by seniors in Medicare Advantage plans sends a clear message from the consumers to even local care market and care infrastructure. Plan selection choices that are made by consumers can actually help to structure local markets for care. But individual consumer purchasing choices, by themselves, generally have no significant impact on either the cost of care or the quality of care as we have currently structured both the marketplace for care and the infrastructure of care.

Employers Have More Leverage -- Much of It Indirect

Employers obviously have significantly more clout than individual consumers. Employers channel a lot of cash to the purchase of care.

Employers who provide health coverage to their employees and their families are also very clearly and directly upstream in the cash flow for care in this country. A lot of money flows from that source of cash into purchasing care. As a consequence of that cash flow, many employers have more leverage over care delivery than the individual consumers have. Employers clearly can have collective influence over care delivery and some of the larger employers can have significant direct and individual leverage over both the delivery of care and the financing of care in some local care settings. But even larger employers still tend to be relatively small in volume as a percentage of the full set of patients who get care from any caregiver in any relevant market setting or local context. Individual leverage by even large employers over significant areas of care is hard to achieve. Individual employers -- like individual patients -- tend to have insufficient leverage to change the basic delivery of care in most settings.

Collective employer leverage over care delivery, however, does exist and collective employer leverage can have a significant and extremely important impact on the delivery of care.

Many employers, for example, use the current NCQA ratings of health plans as part of their specifications for selecting health plans. NCQA is the National Committee for Quality Assurance. The NCQA has created a formal systematic process that measures the quality of care and the level of service for health plans in this country, using about six dozen performance categories.[204] Employers can have a significant impact on the quality of care in their markets by insisting that the health plans they contract with for their employee coverage go through the NCQA reporting and accreditation processes.

That use of NCQA reports by employers actually does change the way care is delivered in this country. That requirement to use NCQA changes care because cash flow is involved for health plans based on the potential loss of revenue for plans that are not accredited. When employers use NCQA ratings as a purchasing factor as they are making their decisions about which health plans to use, then health plans who want to serve that employer as vendors and who want to get cash from that employer will do the work that is needed in areas of targeted quality improvement both to be NCQA-certified and to earn higher NCQA ratings. Care is significantly better in a number of areas in this country because of that indirect but cash flow-related employer influence on care delivery through that market process and though the health plans who have an impact on care.

Indirect Employer Influence Changed Immunization Rates for America

As one example of the impact that NCQA measurement can have on care delivery, before NCQA started measuring the childhood immunization rates for each of the health plans, immunization rates were a lot lower. NCQA required the use of that measurement, compared the results in performance between plans and then reported the differences in immunization rates between health plans to employers. When that measurement process started, this entire country had amazingly and embarrassingly low rates of immunizations. When NCQA started tracking and reporting immunization levels by health plans, every health plan that was evaluated by NCQA set up their own set of individual approaches to work with their contracted caregivers to increase the number of immunized children in their customer base.

The United States was far below almost every country in the world on immunizations when NCQA began to exert their leverage through health plans and their provider networks on that issue. The next chart shows the progress that has happened in immunizations in this country over the past decades, since the NCQA measurement of that particular procedure was introduced.

Figure 5.1

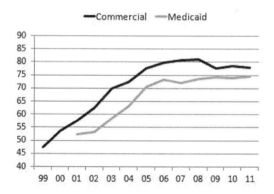

NCQA Childhood Immunization Status

SOURCE: National Committee for Quality Assurance (NCQA), The State of Health Care Quality 2012, Childhood Immunization Combination 2 for Commercial and Medicaid HMO

When NCQA started measuring the rate of immunizations, barely half of the kids in this country were immunized. Health plans made that particular area of care delivery a priority and now the numbers for those plans are closer to 80 percent. That is a major improvement -- created in part because the employers exerted collective influence on care delivery by tying their own cash flow to NCQA certification requirements. Similar results have happened for several other NCQA measurement areas -- including blood pressure control, diabetes care follow-up, and follow-up for mental health care. Those are all areas where care for the entire country has gotten better over time because health plans have been focused on those directions by the NCQA measurement process.

So, even though it is clearly hard for any single employer to directly influence any individual performance area for care delivery -- like changing the immunization rates for children in any specific geographic setting -- employers can collectively influence the quality of care and the overall immunization rates by using NCQA and their certification processes as a tool to make those measurements relevant to the cash flow realities of health plans.

Employers have also bonded together to create an organization called the Leapfrog Group that has created safety measurements for hospitals. The Leapfrog Group measures results and has publicized differences in those safety and performance levels between hospitals. The Leapfrog Group has done some very good and informative work. The influence of that process on all relevant hospitals has been somewhat less effective than the NCQA impact on health plans primarily because most of the buyers who are involved in the Leapfrog effort have not directly connected the hospital performance variations to hospital cash flow by only using hospitals with good Leapfrog safety ratings. The hospital safety reports are informative and useful -- and many hospitals are improving their safety levels because of the Leapfrog measurements and safety advocacy -- but the standards have not had a direct business impact on the actual cash flow of hospitals.

Employers Can Have Major Influence on Providers Through Health Plans, However

It is difficult for employers to have a direct impact on care delivery, but employers can have a very powerful indirect impact on care delivery through the health plans they use to either insure the care for their employees or to administer the health coverage for their employees.

Employers hire plans to run their employee health benefits.

Health plans are businesses. Cash flow is also king for the health plans. Health plans very much want cash flow from employers. So health plans tend to pay very close attention to their customer base -- and employers are usually the bulk of the health care insurer customer base for any health plan.

Health insurers sell services to employers. Health insurers survive if they have customers. Plans who want to keep their customers tend to listen to their customers...particularly their large customers. So employers can change the cash flow for care by literally changing the health plan they use as a channel for their cash. They can also influence care by mandating that the plans they hire to administer or insure their coverage deliver a care product that meets care delivery specifications created by the employer. That set of levers -- focused on specifications about care delivery -- can be fairly effectively used by employers to influence care through the health plans they hire.

If buyers tell their health plans for example, that they want the plans to support and institute the care improvement reforms that are described in this book, that insistence on that support for those care improvements can have massive impact on the priorities and the actions of their health plan vendors. In other words, employers can often significantly extend and increase their own leverage and their own influence over the actual provision of care through their health plan vendors by getting their health plans to do particular things in ways that subsequently influence provider behavior in the community. Employers who use their leverage through the health plans skillfully can have more indirect impact on care delivery than direct impact, and that subsequent indirect impact can be -- in some cases -- both powerful and significant.

Well Leveraged Employers Can Insist That Their Vendor Achieve Those Reforms

As one easy and clear example, employers can insist that the health plans they hire work with patient-centered medical homes. Employers can also insist that their contracted health plans work effectively with appropriate palliative care programs. Employers can easily insist that health plans provide data to individual patients about the heart surgery mortality rates of the hospitals that the health plans use. If buyers insist on that data about death rates being provided, plans can make it available. Employers can insist that the health plans they hire should give their employers access to either a full and complete electronic medical record or to some form of electronic patient profile support tool that provides care support data to caregivers. Plans can use their claims data-bases and their own systems expertise to support that work when full EMRs are not available at the care sites.

Plans will do all that work and will create those data flows to support care if the employers demand that work be done by the plans and by their contracted caregivers.

At a very basic level, buyers can insist that plans report important data about care, and buyers can require health plans to make key pieces of information available to patients. The plans who want to be the vendors for the employers will gener-ally be influenced in significant ways by those buyer demands and buyer specifications. If they are well written, the influence of those buyer specifications will spill over very effectively to the actual delivery of care.

Buyers Have More Leverage Than They Know

Buyers today actually can have a lot more leverage on care delivery in that indirect way than they usually appreciate. That wasn't always true -- but it is true now. The tools exist to do that work now -- and they will be used if buyers insist that they be used. Purchasing of health care and coverage doesn't need to be a passive process for employers. Purchasing of care also does not need to be passive and inert process for our government agencies relative to care improvement requirements. Buyers and the consultants they hire to help them manage both their self-insurance vendors and their insured health plan vendors can build specifications for health plans that specify and insist on better performance in important areas like team care. If buyers insist that the health plans they hire must support team care, the odds are very good that team care will be supported.

Most Health Plans Will Welcome the New Specifications

The time is perfect to do that work.

The truth is -- many health plans and many health insurers in today's health coverage marketplace will welcome a set of requests from their key buyers to have a more effective impact on care delivery. The value of doing that work is becoming increasingly clear to everyone in the health care financing business. In today's world -- at this point in the history of both care delivery and health care financing -- many health insurers are already highly likely to be competing in those areas, and many health plans are working hard on very ambitious care improvement agendas and tool kits today. A great many plans already are intending to build care improvement approaches -- very often in partnership with various aligned caregivers. In many cases, the better and more enlightened health plans have already decided that team care, coordinated care, and even more accountable care should be a key part of their portfolio of benefits and services. Many of those insurers are working hard now to create effective programs and services in those areas and many insurers see the clear value of doing that work in partnership with mutually supportive caregivers. Some of those approaches to align health plans with caregivers to create better coordinated and more accountable care are discussed in more detail later in this chapter. They are clearly a step in the right direction for better, more affordable and more accountable care.

Self-Insured Employers Can Also Use Their Influence Relative to Health Plan Performance

So employers have a hard time directly changing care -- but employer can clearly do their part by becoming better buyers of services from the plans they utilize. That is true whether the employer buys insurance from their health plans or whether the employer is self-insured and buys basically an array of administrative services from their health plan vendors.

Those data-supported team care agendas need to be applied to patient care for both insured and self-insured employer groups. The fact is most major employers in this country are now self-insured. Those self-insured employers directly absorb the costs of care rather than paying a premium and then having an insurer absorb those costs. That self-insurance status for employers doesn't change the employer's ability or need to use health plans as a useful leverage tool to improve care. Almost every single self-insured employer currently hires a health plan vendor -- usually under a very clearly defined contract -- to administer their self-insurance plan. Those health plans who administer self-insurance for those employers also usually sell their own insured products to other buyers. Those plans and typically have a broad array of contracted provider relationships that serve a broad cus-tomer base that includes insured and self-insured employers.

So intelligent purchasing by both insured and self-insured buy-ers to change the delivery of care -- primarily using the leverage they exert through health plans -- is not only possible -- it is desirable.

This book has outlined several ways that care delivery should change to make care better. Buyer specifications can make those care delivery enhancements real for their health plan vendors.

Buyer Specifications Should Be Used More Effectively as a Tool

Specifications are a key tool to achieve those goals.

Buyers can use their own purchasing specifications to simply and directly require their health plan vendors to use care networks that include care teams, medical homes, care registries, electronic medical libraries and the functionality of electronic medical records. Most businesses that buy other supplies or and other services from a wide array of vendors already use and impose detailed purchas-ing specifications in their relationship with those other vendors. Health care coverage and delivery purchasing that has been done by businesses, by contrast, has been almost specification fee.

Specifications Can Strengthen Care Purchasing

That can easily change. It should change. Buyers should begin to specify a few key points -- like team care and safety report-ing -- for their health plan vendors. When buyers set standards and create specifications for those particular performance issues, plans tend to respond well. Plans then need to do the work to be in alignment with those purchasing specifications.

So when you look at the four sources of cash that we use to buy care in this country, it is clear those consumers actually have relatively little leverage relative to using their purchasing power to change the infrastructure of care. But buyers can and do have some leverage...and buyer leverage at this point in time tends to be most effective when it is channeled through the health plans that buyers use as vendors for their health coverage benefits.

We Need To Optimize the Value of Health Plans

That realization points us very directly to the third source of cash for health care in this country -- the health plan or health insurer.

We clearly need to use health plans as functional change agents and cash flow modifiers. Health plans are the third source of cash used to buy health care listed at the beginning of this chapter. The government is the largest single source of cash that is used to buy care, but health plans clearly have the second highest cash flow volume. Plans may have a more immediate and effective cash flow leverage in the country relative to the cash flow of care. Health plans clearly have the most flexibility relative to cash flow. The opportunities to have an impact are becoming increasingly clear and many health plans are now building the needed tool kits and provider relationships they can use to change their individual cash flow for the purchase of care.

Health Plans Have the Second Most Powerful Impact on the Flow of Cash Used To Buy Care

Health plans cover a lot of people in this country. That number of covered people is projected to grow as we roll out the next stages of this country's health care reform agenda. Health plans today channel a lot of cash to caregivers in this country. Those massive health plan steams of cash create their own obvious, high-leverage opportunities for the plans to have an impact on the delivery of care. In fact, health plans in this country not only have the opportunity to have an impact on the delivery of care –- American health plans should have an obligation to have a significant impact on making care better and more affordable.

Sixty to seventy percent of the people who will have health care coverage in America will have coverage that is either insured by private health plans or administered by private health plans.[205] That doesn't count the major role that some health plans now play as the intermediary administrators who do the key administrative work and functions for the Medicare program.

Health Insurers Should Be Held Accountable For Using That Cash Flow Well

A key point of this book is that we will need the health plans of this country to do some well-structured and highly effective heavy lifting if we want to restructure the cash flow for care and make care both more affordable and better. The opportunity for the plans is huge. Health insurers channel massive -- even staggering -- amounts of money to providers of care. We need to use that fact of economic life to make care better. Health insurers ought to add real value to care delivery in multiple ways.

We need to start with affordability. Being affordable is actually one of the key ways for health plans to add value. The entire next chapter of this book is about health plan and premium affordability. The basic whole approach that we are now using as a country calls for us to use our health plans to provide coverage to two-thirds of Americans. That strategy will fail if the coverage offered by our American health plans isn't affordable.

How can plans be affordable?

Being Affordable Needs To Be a Top Priority

Since health care premium is very directly and purely arithmetically based on the average cost of care for insured people, insurers clearly need to do smart things to bring down the average cost of care for the people they insure. The logic of that need for insurers to effectively bring down the cost of coverage is painfully clear. This whole pathway to universal coverage will fail for us as a country if premium is, in the end, unaffordable.

One of the ways insurers can add value and bring down the average cost of care for the people they insure is to use their volume purchasing power to get better prices for each piece of care they buy. When we pay for care by the piece, bringing down the price of each piece of care is a basic, fundamental, almost logistically crude tool that needs to be used more effectively. The price chapter of this book was very clear about how the pricing model we use now to buy units of care works today in this country. The comparative price charts are pretty clear. We have the highest unit prices for care in the world. We also have -- by a huge margin -- the widest range of unit prices of any country in the world. The charts in Chapter Three show the price differences between us and the rest of the world. One of those charts is shown below to make the point that we pay more for each piece of care than all other countries, and there is a very wide range of prices being paid in the U.S. for each service. The premiums that are charged by each insurer in this country are now based -- by law -- on the average cost of care for the people who are insured by each insurer. Prices paid by each insurer for each piece of care obviously create the average cost of care and the premium -- for each insurer.

The arithmetic is clear. Lower prices result in lower premiums. Plans who fail to do their price-negotiating work well will basically fail their customers. Price negotiations need to be a key skill of health plans. Plans need to very effectively negotiate prices for all pieces of care. If all health plans simply paid the full retail prices that are listed by care sites for care in this country, that level of payment to providers of care at full retail prices would create extremely high premium levels, as Chapter Three also pointed out fairly clearly.

The next chart shows the prices paid for an appendectomy. The chart shows the amount paid in other countries, the price range in the U.S., and the amount paid for that procedure by both Medicare and Medicaid in this country. We clearly pay a lot more in the U.S.

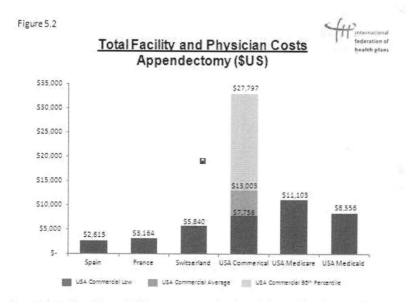

Figure 5.2

As the chapter on prices pointed out, the prices that are paid by consumers who don't have health plans or the government negotiating fees on their behalf are not even on this chart. They are much higher than the $27,797 number. Those charts do not include the pure "chargemaster" prices that are charged by many health care providers to people who don't have insurance of any kind. Those "chargemaster" prices are sometimes so high as to be cruel.

Health insurers obviously need to do a very effective job of negotiating provider prices on behalf of their customers in order to keep their premiums affordable. Being able to negotiate lower prices with caregivers on behalf of plan members creates a stunningly direct and very immediate benefit relative to premium affordability. A health plan that gets a 50 percent discount on all retail prices paid for all pieces of care would have a premium level that is literally half of the premium that would be charged to those same customers by a plan that pays the full retail prices for each piece of care. A fifty percent discount cuts the premium in half. People who buy health insurance in this country would obviously prefer the lower premium level. Plans clearly need to negotiate low prices in order to have lower premiums levels.

Price Negotiations Are Not Popular With Providers of Care

Those unit-priced negotiations that are done by the health plans with providers are not particularly popular with the actual providers of care in many cases. Some care sites, in fact, bitterly protest the price negotiation process. The fairly consistent pattern has been that a number of caregivers will complain with some passion to their patients about the price negotiations that happen with health insurers. The providers of who are complaining to the patients tend not to mention that the prices they charge actually create the health insurer's premiums. In any case, when you look at the price levels shown on those charts, it's pretty clear why those price negotiations are needed by the health plans. It is equally clear why skillful price negotiations by plans directly benefit the people who actually have to pay the premium.

So the absolute first truth to look at relative to health plans and their cash flow impact is that negotiated provider prices clearly bring down premium levels.

We need affordable premiums if we are going to cover most of the people of this country using the tool of private insurance to pay for people's care.

We Also Need To Change the Way We Buy Care

Discounts are not enough.

Simply negotiating lower fees for various pieces of care will not be enough to make premiums better and more affordable. We have been doing those negotiations for years and prices are what they are. We now need a better way of buying care. Lower fees that are negotiated in the context of a piecework business model still leave us buying care by the piece. The last chapter pointed out many of the flaws, the dysfunctional outcomes, and the sub-optimal consequences that far too often result from buying care by the piece. The last chapter also pointed out the savings, the care improvements and the care safety enhancements that can happen when plans and consumers buy care well by the package. The data on both points is clear. Health plans clearly need to have a positive impact on that cash flow issue. The piecework model of buying care is badly flawed.

Like the eye surgery and the heart transplant examples in the last chapter, we need the health plans in this country to be really good at buying packages of carefully defined care from care providers in order to bring total costs down and improve quality and outcomes for those aspects of care. This is important work. It needs to happen. It will not happen on its own.

Buying care by the package will not happen until someone who is part of the cash flow for buying care makes it happen. Who can do that work? The truth is that only the health plans and the key government agencies currently flow enough cash to make a better purchasing model happen.

If health plans -- or the government -- do not make a real and relevant conversion of money to that package purchase of care cash flow model, there is no other element of the care delivery infrastructure of economy that really has the flexibility, the cash flow volume, or even the motivation to use that set of tools to accomplish those goals. We can give all of the speeches we want about buying care by the package and not by the piece -- but if the insurers and the government programs who channel most cash to care don't actually start buying more care by the package, than that purchasing tool will not have much traction and it will not be a factor in the real world of care delivery.

Ideally, a modified cash flow from the private health insurers to buy care more effectively can be set up in harmony with similar agendas being set up by Medicare and Medicaid to optimize the total impact of those purchasing agendas. The next two chapters deal with those issues. In any case, the health plans should now accept the accountability for doing major portions of the work that is needed to create the new business model for care, and people who do policy thinking should be figuring out how best to use health plans to do that work.

Health Plans Need To Support Caregivers Who Want To Set Up Accountable Approaches

So what can and should health plans actually do at this point in our history to make care better and more affordable other than just negotiate lower prices with providers of care?

There are several important things that plans can do. We need to look at the role that plans actually play as a pure function of being really plans. Plans tend to be a major connector between the patient and the infrastructure of care. Plans are natural, functional, in place, fully operational conduits for both cash and data. Plans should improve their role as a channeller of cash and as a channeller of data -- setting up data flow approaches that can improve consumer choices about both care delivery and about providers of care, and they provide data to caregivers that can help them improve care. Health plans can and should tee up and enable a much more robust consumer choice agenda.

As noted earlier, that set of data-related plan functions should be included in the buyer specifications that are used by buyers to select and manage their health plans. Health plans should be required by the buyers to help facilitate choices by patients. Each plan can come up with creative ways of doing that work. Buyers should require that work to be done.

That's not the only business model element we can and should change through health plans in their role as a conduit for cash. Safety and adverse outcomes should also become much more relevant to the way we buy care. No other industry creates a cash reward for vendor screw-ups and no other industry has vendors who make more money when their customers are damaged. That is a very strange business model. It is entirely unique to health care. It should be fixed. It can be fixed. Health plans need to achieve that fix.

Cash flow needs to be channeled away from rewarding mistakes, errors, and inept care.

Health plans clearly very much need to change both their benefits and their payment rules to stop rewarding care delivery screw-ups. Patients with pressure ulcers should not be a source of both revenue and profit for the care sites where those ulcers were created. Having multiple patients with pressure ulcers should result in some kind of financial penalty for the care site and care team -- not a financial reward.

Changing the payment model to address those issues can be done. Simply not paying any additional money for hospital acquired infections is one very simple benefit change that can be implemented by health plans as a better way of buying care.

Medicare has begun to make those kinds of payment decisions about hospital infections, and that is a very good and responsible thing for Medicare to do.

Another very reasonable change in the business model is to say that if a hospital patient has sepsis, the hospital will not be paid additional money for the care of that patient unless the hospital has a formal and functional sepsis response process in place. We can't blame hospitals for patients getting sepsis. Many sepsis patients get that disease in nursing homes or even in their own homes. The payment model for sepsis shouldn't penalize hospitals for simply having patients with sepsis. The payment model should, however, penalize hospitals who don't have a fully organized care team response in place for patients with sepsis.

Sepsis is the number one cause of death in American hospitals.[206] Those care teams can cut the death rate for the number one cause of death in American hospitals in half -- and the right care done quickly can also result in half as many of the surviving sepsis patients from suffering lifetime damage and pain from that disease.

Similarly -- for pressure ulcers -- as noted several times in this book, some hospitals have nearly 10 percent of their patients with those ulcers.[207] The national average is now 7 percent.[208] Each of those ulcers generates an average of $40,000 in hospital revenue for non-Medicare patients.[209] As was also noted earlier in this book, the very best hospital systems have less than 1 percent of their patients with those ulcers.[210] Some very high performing hospitals have not had a single pressure ulcer in years. Not entirely coincidently, as the prior chapter pointed out, the American hospitals that have had zero ulcers success levels have been hospital care sites that have been prepaid for a complete package of hospital care. There is no additional revenue in those prepaid hospitals for any patients if a pressure ulcer happens and needs to be treated.

In other hospitals that are paid entirely by the piece, those same ulcers can generate a lot of revenue. Health plans and buyers can change that payment model. Our payment model for buying hospital care should reflect the need to reduce the number of those ulcers and not pay more when ulcers happen. Simply setting up payment standards that cap payment in some way for hospitals if more than 5 percent of the hospital's patients have those ulcers would give every hospital in America the needed incentive to put processes in place to make care a lot better for those patients. All patients in those care sites would benefit from the quality gains that would result from better processes for those patients. Better care is definitely possible -- and the cash flow we use to buy care needs to be channeled by the health plans to selectively create better care in targeted areas for patients.

Health plans and the cash flow they channel need to be in the heart of the solution set for those issues.

In each of those cases, at a bare minimum, health plans can and should stop rewarding care misfires with rich streams of cash.

Health Plans Can Enrich the Flow of Data

We also clearly need data to make care better. Health plans can also obviously play a key role in bringing better data into existence. Data support should be another key function we expect health plans to play. Health plans need to create and utilize data flows that support the delivery of care.

Health plan and health insurer databases tend to have a lot of care-related data in them now. Health plans have that care-related data now because all providers need to file claims with each insurer in order to be paid for their care. The claims that are filed with the insurer today describe each patient's diagnosis. The claims also are required to specifically list each of the care procedures that were done for each patient in order for providers of care to have their claims paid for that patient. Because that payment process and that data flow exist, health insurer claims databases actually have rich veins of care based data in them now.

That rich set of data is not usually used in any way to improve care. Health plans should be using that data to help caregivers deliver and improve care.

Helping caregivers provide better care should be a major priority for health plans at this point in our history. Some health plans are already tightly allied with care systems. The health plans that are also care systems having great success in both care quality and care costs. We now need to extend that care improvement and data sharing work well past those few fully integrated systems to create similar services and similar data support tools for a broad array of consumers and health plans.

Plans Should Now Help Providers Sell Care by the Package

The most useful and most immediate way that health plans can help to improve care at this point is probably for the plans -- as payers and administers -- to create cash flow options and approaches that support the caregivers who want to set up team care, data-based care, continuously improving care, and to support the care sites who want to deliver packages of care.

Start With Team Care

We need to begin with a very practical and functionality-focused look at the opportunities we have in front of us.

The biggest opportunity we have for making care better and more affordable is to focus on the patients who have chronic care needs.

As this book has noted a couple of times, those patients who have chronic conditions currently drive more than 75 percent of the costs of care.[211] Health insurers should be required by their buyer customers to recognize the obvious need for team care for all of the patients in this country who have those chronic conditions. There should be a particular focus on patients with chronic conditions and comorbidities. We should expect our health plans and our health insurers to work with the infrastructure of care delivery in America to create, support, and build team care in various approaches that can make care better and more affordable for those patients.

Health plans need to be more effective channellers of their vast flow of cash relative to team care. Insurers should be paying providers to set up care linkages and insurers should be paying providers for team care infrastructure support. The current payment approach penalizes providers who stray from the current rigid and inadequate list of approved services that are included and defined on the standard piecework fee schedules that insurance company claims examiners administer today. We should demand that our health plans face up to that task of creating and supporting team care and should modify the way they pay providers in ways that cause team care to happen.

In exchange for the right and privilege of being a licensed health plan in America, health insurers should support needed levels of care improvement data flow and continuous improvement work done for health care and should help create and support accountable care by creating cash flow approaches that fund and reward accountable care.

Plans Need To Work in Collaboration With Caregivers

Selling care only by the piece should end.

To achieve that top-priority goal of continuously improving fully accountable care, health plans should set up various kinds of purchasing arrangements with various caregivers that allow the caregivers to sell care by the package -- with full transparency relative to the quality and the outcomes of the care that results from that approach.

This is clearly an area where employers can be a major catalyst for change. Buyers should insist that the vendor health plans they hire do this work and buyers should define those requirements clearly in their purchasing specifications. Experts exist who can help the buyers build those specifications.

If buyers very clearly have plans to create care teams and if buyers require health plans to use their benefit design capabilities to channel patients to the care teams that functionally can coordinate care, most health plans can now do that work and many will also do it quickly and very well.

A few years ago, those kinds of requests by buyers for more aligned caregiving relationship and levels of team care by their health plans would have been much harder to achieve than they are today. Most health plans could not do that work a few years ago. A decade ago, most care business sites also resisted any threat at any level to their piecework payment cash flow approach. As recently as three years ago, the provider business unit resistance to any change of cash flow in those areas was significant. Today, however, many providers of care are ready and even eager to do that work of changing the way they sell and deliver care.

Care Providers Are Seeking Ways of Aligning To Improve Care

Hospitals, medical groups, community caregivers, and even pharmacy chains are all now recognizing that our current piecework-centered business model is too flawed to get us the optimal results we want for both quality and affordability.

Care delivery is changing. Some of the boundaries between insurers and caregivers are blurring, blending and co-mingling in interesting ways. Caregivers are now beginning to understand that the next generation of care delivery should be more patient-focused and better coordinated. Insurers are beginning to understand that simply being passive conduits for cash is not going to be a successful business model for the next generation of health plan competition. The care delivery goals and vision that was outlined in chapter two of this book are being embraced by a growing number of caregivers and care business units as well as by a growing number of health plans. Hospitals are working to figure out ways of becoming more aligned and better integrated with the physicians who give them patients. Physicians in many settings are looking for linkages that can help create continuously improving care for their patients. Health plans and health insurers can and should build on that new intent, that new interest, and that growing provider momentum...and that new set of priorities should enable the cash flow that is now channeled by the insurers to function as a key tool in core patient-focused care alignments and realignment processes.

New Levels of Alliances and Collaboration Will Be Useful

Some very creative work is being done. At one end of the collaboration continuum, some health care insurers are now buying actual care delivery organizations. Some very traditional, financially-focused health plans are becoming both health insurers and direct providers of care.

At the same time, some of the larger health care delivery organizations are beginning to create the functionality of health plans and some are looking to get insurance licenses to compete with the traditional health plan entities. At both ends of that collaboration continuum, organizations are being created that look in many respects like the classic Kaiser Permanente, Health Partners, or Group Health Plans -- with the goal being to build integrated care delivery and care financing models.

Buying care sites is one possible way for insurers to link tightly with care delivery and to enhance collaboration with the provision of care. Those health insurers simply become caregivers as well as insurers. Likewise, forming insurance companies is a very direct way for large caregivers to gain the full advantage of the entire upstream flow of cash from the buyers and government programs. Those care sites simply become insurers and they then collect premiums instead of fees. It can be extremely liberating for those care sites when there is enough cash flow to fund more innovative ways of defining and delivering care.

Both of those approaches create new challenges. Both approaches can be a very difficult way to succeed unless the entity can acquire an adequate, upfront volume of patients. But both approaches can be done and some organizations are going down those new integrated roads today.

Contractual Alliances Can Create Virtual Integration

Another way of moving in that same direction to achieve new and improved levels of collaboration between health plans and caregivers is to create direct contractual alliances. Contracts are much easier to do than acquisitions or mergers. It's a lot easier to contract with a hospital than it is to buy or build a hospital. Very creative organizations are developing a whole range of very interesting new contractual arrangements between health insurers and providers of care. Pioneering work is going on. This is a time for creativity and learning in many sites for both health care delivery and care financing. There are several versions of those kinds of aligned strategies now being put in place in multiple settings across the country. Health insurers in multiple areas are working with care delivery business units -- often with major hospitals or with hospital systems and their aligned medical providers -- to create a variety of contractual relationships that will allow the caregivers to benefit financially by taking account-ability for key aspects of care.

Those same approaches will allow the insurers who are part of the new collaborative effort to have lower premiums because the average costs of care will be lower for the insured people who get their care from those more efficient, process-enhanced, team-focused care delivery models.

The Federal government has included provisions in the Affordable Care Act for care sites to set up new organizations to do exactly that work for Medicare patients. The new organi-zations are called ACOs -- or Accountable Care Organizations. The intent of the law is to help set up a new set of contracting caregivers that will be able to achieve many of the same coor-dinated and cash flow rechanneling functions for Medicare patients as the old Group Health, Health Partners and Kaiser Permanente fully-aligned care and financing approaches have achieved.

Some Providers Want To Be Accountable Care Organizations (ACOs)

"ACO" is actually a very popular and frequently used name and label in health care circles right now. The use of the phrase and the concept now extends well beyond the Medicare -focused ACOs that were initially teed up by the new law.

There are an amazing number of current efforts to create aligned care teams in multiple settings for private insurers as well. Many of the new collaborative provider organizations that are being built in the private insurance market are also being labeled ACOs or Accountable Care Organizations. At this point in time, the ACO term is being used to describe a wide range of pro-vider-anchored and provider-centered alliances, collaborations, and organizational models that intend to sell packages of care to health insurers and the government. That alignment agenda is a step in the right direction. The basic underlying concepts of the ACO agenda have real value and are very directionally correct. Each of the three words in that label has significant significance, and each is worth a brief discussion.

Accountable -- Care -- Organizations

The term "organization" in ACO indicates that the care will be organized and not just will not be the haphazard piecework, unconnected, and unlinked approaches to care delivery that have been our norm now for this country for a very long time. Organization implies functioning in an organized way -- rather than just creating isolated incidents of care delivery.

"Accountable," as a term, implies a sense of purpose, responsibility, and -- yes -- accountability that also goes beyond just treating isolated incidents of care as isolated instances of care. Accountable for the full care needs of an entire patient is a concept that is new to most of health care -- because most care delivery in this country is incident-focused and not "accountable" for the entire care needs of a patient. That -- accountability -- for an entire patient obviously creates a whole new way of thinking about patient needs and pieces of care.

The third basic term, "Care," is an indication that the primary function of an ACO is to deliver care and not just to provide insurance or coverage. ACOs are not intended to be simply care financing tools. ACOs are intended to focus on actual care -- using an organizational approach to delivery that care that involves being accountable for the entire process and for the results of care for each patient.

ACO means, in other words, an organization focused on care delivery in an accountable way. That is clearly a good thing to achieve and a great aspiration to have.

Many Care Sites Aspire To Be ACOs

Most major care sites in America are currently thinking about how they can each succeed in an ACO-relevant world.

Health care entities all over America are building a general sense and greater understanding at this point relative to the kinds of team-based care delivery approaches that they can set up, design, or create to deliver care in an organized and accountable way for population of patients. The ACO thinking is very much a learning process for those care organizations. It is also a discovery process. The exact nature of the alliances, alignments, and functional processes that will create a new generation of aligned care approaches is in a state of exploration, flexibility, creativity, and learning. That is a good thing. We don't have the final solution for ACO functionality or success yet. We are inventing the best solutions in multiple settings. There are many variations on the ACO model in this country today, and we can learn from each of those variations.

As noted above, Medicare began the process by creating its own very definite set of initial ACO regulations for one version of the ACO approach.

That set of specifications for Medicare ACOs was derived directly from the Affordable Care Act law. The learning process about ACOs was at an early stage when the law was written, so those initial specifications are not perfect. The initial Medicare ACO work needs to be enhanced, as we learn more about how to build and use ACOs.

The good news is that there are now very flexible ways of building even Medicare ACOs because the ACA law gave Medicare the ability to do some experimentation. Medicare is using that ability to learn to be somewhat flexible, at this point, relative to ACO pilot program design.

The full Medicare ACO rollout process also now includes the design and creation of what Medicare calls "pioneer ACOs." The new pioneering ACOs are encouraged and allowed by Medicare to use variations on ACO approaches for care delivery and care funding that varies from the defined model that was embodied in the initial Medicare ACO regulation set. Some of those plans are doing interesting and worthwhile work and could become models for this country.

As noted earlier, Kaiser Permanente already functions as an ACO -- Accountable, Organized, and grounded on the delivery of care. That model works well, and it anchors one end of the ACO continuum -- an ACO on steroids. That model will not be the one that is used in a number of settings because it is not easy to achieve that level of full integration everywhere.

Some of the new ACOs will look like Kaiser Permanente clones, but many will use other ways of creating both organization and aligned accountability.

ACOs Are Intended To Create Team Care

Some of the best new ACO designs, at this point, will probably not be the ones designed by Medicare. Many of the best ACO designs will probably be the ones that are being put together by private health plans and by various alliances of motivated and organized caregivers. In all of the public and private care settings, and in all of the financial variations, the new ACOs are being formed to create a kind of integrated provider team that can focus on -- and be accountable for -- the care needs of a defined population of patients. The new generation of ACOs actually have a variety of owners, funders, and coordinators.

Cash flow will be key. Access to data will be essential.

At this point in the ACO process, it appears that the ACO models that will be most likely to succeed over time will probably be the ones who are linked most effectively to an existing payer -- to Medicare, Medicaid, or to a private insurer -- who has the tools, patient volume, data tools, motivation, and the real and existing cash flow that is needed to make the approach successful.

Most of the ACOs that have been designed up to now typically have hospitals at their core -- or they at least have hospitals as a key partner. The first generations of ACOs also tend to include a full array of aligned physicians -- with primary care physicians usually at the core of the care team. That primary care based model is fundamentally sound. In many ways, moving to a care delivery model that is built around team care and anchored by primary care has some obvious merit relative to making care both better and more affordable.

Medical Homes Also Create Team-Based Care

ACOs are getting most of the publicity right now, but another extremely important care delivery enhancement approach that may actually have a bigger impact more quickly for more patients than the ACO agenda is the creation in many care settings of patient-centered "medical homes." America obviously needs better team care. This book has made that point multiple times. Patient-centered medical homes are an approach to team care that can create a direct care team for each patient. The medical home approach almost always has primary care at its core, and it generally is supported with systems that provide basic care delivery information about each patient to each care team.

That very practical patient-focused approach has been proven to work really well in many care settings.

There are about 400 ACOs that are either being formed or that are already operational as this book is being written.[212] There are now more than 10,000 care sites that are currently functioning and being paid with real cash to be patient-centered medical homes.

Medical homes are growing so rapidly in so many places in this country because they are relatively easy to set up and they fill a huge gap in the usual splintered and unconnected approach to care delivery in this country. Many health insurers and health plans love medical homes because they are a relatively easy and fairly quick way for the health insurer to positively impact care... particularly for patients with chronic conditions.

Medical homes aren't, of course, actually homes. Medical homes are team care models that are set up to create coordinated care for individual patients in a very local and focused setting. By contrast, the full scale ACOs that are being created in most settings tend to be larger, more complex organizations that can involve multiple levels and multiple layers of caregivers. Medical homes are usually much less complicated. They tend to be a very local, nicely-focused, primary care-anchored team care approaches that are usually set up to create and deliver patient-focused care in a very local context. Remember the data cited earlier about most health care costs in this country coming from patients with chronic conditions and comorbidities. More than 75 percent of the care costs come from patients with comorbidities.[213] We usually do a very poor job in this country coordinating and linking care for our chronic care patients and we do an even worse job when the patients have more than one medical condition. Medical homes are intended to help solve that problem.

The best medical homes are set up with the tools needed to provide a set of linked and coordinated services to the people who elect to use them as patients. Those tools are intended to give each patient who needs team care a care team.

Most medical homes are anchored in primary care physician practices. In essence, medical homes tend to be small teams of caregivers with primary care physicians at their core. The teams generally use nurses, therapists and other related health care professionals to deliver a full package of care. The more successful medical homes have already shown that they can improve care, and many have shown that they can also bring down the total cost of care in the process. They bring down the cost of care because the medical home patients tend to have fewer care crises and they generally have significantly lower needs for inpatient hospitalizations.

Medical home patients who get primary care-focused team care also need emergency rooms less often. The best medical homes are resulting in a major reduction in needed hospital admissions for their patients.[214] Private insurers and Medicare and Medicaid programs that pay for hospital care all love having fewer hospital admissions. In various settings, each of those payers has encouraged and supported a whole array of new medical homes to exist and function in various ways. Money is a key success factor.

The primary key ingredient and functional encouragement factor that enables and supports the creation of those medical homes is -- very simply – cash flow. Cash is king. Payers who support medical homes need to create the cash flow that medical homes can use for their full set of care coordination and care-linking activities. The homes exist and succeed because that real world cash flow exists. Because the cash flow exists in those care settings to actually support team care, team care actually happens in those settings. As always, we get what we pay for.

Both ACOs and Patient-Centered Medical Homes Can Improve Care

Why do we believe that medical homes and ACOs might have a positive impact on the cost and quality of care? Both approaches are new for most segments of this county's health care delivery infrastructure, but the basic approach they are both trying to achieve relative to delivering coordinated, data-rich, patient-focused team-based care had been tested, modeled, and proven to work in integrated settings like Kaiser Permanente HealthPartners, and Group Health Plan of Seattle for many years.

Kaiser Permanente, Health Partners and Group Health of Puget Sound, among other similarly organized care sites, have all been leaders in reducing diabetic care complications, asthma attacks, congestive heart failure crises, and the need for emergency room use for quite a few years. Those organizations have very robust sets of tools in place to deliver patient-focused team care, and those care teams have proven over time that patient-focused team care actually works.

Other care sites in this country who have sold care entirely by the piece have not had those same tools to coordinate care. The sad fact is that most other care sites have not had collaborative payers who were willing to pay for coordinated, patient-focused team-based care. But that basic cash flow reality is changing. Many other payers are now willing and even eager to buy coordinated, proactive, team based care. The existence of that new cash flow is causing medical homes to be a growing and highly relevant point of care delivery…because the medical homes have the tools to make care better in those key areas of performance.

Both ACOs and medical homes represent a significant modification in the usual business model for care that health plans need to support. The role of the health plan or government payer as a source of cash is essential to the success of both of those care agendas.

It is an issue of sheer practicality. Cash flow is king.

To succeed, the new care approaches need patients and they need cash flow. A medical home or an ACO with no patients and no money is simply and purely empty, nonfunctional, and irrelevant -- for obvious reasons. So both medical homes and ACOs need both the patients and the logistical support that can only be provided by a payer. They need the cash flow that is channeled by the health plans or by the government to succeed. Health plans and health insurers can and should now provide patients, cash flow, systems support, investment and needed levels of data support and real-time data that are needed to make both medical homes and Accountable Care Organizations viable economic functions.

Medical Homes Are Very Useful Care Coordination Tools

Process engineering and reengineering is a toolkit that tends to be used well by the most successful medical homes.

Those care sites have a package payment cash flow that at least partially frees them from the standard rigidly enforced fee schedule list of services. That package payment allows the medical homes to use their lump sum payment per patient to design care delivery around the needs of the patient.

Medical Homes Tend To Be Anchored in Primary Care

Those care teams can use that cash flow to generally work closely with their nurses and other therapists to provide coordinated interventional and preventive care to the patients who select those doctors and those caregivers as their care anchor.

Most Medicare patients who have multiple medical conditions -- comorbidities -- have upwards of seven separate doctors.[215] One study of hospital patients found that 75 percent of the patients with multiple medical doctors were unable to name anyone when asked to identify the physician in charge of their care.[216] As this book has pointed out several times, those doctors who share patients typically are not linked in any way. They don't share medical information. They don't share information about the drugs they prescribe. They don't share their care plans with each other for their shared patients.

Remember the numbers cited above. More than 75 percent of the costs of care come from patients with comorbidities, [217] and those patients typically have to wend their own precarious and complex way through their own confusing thicket -- even forest -- of care sites and solo caregivers. We too often see many patients who are trying to bring their own basic care data on pieces of paper from one care site to another to keep their entire set of caregivers informed.

That really is a stupid and unfortunate way to deliver care. It is dangerous, dysfunctional and completely unnecessary with modern computer technology. So a major role of a well-functioning medical home is to give each patient a primary care doctor -- or a medical home-centered, care-appropriate specialist -- who has all of the information about each patient in a computerized care registry and who can coordinate all of the care for the patient. Most patients love that level of support. Care is better. Complications of care are reduced. Safety is improved.

That lump sum payment usually pays for all medical home related services -- including phone calls from non-physician caregivers or emails from the doctor to the patient. Most traditional care sites use email rarely or not at all. By contrast, medical homes often email their patients to gain or share information. Patients tend to like being connected by email to their caregivers.

Emails, e-visits, e-coding and various level of e-connectivity between doctors and patients all make huge sense. That e-connectivity tool kit was discussed in Chapters Two and Four of this book.

Care Sites That Sell Care by the Package Do Millions of E-Visits

Patients like the convenience and the connectivity that can be created by e-visits. The best vertically integrated care systems that already sell care by the package and not by the piece currently do millions of e-visits with their patients. Their patients love that level of convenient electronic connectivity. As noted earlier, Kaiser Permanente alone did over 13 million e-visits last year.[218] Kaiser Permanente also sent over 30 million lab results to their patients, electronically.[219]

But most care sites in this country today do no e-visits. None. They do no e-visits simply because they can't bill for those visits without committing billing fraud relative to an approved fee schedule. Cash flow is important to caregiver business units. Care sites all need cash to succeed as a business and even to survive as a business. American care sites can't afford to deliver care to their patients for free, so they tend to turn each patient encounter into a billable face-to-face contact instead of a non-billable e-visit so the encounter can legally generate cash.

The prior chapter of this book made the point that the business model of care clearly defines both the infrastructure of care and the functionally of care. That is very true for the new levels of care connectivity tools. E-visits happen today in care sites when the business model of care allows and rewards the use of that tool. They do not happen when the business model of care does not pay for -- and even penalizes -- the use of that tool. It is very basic economic reality. Health plans in this country need to figure out how to create the cash flow reality for care sites that makes e-visits a widely used tool rather than a tool that the caregivers avoid because it reduces revenue. Both medical homes and ACOs can set up cash flow approaches that encourage and incent the use of e-visits.

Reengineering, Repricing and Repackaging Are the 3 R's

The key to achieving an industrial revolution that improves care and makes care more affordable is to put in place a business model for the purchase of care that encourages and rewards the 3 R's of industry evolution. We need a business model for care delivery that encourages reengineering, rewards repricing, and benefits from the right levels of repackaging. Reengineering works for healthcare when it is done well. Remember the examples from the last chapter of this book of the cost savings that have already been achieved by reengineering care delivery. We cut the cost and price of heart transplants and the cost and price of eye surgery in half in this country by reengineering care for those procedures. That reengineering happened in each case because the infrastructure of care was rewarded for doing process improvement by the business model we used to buy that specific category of care.

Delivering Care as a Package Cut the Death Rate by 50 Percent

This isn't a hypothetical supposition or pure economic theory. As noted earlier, Kaiser Permanente very directly sells care by the package and not by the piece. Kaiser Permanente delivers care from its own care system to more than 9 million people.[220] In the prepaid Kaiser Permanente care system, the reengineered processes that were enabled and rewarded by the business model of selling a package of care instead of selling pieces of care have reduced stoke deaths by 40 percent, [221] reduced HIV deaths to half the national average, [222] reduced broken bones in seniors by over a third, [223] and improved the cancer survival rates for breast cancer and colon cancer patients to some of the highest levels in the world.[224] The model works. Kaiser Permanente has cut sepsis deaths by two-thirds, [225] cut pressure ulcers by over 80 percent, and as noted earlier, the KP hospital system actually has some hospitals that haven't had a single pressure ulcer in over a year.[226] Other hospitals average 7 percent of their patients with those ulcers[227] and those hospitals charge the health insurers $40,000 -- on average -- for each case.[228] Care can be a lot safer when you buy it as a package.

The model of selling care by the package works. All health plans need to be figuring out the very best ways of buying packages of care from aligned care teams.

Chart 5.3 below shows the reductions in hospital use that were achieved in North Carolina when that state started using patient-centered medical homes to support care for their Medicaid patients. Care got better. Care costs went down. Those gains could not have been achieved without the medical homes of North Carolina.

That model works well when it is done well. We need the new medical homes and the new Accountable Care Organizations to build on the best features of those existing prepayment models and we clearly need our health insurance plans motivated and enabled to work closely with the medical homes and with the new ACOs to help them succeed. We also -- as this chapter pointed out earlier -- need to stop paying more when care is bad. The benefit redesign strategies were listed earlier in this chapter. Buyers should insist those benefit changes be made by the health plans they use for their employee coverage.

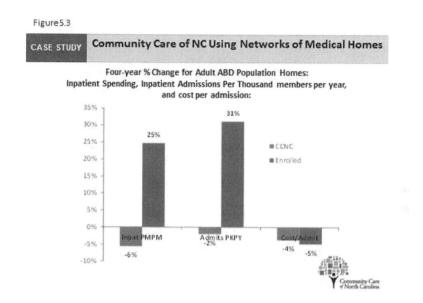

Figure 5.3

Prices Need To Become Relevant -- Not Just Transparent

We clearly need health plans to support approaches that will make care better and more affordable. As part of that total agenda, we need health plans to address the issue of care prices at a couple of levels. Earlier in this chapter, the role of plans in negotiating price discounts was discussed. That is good work for plans to do -- but it is not sufficient to really create a difference and better market environment for care prices in this country.

Some people believe that we can have a positive impact on prices by making more prices transparent -- visible -- easily know-able by the consumer. They believe people will invariably choose to buy lower priced care if prices were known for each piece of care. The people who believe that are wrong. As noted earlier, simply creating price visibility is not enough. Visible, by itself is inadequate. Visibility can even have perverse consequences.

We need prices to be relevant -- not just visible.

Relevant is the goal and relevant is the key word to keep in mind relative to prices.

Prices create huge costs overall, but because of the way we usually pay for care through our deductible insurance plans -- prices are simply not directly financially relevant to individual caregivers for most of our care expenses. Deductibles do make some front-end prices relevant for some pieces of care. It is a very good thing for patients to know what those prices are for pre-deductible expenses. Prices are, however, only relevant for any patient with deductible insurance until the deductible is met and then they become completely irrelevant for that patient.

Look at the actual spending levels and the distribution of costs. The obvious truth is that the expensive ten percent of the population who used eighty percent of all care costs in this country last year blew right by their insurance deductible almost as soon as their care began. A thousand dollar deductible might pay for one CT scan. Then the deductible makes other prices irrelevant. That thousand dollar deductible pays for one-third of one day in the hospital. Then prices become irrelevant for hospital care. In the real world, no one buys hospital care by thirds of days. It is also very rare that the first piece of care that a patient will face in a year is a CT scan.

Once each person's deductible is met, prices become both invisible and completely irrelevant to most patients in this country.

Some People Confuse Visibility With Relevance

As noted above, some people do believe that the major price issue we need to address in this country is price visibility and not price relevance. Those people believe that keeping prices for pieces of care visible to the patient even after the deductible is met will still cause people to be price conscious in a productive way. The people who hold that position believe the pure awareness of price differences will result in consumers choosing less expensive care.

The truth is -- once the deductible is met for any given patient, if prices for any further pieces of care actually do become visible, patients who know multiple prices often prefer to use the higher priced care vendor. Higher prices seem to indicate higher quality. Many patients prefer to get their care from the surgeon who charges $20,000 for a surgery instead of the one who charges only $5,000 for the same surgery. As one speaker at a policy seminar said, "I really don't feel like I want to have a $4,000 appendectomy when there are $20,000 appendectomies available. I want first class care. Not discounted or cut rate care. My appendix is worth the extra money."

That speaker seemed to have no clue that there is a high likelihood that the higher cost care site for that particular surgery might well have more post-surgical infections, more pressure ulcers, and more surgical redos. Studies have shown that the care sites that charge the most for sepsis care tend to have the highest death rate from sepsis.[229] That piece of information is invisible to consumers, and it certainly isn't how people usually think about prices. Prices very much do not link to quality in this country for care delivery. But patients don't know that, and they are somewhat more likely to select the higher priced site if the price difference isn't going to have an actual cash impact on the patient.

Also, the truth is that the patients who do see those high prices for that procedure usually do not know that the same site that is charging $20,000 for patients who have that patient's specific insurance coverage for that particular procedure is probably charging $5,000 or $10,000 for the same exact procedure to another patient who has different insurance coverage.

There clearly is no linkage between quality and price in those settings. The range of prices that are used for each service inside each care site is often amazing. As noted in the chapter on prices, the prices charged by the caregivers at each care site tend to vary by payer, not by patient. So even if you do know some prices as a patient, that information doesn't help you figure out anything real about quality at that site, and it doesn't even tell you very much about the actual prices that are being charged to other patients for care at that same site.

We clearly need to do more than make prices transparent. We need our health plans that pay for care by the piece to make prices relevant. We also need to give consumers value-related care data about each piece of care wherever we can add that data to the design process.

Our health insurance companies need to build much better benefit plan structures and approaches that make both prices relevant and visible when unit prices are the way we pay for our care. Buyers should insist that the health plans they use to administer their coverage should put benefit designs in place that will make unit prices both visible and relevant to both patients and caregivers.

The French Set a Baseline Payment Level

As noted in the price chapter of this book, the French actually have figured out a very nice way to deal with the price relevance and visibility issue. The French don't use front-end deductibles. They use a kind of reverse deductible. The French set a fixed price to be paid from their national health program for each and every individual procedure. So every French citizen actually has first dollar -- or first euro -- coverage for every procedure. That approach doesn't cap prices in France. It sets up a price base payment for each procedure. Doctors in France can then charge patients more than that base payment amount if they want to charge more -- but payment of any additional amount for that care comes from the patients and not from the taxpayer.

The French also insist that each patient pay first for each piece of care. They make people pay first for their care and then the patient must file a claim for that expense -- with each claim paid at the basic benefit level set by the national plan. The French government clearly wants the French people to know what each piece of care costs. They want everyone to have health insurance and they want every citizen to know how much money care costs. The French decided to offer first-dollar coverage -- with a payment approach that makes every patient aware of every price. We do just the opposite in this county. We insulate patients from most care prices. The French make all of their prices naked to each patient.

Doctors Will Compete on Price When Price Is Relevant

Doctors in Paris who do want to charge French patients more than the base fee can simply say to the patient -- "The government fee to deliver a baby is five hundred euro. I charge eight hundred euro to do that work. If you want me to deliver your baby, you will have to pay me the difference between the five hundred euro base fee and eight hundred euro price."

It is a very simple payment approach and a very clear price setting method.

That French approach obviously makes prices relevant. It makes prices both highly visible and definitely relevant. That approach creates market forces for care in a very direct way. The French doctor has to convince the patient that the doctor's service levels or the doctor's expertise or the doctor's office décor or charm or convenience and access levels to care are sufficiently superior in some way to make spending the additional money a smart thing for the patient to do.

The French Model Pays Up Front for Chronic Conditions

If that exact model were used in the U.S. for key pieces of care, and if we also decide that we will simply continue to purchase care by the piece and not by the package, using that French approach here would do several very useful things. It would very much make prices visible. It would make prices relevant. It would create a new market model for a wide range of care that would probably work very much like the market model for eye surgery described in the prior chapter. That new payment approach would enable caregivers in this country to improve their business success levels by having competitive prices.

It also would serve the lovely dual ethical and economic benefit and function of not simply shifting the cost of one patient's expensive care site decision directly to all other patient's monthly premium. In the U.S., we actually -- when all the money is moved around -- simply shift the cost of that higher priced care to other people's money. That high average cost of care is then calculated and collected as a premium that is charged to insured people.

That French approach creates a nice relevance for prices relative to decision-making about caregivers by patients. It also has a nice intellectual elegance to it. A number of health insurers in this country are beginning to use variations of that model to design their benefits for some procedures.

First Dollar Coverage Is Good for Chronic Care Patients

Another good point to keep in mind in thinking about benefit design is that the French payment approach can offer a very nice additional benefit feature for many patients with chronic conditions. That is true because the French model pays up front for all services -- including chronic care -- instead of having a deductible that causes people to pay for their initial services for their chronic condition each year until their personal deductible is met. Chronic care patients in France don't need to pay a deductible before getting benefits. Not having an upfront deductible is a particularly good thing for chronic care patients. Remember where most of the costs of care in this country are -- with chronic care patients. We very much want patients with chronic conditions to refill their prescriptions and we want those patients to have their blood tests and other follow-up care done. When chronic care patients in our country have to pay an upfront deductible each year, there are often delays in getting needed care early in the year. Studies show that the higher deductibles often create financial barriers to some chronic care follow-up for some American patients.

The French model eliminates that barrier by paying first for that level of care without a deductible. The French model might only pay twenty euro for a blood test and a French doctor might charge thirty euro for that test. The patient can either find a doctor who will do that specific test for twenty euro or the patient can pay the difference out of pocket.

Both prices are less than a typical American deductible.

Even if the patient decides to pay out of pocket for the price difference, ten Euros paid out of pocket is still less money than the patient would pay for that service with an American deductible plan where the full thirty euro fee paid would then be charged to the patients and then paid directly by the patients until the deductible is met for that patient for each year.

We Need Better Benefit Design When We Buy Care by the Piece

That is another issue for buyers, employers, and health plans to consider in setting up the cash flow we use to buy care.

Deductibles are actually a highly imperfect payment approach that tends to have multiple perverse and entirely unintentionally negative impacts. Those unintentional perverse impacts can often be avoided as part of the benefit package design when a given insurer's approach to financing care involves buying care by the package and not by the piece. Those perverse impacts can also be avoided by having a fixed first dollar benefit schedule to buy care instead of using a pure up front deductible for all care before payment for any care.

Insurers need to do a better job of designing benefit packages around patient needs -- with chronic care patients having benefit plans that facilitate patients receiving right follow-up care. Insurers also need overall care strategies to improve care. Insurers need to support better care plans and better care approaches to achieve premium affordability rather than simply using increasingly high deductibles to shift increasing levels of costs to patients to keep premiums lower.

We need to get the insurance mechanisms right. We need to do smart things relative to health insurance if we want to make appropriate changes in the actual delivery of care.

The Political Power of Health Care Is Huge

Some basic business model changes are needed -- but in some ways -- for some segments of the current health care infrastructure, those changes will not be easy to do.

We spend nearly two point eight trillion dollars on care in this country.[230] The infrastructure of care in this country is very protective of that cash flow. It results in jobs, health careers, significant local cash flow, and wealth.

The political power and the political connections that result from all of those local jobs and from that local economic strength is massive. Politicians often bemoan the total cost of care but politicians seldom bemoan caregivers. When the political world does look to attack someone for the total cost of care, the usual politically correct target of the cost-related attack tends to be health insurance companies.

This book calls for insurance companies to be a significant positive factor and a major asset in the agenda of making care more affordable in this country. That isn't the role that most people believe that health insurers play today relative to health care costs.

Blaming the Speedometer for the Speed of the Car

Surveys tell us, in fact, that a significant number of people in this country who are unhappy about care costs actually blame insurance companies, themselves, for the high cost of care. Several surveys have shown that belief to be widespread. A high percentage of people literally believe that premiums, themselves, create health care costs. When you understand how premium levels are actually calculated, that's actually a bit like blaming your thermometer for your fever -- or blaming the speed of your car on your speedometer.

But surveys show that the number one factor at the top of most lists when people are asked what causes health care costs to be high in this country is the health insurance industry. Insurers tend to be rated by caregivers to be the top driver for health care costs in this country.

Blaming Your Thermometer for Your Fever Isn't Accurate

In the real world, health insurance premiums are very basically the average cost of care. In the context of true functional economic and arithmetic reality, those premiums are simply the speedometer for runaway health care costs. As this book has stated several times, premiums are based on the average cost of care for any given covered population. When the cost of any insured piece of care goes up, the average cost of care for the insured people goes up. The average cost of care is key. When the average cost of care for any given insured population goes up, insurance premiums for that insured population go up. It is a very direct and almost immediate linkage.

So why do so many people blame insurance companies for the high cost of care? That perception is widespread, in part, because a number of political leaders have chosen to ignore the issues of provider costs and to completely duck any mention of provider prices in the cost debates and to focus instead in a very public and focused way on the issues and visible events that relate to insurance costs.

The New Insurance Laws Make Some Old Practices Illegal

How did politicians come to that conclusion? Why do politicians offer that assessment as the primary cost driver for care? They reached that conclusion, in part, because most political leaders have not wanted to challenge the political power of the caregiver community. Political leaders also reached that conclusion because that sense of insurers, themselves, directly triggering excessive cash flow used to have some situational truth for some insurance companies in some settings.

It is true that some health insurance companies in the past in some market settings did very visibly take some excess profits from some subsets of the health insurance marketplace. The health insurance industry, overall, actually has a lower average profitability level than almost any other industry. The total profit margins for the health insurance industry typically run lower than 5 percent overall. The public -- when asked -- tend to believe the profit margins of insurers exceed 10 percent. That 10 percent number is not true. Two and three percent margins are not uncommon.

Some insurers did, however, make much higher margins in past years -- and some of those margins were visible to the public and policymakers. Those margins are no longer legal.

So it is true that the rules about how insurers calculated premiums were much looser in some settings before the new Affordable Care Act law was passed. Those days of insurer spending very low percentages of the total premiums they collected on actual costs of care are now gone for everyone. To the extent that some insurers actually used those business models, those practices have been ended. The new truth is that the new insurance premium setting laws have simply made those old profit-taking practices and those very low percentages of premium spent on care illegal for insurers. Insurer profits and insurance administration costs are now functionally and legally capped as a total percentage of premiums.

The new law specifies the minimum portions of premium that must be spent by insurers to pay for care. The new maximum loss ratio laws that exist today now define and constrain the calculation of health insurance premiums. So any insurers who might have done any kind of abusive or excessive premium pricing in the past now face strict and rigidly enforced loss ratios laws that keep excessive profits and high administrative cost from being charged to insured people. Those days are gone. They were ended by the new loss ratio laws.

So now, premiums are the thermometer -- not the fever.

Premiums Are Directly Based on the Average Cost of Care

The basic arithmetic reality today is that health insurance premiums in this country are based on the average cost of care for insured people. That is true here and it is true in every other country that also uses private insurance as the key mechanism to make other people's money available when that money is needed to buy care for sick people. The ACA law directly bases the cost of today's premium on the current and actual cost of care for insured people. So the truth is, care costs create premium costs and premium costs do not create care costs.

Another key truth is -- we do need to make premiums affordable at this point in history. This book argues that the best way of making premiums affordable is to bring down the average cost of care for each insured person. As noted above, we can do that in several ways. We can do it by negotiating lower fees -- we can do it by buying care by the package and not by the piece -- we can do it by delivering better care (that has fewer complications and fewer crises) -- and we can do it by improving the health of the insured population.

Those are all important things for health plans to do. As we try to bring down the total cost of care in this country and as we work to make premiums more affordable, all four of those agendas need to be part of the health plan agenda for the country.

U.S. Premiums Could Drop by Over a Third If We Paid Canadian Prices

Some people argue that the administrative cost burden charged in the health insurance premiums today are still too high. Some people argue that we could make care costs a lot lower in this country if we simply used the Canadian single-payer insurance model...and more than one speaker has said that the difference in costs between the U.S. and Canada is actually the difference in expenses that is created by the health plan administrative costs in the U.S. versus the lower costs that exist for administration in Canada.

Is that accurate?

Are the administrative cost components of the Canadian national health insurance model the primary reason Canada spends so much less money on care than we do?

No. Those administrative costs in Canada are lower -- but they are not the primary reason Canada spends less than 12 percent of their GDP on care while we spend almost 18 percent of our GDP on care.[231]

That belief is, in fact, partially accurate. We do spend more money on insurance administration than the Canadians spend, but the total cost impact is not as high as people believe it to be. Look at actual numbers.

The relative impact of those administrative costs and the relationship between care costs and insurance costs can be seen pretty easily if we compare the key elements of health care costs in the U.S. and Canada. Remember the chapter of this book on care unit prices. Look back at those price charts. Canada spends a lot less on each piece of care. If we used actual Canadian care unit prices to buy each piece of care here, and if we kept our entire private insurance plans intact, our insurance premiums in this country would actually drop overnight by about 40 percent overnight.

Premiums are based on the average cost of care.

The average cost of care purchased by American insurers would be a lot lower if American insurers paid Canadian prices for each piece of care. Look again at the prices for pieces of care in Canada that are shown in the price chapter of this book. Check the chart for Canadian care prices. That forty percent reduction insurance premium in this country would happen with no change in the amount of care delivered in this country if we just paid for each piece of care using Canadian prices. That lower premium level would happen because the American insurers simply could pay for each piece of care using Canadian prices.

How much of that difference is due to the difference in administrative costs?

If we moved to the Canadian single payer administrative costs model and if we eliminated all insurance company administrative expenses for this country and if we replaced them with

Canadian administrative costs that they incur for running their program, we would replace nearly 15 percent[232] insurance company administrative charge in this country with the 7 percent total administrative expense level that is now charged in Canada.

The numbers are clear. Replacing our 15 percent with their 7 percent would reduce our total health insurance premium levels by 8 percent.

Eight percent is a big number -- but it is a lot smaller than the 40-percent reduction that we would get if we paid for care using the Canadian fee schedule.

The Canadian government fees for each piece of care are all set by the government. They look very much like the fees we pay when our fees are set by our government. As noted earlier several times, states set the Medicaid fees in this country. Those fees in some states are very close to the fees that are set by some of the Canadian provinces.

It probably is not coincidental that when government legislative bodies in each country have to decide whether to set low fees for pieces of care or raise taxes to pay for that care, the decision that results from the political process and the government officials is to set low fees on both countries.

If that is actually why Canada spends so much less money on care, why don't we simply follow the Canadian model and have our own government impose its own set of prices on all care?

That is the logical final question in this chapter on using the business model to change the way we deliver care. Setting fees by government edict is clearly a business model option we can consider.

Why isn't it the recommendation of this book?

The answer to that question was given at the end of Chapter Three. We would financially destroy the health care infrastructure of this country if we used Canadian fees to buy all care here.

We would also be continuing to buy care by the piece.

Chapter Three also explains how dysfunctional it would be for us to cut prices and also to continue buying all care by the piece. So even though that solution would work at one arithmetic level, it would be disruptive, damaging and even destructive at multiple other levels.

We have better solutions. We may want to write some pricing laws that do prevent providers from using truly abusive pricing for uninsured people. We may want to set up pricing rules that say people without insurance could cap their payments at prices that are double or even triple what Medicare pays for a piece of care. That could end some obvious pricing abuses. But we do not want to have the government simply set all prices because the consequences of doing that would keep us from continuously improving care.

We Will Not Use a Canadian Fee Schedule or Insurance Plan

If we are going to change the way care is delivered in this country, we need to change the flow of cash that goes to the infrastructure of care in some important ways.

There are four major sources of cash in this country that create that flow of cash. The four sources are patients, employers, health plans, and the government. This chapter explained why the consumers currently have relatively little leverage in changing the way we buy care -- and it explained that employers clearly have better leverage than individual caregivers. It also explained that the two best mechanisms for charging the flow of cash are the health plans and the major government programs that buy care.

Chapters Seven and Eight of this book explain what Medicare and Medicaid can do to bring down the cost of care.

This chapter has basically focused on the role that health plans need to follow to help caregivers improve the way care is delivered.

As we look at the total business model of care to see where we could make changes that can help bring down the cost of care and reduce the premiums that are needed to pay for care, it is clear we need health plans to serve as the tools we use to get that job done. We know that health plans need to be buying care more by the package and less by the piece. We know that health plans need to modify the benefit design to make prices more relevant when prices are the way we pay for care. We know that health plans need to support caregivers who are reengineering care to make care both better and more affordable. That approach of working with caregivers and using the cash flow of health plans to modify the way we deliver care is a very useful strategy that has a high probability of actually succeeding if we do it well.

That entire agenda will fail, however, if we don't make the premiums that are charged by the health plans affordable. Premium affordability is the topic of the next chapter of this book.

CHAPTER SIX

USING PRIVATE HEALTH PLANS TO COVER EVERYONE WILL NOT WORK IF WE CAN'T MAKE COVERAGE AFFORDABLE

Using private health plans to provide health coverage for most Americans will only succeed for us as a country if the coverage that is sold by the private health plans is affordable. Affordability is essential. This strategy will fail if we use private insurers to provide health coverage and the premium that is charged by the plans for their coverage is so high that people can't afford to buy the coverage.

This Strategy Will Fail If Premiums Are Not Affordable

We need to make premium affordability a top priority.

So what can we do to make premiums for health insurance more affordable in this country?

Some of the necessary strategies to keep premiums affordable have been described in the prior chapters of this book. Insurers in this country need to perform several key roles relative to affordability and they need to perform each of those rules increasingly well.

For starters, if we want premiums to be affordable for Americans who buy insurance, we need our insurers to negotiate good prices with the caregivers who take care of their patients. That strategy was mentioned in two earlier chapters. Premium for health insurance is, of course, based very directly on the average cost of care for insured people. We need insurers to help bring down their needed premium levels by successfully reducing the average costs of care for the people they insure. Reductions in the fees paid to providers of care can obviously help reduce premium levels.

Cash Flow From Insurers Should Encourage Continuous Improvement

Negotiating better prices for each of the pieces of care that are being purchased by the piece is clearly an important thing for insurers to do to bring down premium costs. Those fee negotiations are actually not, however, the very best and most useful thing that insurers can do to help bring down the cost of care for insured people.

The most useful way for insurers to bring down the cost of care is to buy care differently -- buying care, wherever possible, by the package and not by the piece. This book has explained multiple times why that approach to buying care is a good idea.

Insurers very much need to work with caregivers to create better cash flow mechanisms and more process-focused business models for care providers. The business model we use to buy care needs to free the caregivers from the rigid controls and the functionality tyranny that is created by our standard fee based approach of paying for care entirely by the piece. As earlier chapters of this book have explained several times those standard insurance company lists of approved procedures limit, inhibit, penalize, and even cripple process improvement in care delivery. Health plans can help make process improvement happen for the business units of care by using business models and payment approaches that incent and reward better processes. We need creative and enlightened payers to work with creative and collaborative care delivery entities to create better care business models. We need business models that will allow the caregivers to reengineer care and bring down operational costs without suffering revenue loss and financial damage. We can easily create a functional industrial revolution for care delivery if we do that business model redesign work well. We need that industrial revolution to happen -- and it cannot and will not happen as long as care is purchased only by the piece.

ACOs and Medical Homes Both Sell Care by the Package

The good news is that there is actually a growing list of ways we can buy care by the package. ACOs and patient-focused medical homes were both described in the last chapter of this book. Both of those care delivery approaches sell care by the package in ways that enable caregivers to do a better job of team care and a much better job of care coordination. ACOs and medical homes are high potential care delivery models. That potential will only be triggered and realized if both health plans and government purchasers decide to support those care approaches with real cash flow. Cash flow is the key. Those steps in the right direction by the business units of care need cash flow support from key purchasers of care to survive and thrive. Caregivers can't take the steps to implement and run either ACOs or medical homes without sufficient cash flow support.

Having the purchasers of care and the providers of care working together in alignment to perform those functions makes huge sense.

The Primary Function of Insurance -- Spread Risk

There is an obvious opportunity to use the vast river of cash that flows in our country more wisely because that massive cash flow exists now and much of it is being channeled through health plans today. Health insurers are the conduit for cash used to buy care for the majority of Americans. They will not be able to succeed in those efforts if the premiums they charge people to buy coverage are unaffordable.

Insurers Exist To Spend Risk

All of those efforts to make premium affordable will fail if we don't succeed with another major element of the business model we use to maintain and sustain the basic product sold by the health plans and insurers. That basic product is -- in a word -- insurance.

That topic is particularly relevant right now because the Affordable Care Act has made some changes in the traditional business approaches of health insurance for a major piece of the insurance market. For the individual insurance market and for the small group insurance market, the new law makes it illegal for insurers to exclude people from coverage for being ill or high risk.

Most of the insured people in this country have "group" coverage -- with insurance purchased through employer groups. That coverage accepts all applicants inside each group and doesn't health screen anyone. But roughly 10 percent of insured people have purchased individual coverage directly from an insurer. [233] The insurers who have sold individual coverage have been allowed to do health screens and have been able to refuse to sell individual insurance to people who are in poor health or at significant risk of being in poor health. That ability to reject people for those reasons is now gone for health insurers.

The most basic role of health plans is actually very simple and very clear. We use the plans to create "insurance." We basically pay billions of dollars to our health insurers so they can perform a very basic and fundamental cash flow function. Their basic job and their most foundational function for the bulk of their customers is to be insurers -- to spread risk and to spread care expenses among insured people.

We Buy Care With Other People's Money

Spreading risk actually is their primary reason to exist. How do the insurers spread risk? The process is pretty simple. The insurers only have one source of cash. Customers. They each collect money from their customers in premiums. The premiums are paid to the insurer by all of the people they insure. The insurers then use that money to buy care for the people they insure who actually need care. That cash reallocation process between insured people is their core function and most fundamental value. The insurers create a functional and practical cash flow mechanism that allows all of their insured people to use other people's money to pay for their care when that money is needed to buy care because the care itself is needed by that insured person.

Some people need a lot of care. When people need care that costs a lot of money, then people very clearly need access to other people's money to pay for that care. Having secure access to other people's money is a very valuable financial reality for all of the people who need that money to pay for their care. That's where risk spreading by the insurers becomes relevant. Insured people actually have access to that needed money only because their insurers have been successful in spreading risk and because the insurers have collected the money from other people and then have it on hand to pay for insured people's care.

To make that risk-spreading financial model work, the insurers need to collect premium from a large number of people who aren't currently using care so they can use the money they have collected from those people to buy care for the insured people who actually are using care at any point in time. As this book has also noted earlier in a couple of places, when we are ill, we have three ways of getting access to other people's money so we can use it to pay for our care. We can use tax money -- or we can use money collected in premiums -- or we can use money paid by our employer as part of our employee benefit package. Taxes and premiums are the two key mechanisms we have to get access to other people's money. If we are covered by one of our government programs, the other people whose money we use to buy our care are the taxpayers who pay taxes and who generate the government flow of money used to buy care. When we have private insurance, the money we use from other people to pay for our care is the money that those other people have paid in their insurance premiums to the insurer we share.

The job of each insurer is to collect enough money from all of their insured people so that there is enough money to buy care for the people they insure who need that money to pay for their care.

This book is also, obviously, recommending strongly that our health insurers now should not only spread risk -- they should now also take on multiple additional functional roles that can help improve both the quality and cost of care. As noted earlier, only insurers have the tools, the leverage and the cash flow to do important parts of that quality improvement and care redesign work. We obviously need our insurers to do some key pieces of improved quality work and some key pieces of cost mitigation work or that work will not be done. Those are good and important roles for insurers to play -- but if we cut to the essence of the pure insurance model, that risk-spreading function is clearly the basic role that insurers must play in order for that money to be available by the insurer when it is needed to pay for people's care.

This Model Will Fail If the Risk Pools Are Destroyed

In order to spread risk, the insurers need to have a number of customers who are paying premiums but not using much care so the insurer can use their money to buy care for the people who are also paying premiums and who do currently need that insurance cash flow money to buy their care.

In the group insurance market, everyone in each group buys the insurance -- so the risk selection issues are relatively small. In the new individual insurance market, we now have a situation where individuals who are at significant risk or who are already using expensive care can now buy individual insurance. The concern, of course, is that most of the new people who will buy individual coverage may now be very expensive users of care dollars.

At the essence of the issue, we need to recognize that the premiums that are charged to buy coverage will become either highly unaffordable or completely unavailable -- if the business model and the market reality we use to fund our health insurance premium cash flow for that individual marketplace doesn't allow each of the insurers who sell insurance to that set of people to have enough non-sick customers so that they have viable risk pools and they can pay for the care costs of their insured sick people.

Viable is a very important concept relative to risk pools. If the insurers of this country each end up with risk pools for the individual market that are made up entirely of sick people -- then those risk pools will collapse. That is a real danger. If the people who buy individual insurance are too heavily based on the subset of possible customers who are sick people, then the average cost of care for the people who are covered by each insurer to buy care for those sick people will be very high. Arithmetic becomes very relevant at that point. When the average cost of care for an insurer is high, that of course, creates premiums for each insurer that are very high. When premiums for any insurer are high, very nasty and dysfunctional things can happen to that insurer and to that insurers risk pool in any market-based insurance environment.

Why can dysfunctional things happen to those risk pools?

People Make Intelligent Choices

People are intelligent. People also tend to make decisions that meet their own self-interest. Both of those facts are relevant when the purchase of insurance is voluntary. People who voluntarily buy health insurance are capable of making very intelligent choices relative to their own costs and expense levels. Those choices made by individual people based on their own direct costs of premium and care can sometimes potentially damage the new risk pools. That is not a new phenomenon.

When premiums go up for any given insurer, the people who buy that specific insurance react individually and personally to each price increase. People make very real choices about whether or not to cancel their insurance coverage when their premiums go up. The decisions about continuing to be insured are made at that point by each person based on each person's individual financial status and health care reality. The healthy people who have that insurance who have no immediate personal health care needs may decide that they don't want to continue to pay the higher premiums when they have no current or anticipated use of care.

So when premiums go up too much for currently insured healthy people, those low-cost currently insured people may simply cancel coverage. Each insured person can make that individual choice based on their own judgment and their own circumstances. When a number of healthy people make that choice to cancel their insurance coverage, those healthy people immediately stop being part of that specific risk pool.

Insurers tend to panic when that happens. Panic is an accurate description of the insurer's reaction to a risk-pool deterioration situation. Insurers know that when the healthiest people are leaving their risk pool, that will cause the remaining risk pool of less healthy but still insured people to have an even higher average cost of care. If that higher cost of care happens for that remaining risk pool, then the premiums for that insurer also simply go up again to reflect the new average cost of care for the people who are still insured. When a next rate increase happens for that same set of people, there can be additional consequences. The usual pattern that follows additional rate increases is that more healthy people will leave the risk pool each time the rates go up. That set of consumer decisions is obviously not good for any risk pool. That sequence of events and those choices to cancel coverage by insured people can far too easily create what insurance actuaries call a "risk pool death spiral." A risk pool death spiral very much is not a good thing for an insurance company.

The need to have a sufficient number of healthy people in each insurers risk pool is pretty clear. That is going to be particularly true for the new risk pools that will be created by the new law that allows everyone to purchase insurance, regardless of their health status.

When the opportunity to buy health insurance is fully activated for currently sick and uninsured people, it is clear that anyone who has cancer or who has diabetes and its various complications would be making a mistake not to buy that newly available insurance. The number of people with cancer who do not enroll will be fairly low. The challenge will be to get additional people who don't have cancer to also enroll.

Affordability Is the Goal and the Key To Success

Insurers, of course, understand those sets of risks very well.

Insurers very much want the premiums they charge to their customers to be affordable. Insurers have traditionally wanted premiums to be affordable not because the insurers want to charge less in premiums but because the consequences to an insurer of significant risk pool deterioration can be so grim, painful, and financially deadly.

A major business goal of the people who manage operations for voluntarily purchased health insurance premiums risk pools always needs to be affordability because actuarial death spirals can be triggered far too easily and far too quickly by unaffordability.

What does that set of financial realities tell us?

It tells us that the strategy that we have chosen as a country to use private insurers to insure people in the individual market who do not have group insurance coverage cannot succeed if the premiums charged by the insurers for those individually purchased insurance policies ends up becoming unaffordable. The premium that will be charged to people in the individual market needs to be low enough so that people who already have that insurance coverage will not cancel their coverage. It is a very circular situation. Premium affordability cannot happen if the average cost of care for any given insurance risk pool is too high. If any given risk pool deteriorates and if all of the healthy insured people leave a risk pool, the remaining insured population in that risk pool will have a very high cost of care and premium for that set of insured people will become unaffordable.

Access To the Risk Pool Will Now Change

We are in the process of changing a significant part of the business model for health insurance in this country. Those changes are making health insurance more accessible to many people in the individual market. Those changes also are increasing the risk that the people who buy insurance and who retain insurance will be less healthy than the people who are in the current risk pools for individual coverage. This change in the law will not affect the people who now have group insurance in the U.S. As this chapter explains, we have always allowed all people with group coverage to enroll in health insurance plans regardless of their personal health status. Group coverage is a huge part of the insurance market. The group coverage model has always fundamentally included all members of each group with no health screening for any applicants and with no individuals in each group refusing to buy coverage.

But for the nongroup or individual insurance marketplace in this country, the insurance companies have always been allowed to reject individual applicants for coverage who fail each insurer's health screening criteria. The insurers used the health screening approach to keep premiums lower for the individually sold portion of their insurance business.

The Individual Market Will Now Outlaw Health Screening

We have chosen as a country to now require all health insurance companies who sell coverage to individuals to stop doing health screens for a couple of months each year and to simply accept for coverage any person who applies for health insurance coverage during that enrollment period. That represents real progress at a very important level for the insurance marketplace in this country. Under the old approach, people who had health care problems -- who really needed other people's money to pay for their care -- could be rejected for coverage when they applied for that coverage. The old laws allowed American insurance companies to require people who applied for individual insurance coverage to fill out health history forms outlining all of their health care diagnosis and their entire history of care. The insurers then used that information about each person's care to figure out whether or not to sell health insurance to that person. That process often wasn't a good thing for sick people for obvious reasons. Most insurers tended to reject the sick and unhealthy applicants for insurance. So -- in a nutshell -- sick people who really needed insurance often could not buy that insurance.

As noted above, that business model for the individual market is changing right now for January 1, 2014. There has been an open enrollment period to start the process. Insurers cannot reject applicants during that open enrollment time frame based on their personal health statuses.

Insurers now have to accept every applicant for individual coverage, regardless of the applicant's immediate health care expenses or needs and also they will need to accept them regardless of their historical use of health care. That will be of course, a good thing for many applicants who might have been rejected for individual insurance in the past. But that process does create a possible risk for the health insurers that we all need to understand.

The Risk Pool Challenges Do Not Exist for the Group Insurance Business Model

It is important to understand that the new risk pool changes for the insurers really will only be created for the subset of the insurance market that provides non-group coverage to individual purchasers of insurance. As noted above, group health insurance coverage will not be affected by these new agendas.

The non-group insurance market is not the biggest portion of the health insurance marketplace. Roughly 10 percent of the people with health insurance in this country buy that insurance now through the individual insurance marketplace.

Far more people in this country get their health insurance coverage by being part of the group insurance marketplace -- usually getting their insurance from their employer.

In the much larger group insurance market that exists in this country, there will be no new danger to insurers relative to risk pool collapse. There is no new risk for the existing group insurance risk pools because in the existing group market, everyone in each group is already simply enrolled and in the group insurance marketplace everyone in each group is already insured. People with group insurance do not make individual choices about being insured. Entire groups are insured as groups. There isn't any danger from the new law for the existing group insurance coverage that provides insurance today to most Americans because there are no selection issues today inside the groups. Those issues existed to some degree at one time in the early days of group insurance, but they were resolved years ago by creating basic underwriting rules that simply enroll each group as a group with no significant individual choices.

So we will not see any new level of risk pool deterioration threat for group insurance coverage in this country because people in each group have no choices now about whether or not to keep coverage. People enrolled in those groups will have no new choices on January 1, 2014. Group insurance has a built-in risk selection safety net that exists in practical reality because the employer groups in this country typically cover all group members. Everyone in each risk pool is permanently covered as part of that insurance business model.

People Who Buy Individual Insurance Can Make Individual Decisions

That level of stability and inclusiveness is not true for the purchase of individual insurance coverage in this country. Individuals in that insurance market approach each buy or cancel their own health insurance coverage and the people who buy individual coverage make those decisions as individuals. That is a very different business model for the health insurance companies. To survive financially in the individual portion of the health insurance market, the insurers clearly each need to have and maintain viable risk pools of individual customers.

Insurers have kept premiums lower historically by not enrolling people who are sick at the time of enrollment and by not enrolling people who had a history of being prior users of health care services. Rejecting those people for coverage was sad and very unfortunate for the rejected people, but it functionally kept the premium levels for individually purchased coverage lower for those insurance companies than the premiums would have been if people could have waited until they had cancer or a stroke and then purchased an individual insurance plan.

To understand the impact of those new rules on the individual insurance marketplace, it makes sense to consider briefly how other insurance markets might react to similar rules about not screening applicants.

Some people object very directly to the fact that the open enrollment period each year is only a couple of months. Those people would like the open enrollment period to be continuous -- allowing enrollment by any person at any time.

If anyone who wants to buy health insurance could buy insurance with no health screening at any time, it would be a little like implementing a new law for car insurance that would allow people to not buy their car accident coverage until after they had an accident. The car insurance version of that open enrollment law would allow any person who actually had a car accident to simply call their car insurer after the accident to sign up for their car insurance coverage on the spot from the site of the accident.

What would be the consequence of that model for car insurance? Figuring that impact out doesn't require an economist or an actuary.

Insuring Burning Homes Is Not Optimal

If people could wait until they had an actual accident before buying their car insurance, the premium levels for car insurance would go up. The premium level for that insurance would need to climb to the point where the premium charged by the insurer to insure each car exactly equaled the insured cost of each accident. If people could buy car insurance after the accident, then premium for a $20,000 car accident would need to be $20,000 -- plus administrative expenses -- so the insurer could have enough money to pay the claim. That kind of post-accident enrollment in collusion coverage would be a very tough business model for car insurance. Who would buy car insurance if the premium price was that high?

Having a regulatory body of some kind use rate regulation mandates to arbitrarily cap those car insurance premiums would not help solve that problem. Arithmetic is arithmetic. Requiring a car insurance company to charge only $1,000 in premium and then require the company to pay for a $20,000 wrecked car that was already wrecked before the insurance was purchased obviously would financially destroy any car insurance companies that continued to sell that insurance.

That market would disappear very quickly if a regulator of some kind simply imposed rates on the car insurers that were less than the cost of the wrecked car. What insurance companies would sell car insurance if the premiums for that insurance were capped by the law and if the premium caps were far below the cost of paying for each wrecked car?

This is a very basic, common sense issue. If the maximum allowable premium that could be charged for insuring a $20,000 wreck would be $1,000, what sane insurer would sell $20,000 coverage for that market? Again --any insurer that would agree to take on $20,000 in expense in exchange for $1,000 in regulated premiums would have to be questioned and challenged relative to their basic math skills, their business judgment and their common sense.

Selling Life Insurance To Dead People Is a Tough Business Model

Likewise, it would be hard for fire insurance companies to survive financially if people could wait until after their homes had burned before buying fire insurance. It would actually be even harder for life insurance companies to survive as viable business entities if a law was passed mandating that life insurance could be purchased for an individual by some family member after the person who is named on the insurance contract as the insured person had already died. The life insurance industry would be destroyed as an industry if a regulation uses magical thinking to require the life insurance companies to sell a million dollars in life insurance to dead people for $100,000 -- or some other lower number -- in order to "make life insurance affordable."

The truth is -- fire insurance works as a business because people whose houses are not burning buy fire insurance. The people whose houses are not burning pay their premiums for that insurance every month. The premiums are affordable because many people buy that insurance whose houses never burn. Their collective collected premium money is then used by the insurer to pay for the houses that do burn. People use other people's money to pay for their burned homes. If other people don't pay their premiums to fire insurers, that money isn't available to pay for the burned houses that do happen.

So obviously, those kinds of risk pool issues are very real for every kind of insurance. Health insurance isn't unique in facing those realities. To make any insurance business model work, there needs to be a sufficient number of people in each risk pool who are paying their premiums and who are not immediately using the benefits of the insurance. To protect the health insurance risk pools somewhat, the open enrollment period for health insurance is limited to two months. If car insurance had only a two-month period when people could wreck a car and still buy insurance after the fact, that rule would still cause a lot of people to buy car insurance at other times in the year to be protected against an accident in the other ten months of the year when there was no guaranteed issues of car coverage.

The new law for individual health insurance went into effect on January 1 of 2014.

We actually do not know yet whether we have inadvertently chosen to use an insurance model for individual health care insurance for this country will have on affordable average cost of care or if we have set up a business model that functions much more like a car insurance approach that will allow people to buy collision coverage after the accident.

We Want Everyone in the Risk Pool for Health Insurance

Our goal as a country is very clearly to get everyone in the risk pool for health insurance.

There is actually a penalty in the new law that says anyone who does not buy coverage must pay a fine for not having coverage. That penalty is not huge -- but it is real and it will at least draw attention to the enrollment issue for uninsured people in the individual market. The government is also setting up insurance marketplaces called insurance exchanges in every state. The new insurance exchanges will provide premiums subsidies to low income people who will be buying individual insurance. That will obviously increase insurance sales. For many low income people, those subsidies will pay most of the premium. That is an extremely important financial reality. The affordability issues that could cause risk pools to deteriorate are being softened a lot by the fact that many people's premiums will be subsidized -- health coverage will be much more affordable for many people. The exchanges, if they are run well, will also give consumers an easy way of buying individual coverage and getting access to available subsidizes. The subsidies that will be available through the exchanges will make care more affordable for significant number of low income people.

One stated goal of the exchanges is to create competition between health plans for individual insurance sales. Consumers will be able to choose between competing health plans in each exchange. Informed choices will be available in the best exchanges. The new features are all good -- but the very best feature of the exchanges relative to the issue of keeping risk pools intact and viable is that low income people will have their premium levels subsidized in the exchange.

Lower income people who buy coverage in the exchanges will have premium subsidies that are based on their personal financial situations. That should be a major positive factor that will help set a wide range of people enrolled. The new subsidies will reduce the affordability barrier hugely for many people. Experience has shown that premium affordability is the primary reason people either do not buy health insurance or cancel health insurance. Premium subsidies obviously can mitigate that barrier.

If a significant number of healthy people who have low income levels decide to enroll in the individual market plans, then the risk pool issues for the individual insurance coverages can be significantly reduced.

If, however, only the low income people who actually have high health care needs enroll in the plans though the exchanges, then the risk pool issues that result from that process could be highly problematic and catastrophic for some organizations and markets.

We don't know today how well that process will work. We don't know how many healthy people will enroll in the new guaranteed issue insurance plans. We do know that we will need enough healthy people to enroll in those health plans and to contribute to be insured by those plans to keep the risk pools for those plans from deteriorating. If the only people who decide to buy insurance from a plan after January 1st of next year are the sick people in each market, then the average cost of care for the insured people in each existing risk pool will go up.

The math is actually pretty simple. Look at one very simple but very possible hypothetical outcome. If the people who end up buying insurance from a given insurer have care costs that are twice as high as the community average, then the premium that will be needed to pay for their care will be twice as high as the premium that would be needed to buy care for that risk pool if the people who are in the pool and who are insured actually had average costs of care.

The Risk Pools Are Viable in Europe Because Everyone Is in Them

That simple fact of arithmetic truth about the average cost of care is true everywhere on the planet. In Europe, where so many countries today use private insurance companies as the only way they insure people, the risk pools for the insurers are all viable. Why haven't those European countries seen a massive risk pool deterioration problem if the health insurers are all required to take all sick applicants for care? The risk-pool situation in Europe requires every single person to buy insurance -- and that works for individual insurance sales in Europe just like the group coverage risk pool that covers the entire group works today in our country.

Everyone in each European country who sells private insurance is in the mega group for the country. Everyone in that mega group now chooses an insurance company. Insurance companies can cover people at affordable premium levels in those European settings because the insurers have everyone in the country absolutely insured. Those countries have a pure mandate. Coverage is not optional. Everyone in those countries must buy private insurance. Those countries do not have just sick people buying health insurance. There are no exceptions. Europe has no "free riders" when it comes to people not making their contributions to the shared risk pool.

The governments in each of those European countries understand the basic arithmetic realities of risk pools. The purchase of health insurance is simply mandated for all citizens in those countries. The Dutch, Swiss and Germans all join private health plans. That "individual mandate" keeps everyone in those countries in the risk pool and that keeps the premium levels affordable in those countries.

Care Costs Are Not Evenly Distributed

The people who make the laws in those European countries understand, clearly, the cost distribution realities that are shown on the next charts.

They know that care costs are not evenly distributed. Care costs are not evenly distributed in our country and they are not evenly distributed in Europe. Remember -- in any given risk pool -- about one percent of the people incur about 20 percent of the cost. Five percent of the people incur about 50 percent of the cost. And ten percent of the people incur about 70 percent of the cost.[234]

In every country, small numbers of people incur most of the costs. Most people incur very few costs. The eighty percent of the population who incurs very few costs are the people whose premium dollars are needed and used to buy care for the people who need care.

This is very important chart to understand.

Figure 6.1

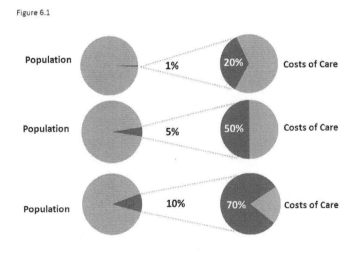

That disproportionate distribution of costs for care across populations is true in the U.S. and it is true in every other country where data is available.

When you look at that distribution of costs from the perspective of health insurance functionality, and risk pool viability, it means that some people in each risk pool will use care and others who are in that same pool will pay their own personal premium but those people will use little or no care. The secret of success for any risk pool setting is to collect regular premiums from all of the people who are not using care so their money can be used to pay for the costs of the people who are actually using care.

The 50 percent of the population in each European country who uses no care in any given year all pay their premiums continuously in those countries so that the 1 percent of the population of Germany or Switzerland or Holland who use 30 percent of the total care dollars can have their care paid for with that premium money that was paid into the pool by everyone.

Having everyone in the risk pool obviously makes premiums much more affordable. When you calculate the average cost of care used by insured people to determine your premium, that average cost of care is a lot lower if half of the people who pay premium personally used zero care dollars.

No One Can Predict the Outcome

So what will be the final impact on individual insurance risk pools in this country from all of these changes?

No one knows.

At this point in time, that impact of all of those factors on future risk issues is both unknown and unknowable. Under the right set of circumstances, there will be more people covered next year and they will have better benefits and more financial security. Under a worst set of circumstances, the result of those changes and those resultant premium adjustments could be risk pools that deteriorate, collapse, and even meltdown -- with extremely high premiums charged in a year or so to the people who still buy insurance. That scenario would leave us with even fewer people insured than we have today.

The jury is out.

The Medicaid expansion created by the new law is not affected in any way by these risk pool issues. For those states who are expanding their Medicaid coverage, the Medicaid expansion population is defined and inclusive, and Medicaid coverage under the new law in those states doesn't involve consumer choice about whether to pay premiums or to be insured.

Likewise, the Medicare future marketplace and the Medicare risk pools are not at risk from any changes made in the law.

The group insurance marketplace in this country is also not at risk. That is a very good thing. We really do not want our group health insurance marketplace to be at risk. Most people who have private health coverage in this country today get their coverage through their employer. These selection-related risk factors are not relevant to employer group coverage because everyone in each employer group is simply covered -- and the chances for people to make individual decisions that could cause group risk pools to meltdown do not exist.

But for the individual insurance market -- for the type of health insurance that is purchased directly by private individuals -- we can expect that the new rating, pricing and coverage rules will trigger a whole set of potentially problematic issues -- and we will see the impact of all of those factors beginning in January of 2014 and then rolling through the next couple of years as the process unfolds.

So what do we know for sure right now?

We know that premiums will go up for some people and we know that premiums will go down for other people.

We know the rate changes for some people will be significant... and that those rates will be different for individuals.

We do not know what the total consequences of the new rule sets will be on the market for individual health insurance in America.

We will be a lot smarter 24 months from now.

The New Insurance Exchanges Can Create a New Marketplace for Coverage

The individual marketplace has been transformed as of January of 2014. In addition to the laws relating to the guaranteed sale of insurance, the current law requires every state to set up health insurance exchanges that will function as a marketplace for competing health insurance companies. As this chapter pointed out earlier, those new individual insurance market exchanges may be a wonderful and brilliant thing to do. Done well, the new exchanges could give consumers a chance to make informed choices between competing health plans and health insurers.

If the exchanges are well designed, they will facilitate informed choices, care system competition, team care, and benefit packages focused on the consumer and not the insurer or the business needs of the insurer.

The exchanges will not have an immediate impact on the people who get their coverage through larger group. The exchanges will, however, be the only place where all of the people who buy individual coverage and who have income levels that are low enough to qualify for a government premium subsidy will their coverage.

Exchanges Could Mandate Team Care

The existence of the exchanges gives the government a wonderful opportunity to make a real difference in setting up a context for purchasing both coverage and care. Since we know that we want team care for people who need team care, the exchanges in each state could set rules that say every health insurer who sells coverage through an exchange must have products available to the consumers that that feature, support and utilize team care.

Each exchange could also mandate that participating insurers make quality data available to consumers who are choosing between health plans and providers of care. Well-structured exchanges can help significantly with the evolution of American health coverage and health care. All of the goals identified in the cash flow chapter of this book can be implemented as specifications for health plans under the exchanges. Some state exchanges are doing that kind of work now. The others could and should do that work in the future.

We Need Affordable Coverage

We need coverage to be affordable.

This model will fail if premium isn't affordable.

We need coverage linked to the care delivery models we want to encourage. We need coverage from viable insurers who will have both the risk pool stability to survive and the provider delivery competence to be both high quality and affordable.

For the business model of care to thrive, we also need the business model of coverage to thrive. We need the business model for both health coverage and health care delivery to be high performance and thriving.

The single biggest leverage point we have to make care better for the country is all the care we buy through the government.

Having the government became a better buyer of care is the topic of the next chapter.

CHAPTER SEVEN

WE CAN'T ALLOW GOVERNMENT-FUNDED HEALTH CARE TO CRIPPLE OUR ECONOMY

We really cannot afford to allow the health care costs that are being incurred by our Medicare and Medicaid programs destroy our state and federal budgets and seriously damage our economy. That is the path we are on today. It is clearly the wrong path to be on.

The biggest strains and the biggest financial burdens for our state and federal budgets are currently the cost increases that are projected for those two major government-purchased health care programs. Medicare and Medicaid expenses are literally squeezing other key functional priorities -- such as education and infrastructure repair -- out of our governmental budgets at multiple levels.

We should not allow those projected spending increases to happen. We should do sane and reasonable things to restrain the rate of growth in both programs and we should hold those expenses to levels that do not destroy our budgets.

This pie chart below shows the projected impact on the federal budget of both programs for just this decade.

Medicaid is not only a major federal government expense -- it is also the largest single expense item in most state budgets.

The next chart shows the impact in state budget spending levels that happened a year ago because of increases in the state Medicaid budgets. As you can see, Medicaid spending grew at the expense of all other major categories of spending.

Figure 7.1

Medicare & Medicaid as a Share of the Federal Budget

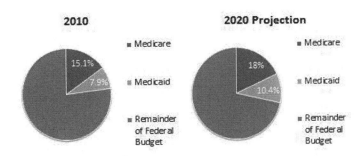

2010

2020 Projection

SOURCE: Historical spending for 1980 – 2010 from Congressional Budget Office (CBO) Budget and Economic Outlook: Historical Budget Data (January 2011); projected spending for 2020 from CBO Update to the Budget and Economic Outlook: Fiscal Years 2012 to 2022 (August 2012).

Figure 7.2

Changes in General Fund Spending by Category Between Fiscal 2011 and Fiscal 2012

Health Care Spending Continues to Drive General Fund Growth

Fiscal 2011 data is based on enacted budgets and fiscal 2012 data is based on governors' proposed budgets

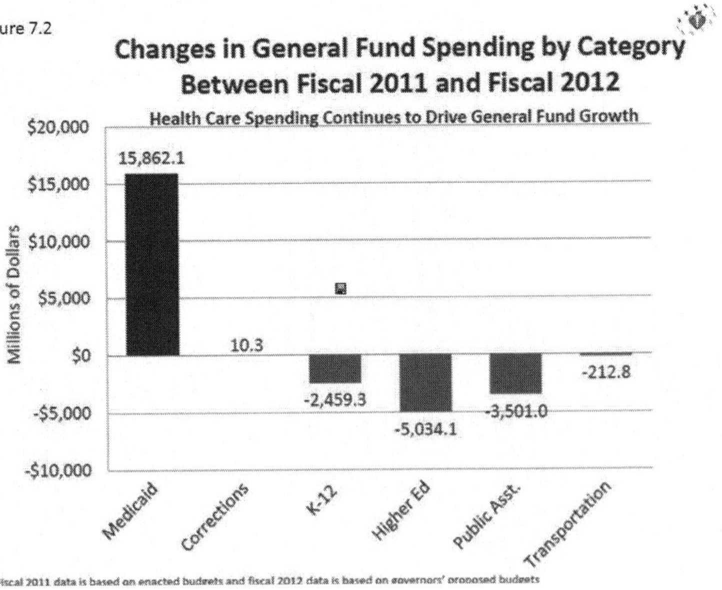

It is not a good thing to spend that much taxpayer money on healthcare. It is not a good thing to have health care costs eating up other governmental programs. The truth is -- we can do better. We can take steps that will reduce the projected rates of increase in both of those programs and we can improve the effectiveness and the quality of the care delivered by both programs at the same time.

It would be bad enough if we were paying those growing health care costs with current tax dollars. The truth is, we are actually borrowing money as a country to pay some of those health care bills.

Using debt financing to pay for current health care costs means that we are using health care services for ourselves and for our fellow Americans today and then we are simply sending the bills for much of that care into the future to be paid by our children and our grandchildren. Our children and grandchildren will literally need to pay taxes in the future to buy our care today. Their paychecks and their bank accounts will be reduced by those taxes.

Spending their tax money to pay for our current costs of care will prevent them from being able to use using their own tax money to deal with the actual issues that they will face themselves at that point in time. That is not a good thing to do to our children and grandchildren. We need to do sensible and reasonable things now so we can to spend less money on those programs today and not have to borrow money to buy that care.

We should have the insight, the skill, and the political courage to deal effectively with health care costs today. If we can't reduce those costs today, we should at least decide to simply pay for today's care with today's tax dollars. We have two fully ethical choices about how to avoid creating that debt burden for our children. We could avoid that burden by raising taxes today to pay for that care with our own money, or we could avoid borrowing that money by cutting costs. Both of those solutions are preferable to the path we are on. For us to duck, avoid, hide from and ignore difficult issues today relating to health care costs and for us to choose instead to have our children use their future wages and earnings and their future tax cash flow to pay -- with interest -- for our current care is not a good thing to do. We should be apologizing to our children for making that choice. We definitely should stop doing it.

The very best way to stop using their money to pay for our care is to do the things now that are necessary to bring today's costs for those major programs down to the levels where the costs can be funded with today's dollars.

Debt Financing Can Be an Intelligent Strategy for the Right Expense

That is the key message of this chapter.

The point being made here is not that debt financing for government expenses is inherently a bad thing to do. Debt financing can be a very good thing to do. Speaking as a business head who has been the CEO of one functional, operational and successful multi-billion business or another for more than three decades, the pure business truth is that debt financing can be a brilliant thing to do. Businesses use debt financing all the time in very intelligent ways. Businesses that need capital can use debt in highly productive ways to build factories, to buy stores and expand work sites, and even to train workers. Businesses that have been managed by the author have literally borrowed multiple billions of dollars over the years. Raising money appropriately through debt financing can make wonderful practical and functional sense for a business. If the borrowed money is used wisely and used well, that borrowed money can significantly increase, enhance and improve the future success levels for a business. The factory or the hospital that is built today with borrowed money can allow the business who borrowed the money to build the products to sell and deliver the services that are needed to be a successful business far into the future. Smart debt can be a good thing for a business to do when smart debt improves future success levels for the business.

Likewise, when governments use debt financing to build streets, roads, power supplies, schools, and to create appropriate workforce availability -- and when governments use debt financing to buy expensive and durable pieces of long lasting functional and operational equipment and infrastructure, the future functional gains that result for society from making those kinds of investments can make debt financing a very legitimate and desirable way for the government to create and channel cash flow. That money can be used in very productive ways to good purposes with legitimate results and with valuable returns and consequences.

Building a Bridge With Borrowed Money Can Be a Smart Thing To Do

In a nutshell, borrowing money as a government to build a needed bridge can make great sense. The new bridge can improve societal and economic functionality today and the actual bridge that is built today can extend that functionality far into the future. It is clearly both fair and appropriate to use debt financing mechanisms to transfer some of the cost burden of building a bridge to future generations of taxpayers because those future taxpayers will also get good use of that bridge.

We Are Not Using That Debt Money To Build Health Care Bridges

That approach to debt makes significant sense. It is a fair and practical way to think about debt. That is not, however, what we are doing with our current debt financing for health care services.

We are not borrowing money from the future to build the functional equivalent of a health care bridge. Borrowing money as a government and incurring significant levels of long term governmental debt to generate the cash needed to pay off current situational, incidental, ephemeral, transitory and entirely transitional health care costs for today's patients is a very different thought process and a very different financial equation than paying with future money to build a bridge. We should be very conscious about using the money raised by future taxes to buy things that the future taxpayers will not benefit from in any way.

We Do Not Need To Spend This Much Money on Care

Using debt to finance today's care is particularly inappropriate when we are actually spending money today on care that we do not need to spend on care. We are spending too much money for the care we are buying today. Using debt to finance excessive and unnecessary current spending is operationally inept. We need to address current costs. Current costs should be reduced. We should be spending less money on today's care.

Can that be done? Yes.

The truth is, there are multiple alternative strategies that we could use now to cut current health care costs for both of those major government programs to spending levels that do not require us to pass our current care costs off, down, and on to our children. Unfortunately, we have chosen -- for what are often short term political reasons -- not to look closely and seriously at those approaches and at those cost-mitigating strategies.

Care delivery will actually benefit from Medicare becoming a better purchaser of care if the purchasing process that is used is well designed, stable, predictable and set up to support care improvement rather than penalize caregivers for making care better and more effective.

The Strategy Will Need To Satisfy CBO Rules

The Congressional Budget Office (CBO) is the official scorekeeper for the costs that are either projected or reported for any given legislation or regulatory approaches. We need a strategy that will be scored by the CBO as achieving the goals we want to achieve or the plan is irrelevant.

We also very definitely need to turn the providers of care in this country into allies for this approach rather than enemies. We need to make some politically challenging decisions now that will actually control the cost of care today and we need to do that in a way that providers of care can benefit from the new approaches. The good news is that we should be able to achieve both of those goals. We need to build a model that will have the infrastructure of care evolving to take advantage of new opportunities rather than mobilizing to resist changes in their basic funding. To get the needed levels of provider support, we basically will primarily need to do what this book recommends at multiple levels and that is to move away from buying care only by the piece and put in place approaches that will purchase care for Medicare patients more by the package...and we need to do that in ways that will allow caregivers to benefit from that financial model.

This book has pointed out repeatedly that the business model we use now to buy most is primarily driven by the collection of fees. Business strategies for caregivers who treat Medicare patients today focus on optimizing volumes of those fees. And care for fee-for-service Medicare patients today is limited almost entirely to the specific pieces of care that are included on the Medicare fee schedule. We need the business models for the caregivers who treat Medicare patients to be focused on approaches and care delivery processes that will make care outcomes better without being handicapped by that piecework business model for buying care. We need purchasing approaches that can both bring down care costs and create financial benefits for caregivers.

Two Funding Tracks for Medicare

To achieve those goals, this book proposes that we now should set up two funding models and tracks for Medicare. One track should build off the current Medicare Advantage program. The second funding should continue to pay non-Medicare Advantage caregivers directly from Medicare -- but track two should build heavily on the new ACO, medical home, and bundled packages of care that Medicare is learning to use to buy care.

Both tracks of Medicare funding that are proposed in this chapter can and should help make care better for Medicare patients. The Medicare Advantage channel for cash can be set up to encourage the Medicare Advantage plans to work even more closely with their provider networks to improve the quality and affordability of care. Likewise, the track two funding approach should be set up to provide support for the caregivers who want to provide team care, data-linked care, and continuously improving care.

Medicare Advantage is listed as the first component of that two path strategy because Medicare Advantage is already set up to deliver care and Medicare Advantage already is a fixed payment model with a government defined and controllable cap on annual expenses. The government can easily cap care costs for Medicare Advantage every year by simply capping the amount paid to health plans for each senior who chooses to be a Medicare Advantage member.

Medicare Advantage currently caps the expense levels for the government for enrolled seniors very directly because Medicare now pays each of the Medicare Advantage participating health plans a flat payment every month per senior rather than continuing to buy care for those seniors by the piece. The Medicare Advantage plans already have the flexibility to use that flat monthly payment from Medicare to buy care in different and creative ways from the existing care delivery infrastructure.

The program has its critics, but it has had notable successes.

The results to date have shown that the care delivery levels have been improved for seniors who have enrolled in Medicare Advantage plans.[235] Basic quality of care levels are measured for seniors who enroll in those plans. The quality levels are measurably better for Medicare Advantage patients in all areas where comparative measures exist.

The Medicare Advantage plans have received far greater levels of regulatory oversight than the traditional Medicare care infrastructure. The Medicare Advantage enrollees are currently protected by tens of thousands of pages of regulations about various Medicare Advantage operational issues.[236]

Having people enroll in Medicare Advantage is track one of this proposed strategy -- and that track is explained in more detailed below.

Track Two Is Built on the Traditional Care Delivery Component

Track two for funding Medicare is to continue giving people who don't enroll in Medicare Advantage an enhanced extension of their traditional Medicare coverage. Track two continues using all American care providers who voluntary choose to be Medicare caregivers as the track two care network. That approach protects Medicare patient access for all caregivers who want to treat Medicare patients and who do not want to see those patients as part of one or more Medicare Advantage provider networks. Track two would allow Medicare beneficiaries who want to continue in the piecework care model to select their caregivers and their care sites from any and all caregivers who chose to be part of the traditional Medicare network of providers.

So what would cause the CBO to now give cost control credit of any kind for the expenses that would arise from the seniors who would elect to get their care from the track two traditional network of caregivers? We clearly have not been able to achieve targeted cost levels for the patients who get care from those caregivers in the past. Why would we be able to guarantee the cost for those care sites now? The answer is -- for track two spending levels -- the government should set spending targets by geographic area and should annually make up for any expense overruns in each area by adjusting future fees for caregivers in that area to make up the difference.

To control future spending levels, Medicare would set a fixed per senior cost target for each geography. Medicare would guarantee that those spending targets would be met for the track one, Medicare Advantage patients by controlling the per senior payment level that is made to the Medicare Advantage plans. Medicare would guarantee that those same per capita expense goals would be met for all patients who chose the track two Medicare extension approach and track two care network by adjusting the fees and the payment levels downward in future years in areas when the cost targets are missed.

Medicare actually has had a somewhat problematic version of that retrospective fee-adjustment approach in place in this country today. The current program is called Standardized Growth Rates or SGR. That program has not been a success. The current SGR program also calls for the fees that are paid by Medicare to be adjusted downward whenever Medicare misses annual cost increase targets. The current version of the SGR program has actually been a clear and absolute failure up to now for three main reasons. One reason for the failure of the SGR approach is that the payment reduction approach has not actually ever been activated as a fee reduction tool. Instead of adjusting future fees downward each year to make up for annual Medicare costs that have exceeded targets, the fee cuts that were needed to do that work have been ducked, deferred, and delayed every year...for both political and economic reasons.

Wishful Thinking Was Not a Good Cost Reduction Plan

The second reason the current SGR approach has failed is that it was far too broad in its scope and target setting. The current SGR approach was set up as a national goal with national penalties. That financial mechanism was far too crude and too macro to be an effective leverage tool or functional behavior motivator in any local care setting. The current SGR did not and could not reflect any local cost realities or any local cost and expense level achievements. It was pure wishful thinking to believe that local caregivers across the country would change their behaviors or their care plans to somehow try to influence a national cost number. By contrast, the SGR-two model that is proposed by this book would be to set up and create very local cost targets and then do very local retrospective fee adjustments that are based on local performance levels. Local successes are possible.

The macro target that was set for the current SGR approach was so broad and so distant that it did not directly affect the behaviors of any actual caregivers. The likelihood of a local doctor becoming more efficient in some way with their Medicare patients in order to prevent a future national SGR fee adjustment from happening for the entire country is obviously pretty remote. It was really wishful thinking in one of its purest forms.

The current SGR approach has obviously failed entirely as a functional macro or micro motivator of either physician or hospital behavior.

By contrast, under the proposed SGR-two approach, the use of more local geographic area adjustments could actually be very motivating for local sets of caregivers. Using local fee adjustments could motivate good performance in collaborative ways on the part of local caregivers relative to both care costs and care volumes. The caregivers in a city could collectively decide that basic science-based standards for CT scans should be jointly used, for example. That kind of collaborative care improvement work would make care better in local settings and it could help bring down local care costs. The likelihood of those goals having a local influence on collective behavior are obviously greater than the likelihood of a national SGR creating any collaborative local behavior or any changes in caregiver behaviors.

Magical Thinking Was the Third Reason for Failure

The third reason the current SGR-one approach has failed is that it had no strategy of any kind embedded in it. There was no related strategy to reduce costs or to make care more effective or efficient in any way. SGR-one was purely magical thinking -- with no functional attempt by Medicare to help caregivers improve the costs or quality of care in any setting in any way. The SGR-one proposed impact on care delivery was a wish and a hope -- but it was clearly not a plan or a strategy.

By contrast, the newer SGR-two approach can benefit from some new tools that are being used to mitigate the costs of care.

SGR-two could build on all of the new tools that Medicare is making available for care improvement -- the new ACOs, the new medical homes, the new bundled payment approaches, and the new "meaningful use" rules for connecting electronic medical records between care sites. All of these approaches can help bring down the costs of care. ACOs are not magical thinking. Medical homes are not magical thinking. Local caregivers would be encouraged and incented to use all of those tools because successful use of those tools could help local caregivers achieve the annual cost constraint goals and avoid having future fees reduced by the SGR-two fee reduction formulae.

The cost calculation model for SGR-two could be relatively sophisticated in the application of the local goal to individual local care sites.

In cases where any of new ACOs are set up by the caregivers to accept the equivalent of a prepayment amount for their care, those sites could even be measured separately from the SGR adjustment used for the entire local geographic area. Those sites could be excluded from the regulation and fee-adjusted process if those sites that are ACOs and medical homes are achieving the targeted goals directly through their own performance levels.

That process would be a little more difficult to administer than a flat regional adjustment but it could be done because those sites already will be tracking relevant cost information as certified ACOs. The reason to use that approach is that using that kind of SGR-two approach could functionally guarantee scoreable savings for track two of Medicare for the federal government. Those saving will actually happen if the government has the will to actively implement the SGR fee rollbacks in those settings where those rollbacks are earned by higher than targeted local Medicare costs.

If we set the cost target levels for both tracks at the right levels, the combination of the two tracks would give us the absolute ability we need to protect Medicare payments and expenses forward and to guarantee that overall cost targets will be met. If those cost targets are set low enough, they could end the need for the government to borrow money to fund Medicare deficits. Because the costs for both tracks are functionally capped, the borrowing could cease as soon as the program effective date for track one and track two happens.

Medicare Advantage Has a Great Set of Advantages

Medicare Advantage actually has the potential to stop the cost trend explosion for Medicare all by itself. Medicare Advantage plans are already strongly incented and empowered to use care-enhancing tools like medical homes, subcontracting ACOs, expanded quality reporting and continuous improvement approaches for various elements of care. Our country will not ever mandate full Medicare Advantage enrollment or order a full enrollment in Medicare Advantage to happen -- but if every single senior in this country was enrolled tomorrow in a Medicare Advantage plan, the defined contribution strategy of a fixed payment per month per senior that the government already uses to fund Medicare Advantage would give the government full and immediate control over all Medicare costs in one fell swoop. If every senior in America was a Medicare Advantage enrollee, the government could control per person costs for Medicare by simply controlling the per person payment that is made to Medicare Advantage plans and we would not need to borrow from our children to pay for Medicare expenses today.

Medicare Advantage Works Very Well Now

So what is the status of the Medicare Advantage program today?

It is a popular program.

Roughly, 30 percent of Americans seniors have already voluntarily chosen to enroll in Medicare Advantage plans.[237] In the long-established Medicare Advantage geographic markets, the percent of voluntarily enrolled seniors can range up to 70 percent. For all of those seniors, Medicare has already stopped buying care by the piece. The government now buys the full package of care from Medicare Advantage health plans for a fixed price using the Medical Advantage payment approach. It is a relatively simple financial arrangement. The health plans who sell Medicare Advantage coverage must offer a defined package of benefits to seniors. Those plans are then paid a flat amount of money every month by Medicare rather than being paid fees on a piecework basis by Medicare.

When a senior enrolls in a Medicare Advantage plan, the government has no financial expense or exposure beyond the premiums that are paid by Medicare to the Medicare Advantage plans. Each Medicare Advantage plan takes all risk for care costs. The plan is responsible for the cost of care.

The plan also has to deal directly with all payment and financial issues related to problems like fraud and misbilling by providers of care.

The key difference between Medicare Advantage and traditional piecework Medicare payment approach is the cash flow.

Medicare Advantage gives the government a tool to buy full packages of care -- not just pieces of care -- from health plans and related care systems. The Medicare Advantage package price for each year is both fixed and guaranteed for both the government and the caregivers. Because the government pays a package price per member for Medicare Advantage enrollees, there is no chance that volume increases, fee increases, or perverse care decisions by any caregiver or any caregiver business entity will increase government costs. The Medicare Advantage program payment approach insulates the government from all of those cost drivers because the plans become the entities accountable for managing all of those issues and costs. That per capita cash flow model gives the plans great flexibility in dealing with caregiver business units. Medicare Advantage plans can be very creative in their contracting with their provider networks. Medicare Advantage plans can set up and fund medical home relationships or can help care sites organize into Accountable Care Organizations. In the process, Medicare advantage plans can set up cash flow arrangements with caregivers that are liberated from the traditional Medicare piecework fee schedule.

Medicare Advantage Insulates the Government From Provider Fraud

The Medicare Advantage payment model allows the plans to do creative and innovative things with caregivers in ways that can never be achieved under the standard, rigid, Medicare piecework payment model.

Interestingly -- and very few people recognize this fact to be true -- the Medicare Advantage program payment approach also insulates the government from provider-level fraud.

Many people who look at health care policy issues literally do not know that particular benefit to be true. But that protection for the government cash flow against provider fraud is inherent to the Medicare Advantage fixed payment cash flow model. Fraud is a major and growing problem for the rest of traditional fee-paid Medicare today. One of the major operational priorities for the current piecework Medicare payment program is to reduce the hundreds of billions of dollars in provider business unit fraud that exist today. The government has been building extensive programs of auditing and payment review to help mitigate that fraud -- and yet the fraud levels for Medicare fee-for-service piecework payment programs continue to increase.

The fee-based payment business model that is used by traditional Medicare to buy care by the piece is obviously at the heart of the fraud problem. The temptations to commit fraud that are created by a piecework billing system that pays out billions of dollars by the piece are too great for too many healthcare business units to avoid. By contrast, the flat monthly payment that is made by government to Medicare Advantage plans insulates the government from that fraud. If fraud happens, the cost of the fraud is absorbed by the health plan and it is not passed on to the tax payer or to the federal debt through the Medicare fee-for-service cash flow. The plans, therefore, obviously each have a very strong incentive to do their own fraud detection and prevention. It is often easier for the plans to do that fraud protection work, however, because almost all of the care providers for the Medicare Advantage plans are both in networks and under contract and that set of relationship helps mitigate fraud.

Medicare Advantage Has Robust Quality Reporting

Medicare Advantage also has a much more robust quality reporting mechanism compared to fee-based Medicare. Fee-forpservice Medicare has a weak and woeful record of quality reporting and quality improvement. There are no quality reports, very little data, and very weak quality improvement agendas for traditional piecework Medicare. As this book had pointed out multiple times, quality screw-ups and care misfires increase the cash flow for many fee-paid Medicare provider sites.

By contrast, Medicare Advantage has a robust set of quality reports and quality improvement agendas. Solid quality reports exist today for Medicare Advantage patients for diabetic care, hypertension, heart disease and a whole array of other conditions -- with 55 separate measures of quality[238] and service now used to track care for Medicare Advantage members.

Paying attention to quality makes a difference. Overall, quality of care tends to be significantly and measurable better for Medicare Advantage patients compared to patients who get their care in the piecework Medicare payment approach. Some people had some initial concerns about quality for the first generation of the Medicare Advantage programs -- so extensive quality reporting has been embedded into the Medicare Advantage program in a way that has no parallel or equivalent function anywhere in the piecework Medicare payment model. Quality is reported, measured, tracked, guaranteed and transparent for Medicare Advantage patients and members.

The federal government has written thousands of pages of regulations about the operations of Medicare Advantage plans and Medicare Advantage members have clear mechanisms for reporting concerns about either quality, service or access to care.

Piecework Medicare Has Almost No Quality Reporting

That is very different from the quality agenda that this country uses for piecework Medicare. There are almost no quality measures now for the piecework payment approach that is used today by traditional Medicare. Basically, none. Medicare Advantage, by contrast, has grown to include nearly five dozen separate and relevant measures of quality and service. That entire quality agenda is a valuable asset that the government should utilize and build on as we look at how we can improve care and reduce costs for Medicare patients. It has taken decades to build up that robust quality reporting infrastructure for Medicare Advantage. The quality of care for Medicare Advantage enrollees is known, measured, reported, and comparative quality data is part of the decision-making process for consumers who are selecting their personal health plans.

The ACO Quality Measures Echo Medicare Advantage

The people who designed the new ACO quality measurement provisions for the new set of ACO regulations have built much of their quality reporting around that Medicare Advantage template and thought processes. When the ACO regulation designers looked for an approach to use to track and monitor quality, some of the existing Medicare Advantage quality reporting advantages were pretty clear. The standalone rules for ACOs ultimately settled for a "lighter version" of those MA quality requirements and changed some measurements because piecework paid providers often have a very hard time delivering good quality data.

The whole ACO effort is, however, as stated earlier -- very much directionally correct. But that whole ACO approach is just being constructed. Medicare Advantage, by contrast, doesn't need to be built, constructed, invented or even reinvented at this point in time. The whole MA quality agenda isn't theoretical or hypothetical. It's very real. All of the infrastructure needed to run Medicare Advantage is in place, tested operationally and fully functional.

There Is No Way of Knowing That Quality Standards Are Met for Piecework Medicare

As we take steps now to figure out how to figure out how to improve care and bring down the costs of care for Medicare recipients, we should be very aware that very few of the quality and service level oversight and data reporting approaches that are used for Medicare Advantage today exist in any way for the fee-for-service component of traditional Medicare. For most components of traditional piecework Medicare, the government literally has no idea if any care standards are being met. The new medical home- and ACO-reporting approaches will begin to provide some of the data, but at its core, the current piecework Medicare payment approach has no tracking mechanisms for the Medicare patients who have diabetes, hypertension, depression, or any other chronic conditions. Accountability levels for the care for piecework fee-based Medicare funded care approach have always been almost non-existent. It will not be easy to change in that piecework payment model. Creating any level of accountable care tracking for seniors who are not enrolled in Medicare Advantage plans will be extremely difficult. The new SGR-two proposal that is described in this chapter is intended to help improve that situation by steering as many fee-paid Medicare patients as possible into either certified patient-focused medical home settings or into federally certified ACOs -- places and settings where some new quality standards and reports are being built and implemented. Enrolling all seniors into either Medicare

Advantage plans or into SGR-two care sites with quality reporting will create better transparency for everyone about the quality of care, and it will trigger a more robust set of care delivery regulations.

The cash flow for the seniors who enroll in either track should be adjusted to reflect the health status of the seniors in each track. It is a good idea to adjust the payment level in actuarially legitimate ways to reflect the health care "risk" levels for each senior. Medicare Advantage already uses that payment approach to reflect the differences in enrollment between health plans. The specific amount of money that is paid to health plans for each senior enrolled in a Medicare Advantage plan is basically based on the age and the gender of each senior. There is, however, also a significant adjustment made to the Medicare Advantage payment to reflect the health risk level of each member.

In other words, a Medicare Advantage plan is paid more money each month for a diabetic or hypertensive senior than that same plan is paid for a totally healthy senior. That risk adjustment payment model works for the government because it encourages health plans with good care quality and solid team care to enroll diabetic and other high risk seniors. That payment approach also doesn't encourage health plans to duck patients with chronic conditions and try to focus their sales efforts on enrolling healthy seniors. That health status adjusted business model works well for health plans because it encourages the plans to deliver great care for each diabetic member because the plans can keep their overall costs down by delivering better and more effective care to those patients.

Overall -- when care is delivered as a process and a package, care gets better. Diabetes is now -- in the standard piecework payment model -- the number one cause of amputations.[239] Diabetes is also the number one cause of kidney failure for Americans.[240] In the current fee-based payment approach, patients with diabetes consumes over 40 percent of all Medicare costs.[241] Forty percent is a lot of money. It's easy to see how that high level of expense happens for standard Medicare piecework patients. In the piecework approach, all care is incidental. Crisis care is rewarded rather than penalized in that payment model. Fees are piled on fees when crisis happen. Bad outcomes create even more fees in that payment model. Outcomes and care quality are highly problematic for far too many people under that piecework payment care approach.

The truth is that paying a package price for diabetic care makes a lot more sense than buying many separate pieces of care for diabetic patients. A package payment for diabetic care does not reward the failure of care. The business model and the care delivery model that results from buying care by the package rather than just buying pieces of care has an economic elegance that works very directly in favor of optimal health and continuously improving care outcomes.

Medicare Advantage Sets Up Health Plan Competition Now

Quite a few health care economists have called for the creation of real competition in various elements of health care. The economists want competition so that the health care marketplace can achieve the benefits that typically result in other markets from real competition. Real competition in health care could involve buyers being able to choose between legitimate competitors based on value and price. Real competition clearly and obviously does not happen today in any real way in the piecework portion of the Medicare economy. Neither value or price competition happens for those providers of care.

Real competition does happen, however, between Medicare Advantage plans.

Medicare Advantage plans compete fiercely with each other today. The competition between the plans is set up in a context where seniors actually benefit from the competitive performance of the plans.

Medicare Advantage plans compete with each other in a safely regulated marketplace for senior enrollees. They compete today on the basis of functionality, service levels, benefits and prices. Those are excellent categories for competition. The per-senior monthly payment cash flow model works well to allow, enable, and incent real competition to happen between the health plans. The Medicare Advantage program currently engages market forces on behalf of seniors. That is a good thing. We really do need the energies that are created by competing businesses situations to be at play for our Medicare patients. Medicare Advantage uses health plans to be the competing entities. That competition happens in a clearly constructed and carefully managed market environment.

Seniors who are enrolling in Medicare Advantage plans already have a lot of information to use to make choices relative to both benefit sets and health plan care networks. Medicare has very effectively set up an exchange -- that approach now for Medicare Advantage that allows seniors to choose between competing health plans based on service levels, quality and price.

This country is in the process of building new insurance exchanges in every state that will be used for the individual insurance portion of our non-governmental insurance market. One reason for us all to believe that new exchange model can work for that states and for that market is that a focused exchange approach works now for seniors and Medicare Advantage plans.

Medicare Advantage Cash Flow Encourages Plans and Providers To Work Together in ACO-Like Ways

One very important and extremely useful function of the current Medicare Advantage structure and cash flow is that it encourages health plans and caregivers to work together to serve seniors. Plans are learning to do that collective work with care sites and are doing it better every year. Plans can channel the Medicare Advantage cash flow into medical homes and ACOs with significant flexibility. Because the plans all sell entire packages of care to Medicare rather than just selling Medicare a list of fees, the participating health plans all have their own incentives, tools, strategies, opportunities and good reasons to work in increasing levels of partnership with an array of contracted providers to create team care and integrated care and variations on patient-focused care. That is happening today in multiple settings. Medicare Advantage plans are using a wide variety of creative care system linkages, allowances, and strategies to improve their Medicare Advantage product. Once again, a well-directed business model design is having a positive impact on both care and provider cash flow.

We May Need New Medicare Advantage Competitors

Some additional opportunities to extend competition even further for those patients could arise from inviting additional care organizations to become competing Medicare Advantage plans. The Medicare Advantage set of competing plans could be expanded if some of the traditional care systems that are not currently health plans could be helped to function directly as Medicare Advantage plans. There are a number of hospital system and medical care sites that could effectively organize and build the additional capabilities needed to do that work and play that role.

There are already 563 competing Medicare Advantage plans.[242] That is more competition than exists in most areas of the economy. But in some markets, there are relatively few competitors. Allowing local care systems who have the right functionality to become direct MA plans might make real sense in some markets.

Health care organizations that already aspire to ACO status and who are building ACO capabilities and infrastructure might have a particular interest in evolving one additional step to be able to take on the direct Medicare Advantage plan role as well. Having additional competition in that market could be a good thing for some portions of the market.

A New Competitor or a New Monopoly or Oligopoly?

The impact of changing the competitive situation for caregivers is almost always very market specific. Organizing local care providers into a new freestanding Medicare Advantage plan could create a new competitor or it could create a new local monopoly or solidify a local oligopoly. Monopolies and oligopolies are not good. Thriving competition is good. So the issue of whether or not additional local caregiver organizations should become a Medicare Advantage plan is very site specific. There are more than 500 health plans that now compete for Medicare Advantage patients across the country today.[243] That number is sufficient to create significant competitions in most markets, but having additional competitors in a number of markets could be good for both seniors and the market.

So there are a number of reasons why getting people to enroll in Medicare Advantage plans makes sense for the government. Budget control tools would suddenly exist for the government for those seniors. Expense caps become very real for that program. The government can very easily set a cash flow target for its own total expenses and they can achieve that target perfectly by simply setting up the annual Medicare Advantage payment level at a number that meets their cost target.

When you look at all of the relevant elements -- cost control, quality transparency, performance improvement incentives, fraud control, etc., -- it's obvious that the government would be more competent purchasers of care if Medicare recipients were enrolled in Medicare Advantage plan. It isn't a theoretical proposal or a hypothetical care model. The Medicare Advantage program plan is in place and it works.

How Can We Encourage Additional Medicare Advantage Enrollment?

So how could we get many more people to enroll in a Medicare Advantage plan? We are not likely as a country to issue a mandate and simply require every Medicare member to join a Medicare Advantage plan. That would work logistically, but it would have political ramifications. The plans are popular and growing -- and a majority of seniors in each mature Medicare Advantage local market do tend to voluntarily enroll in the plans -- but the abilities of our government to require a mandated enrollment in that program for all seniors is problematic.

Longer Open Enrollment for Three-Star Plans

Since that is true, what approach could be done to get seniors to either migrate to Medicare Advantage plans or to cause Medicare recipients to get their care in a way that doesn't continue to cause Medicare costs to explode? There is actually a way to achieve that goal.

We Need Plans in All Markets

To go down that path, we would first need to be sure that Medicare Advantage plans exist in all markets. We also should to expand the enrollment windows for Medicare Advantage plans for a couple of years to make enrollment easier for seniors. At the current time, only the Medicare Advantage plans with the very highest quality scores are allowed to enroll seniors 12 months of the year. Only 11 of the 563 Medicare Advantage plans have achieved that five-star quality rating, [244] so most seniors are now banned from enrollment in Medicare Advantage 10 months of the year. That enrollment opportunity in Medicare Advantage plans should be opened to 12 months for at least a couple of years for all plans who have three or more stars on the quality measurement level. It makes sense to make enrollment easier for a while for all plans that have earned three stars or higher. With the right enrollment programs, the number of seniors who voluntarily move to Medicare Advantage could grow significantly. Most seniors would probably voluntarily enroll over a couple of years if Medicare created the right marketing agenda for Medicare Advantage and then allowed the plans to run aggressive market based enrollment programs.

We Need To Also Control Costs for the People Who Don't Enroll in Medicare Advantage

As noted earlier, for the seniors who don't choose to join the Medicare Advantage program, we will need to offer the track two extension and continuum of the current set of providers that was described above.

The strategy for track two should be to help the caregivers who continue to work directly with Medicare with approaches that will improve their quality and their care. Obviously, having Medicare support patient-centered medical homes and ACOs should be a key element of that agenda.

We need the current infrastructure of care in this country to make active use of patient-centered medical homes, ACOs, and other forms of patient-focused, data-supported team care and we need Medicare cash flow to make that happen. This approach will only succeed if caregivers derive benefit from the new approach.

We need the existing infrastructure of care to benefit financially and operationally from using the new ACO and medical home tools for those patients. The SGR-two part of the track two strategy will be key to its successes. We can continue to pay for local care for local care from a wide range of caregivers on a piecework basis as long as we periodically adjust the fees if the total costs of care for any geographic area exceed the targets for that area.

If an area misses their cost target, we can simply adjust the fees in that area for each piece of care. As noted earlier, can move the fee levels in that area down as needed each year to allow each geographic area to achieve its own piecework model total payment cost target.

Other Countries Ration Cash, Not Care

We can and should implement all of the new care improvement tools in each setting to help make care better and more affordable. The real control and the absolute mechanism that CBO will recognize for limiting costs will, however, be the fee subsequent fee schedule adjustments. The truth is, we would not be the first country to control government program costs by controlling provider fees. Controlling fees is what most other governments in industrialized countries do now to control their costs of care.

Most other countries adjust the fees paid to providers each year to help achieve each country's annual health care cost goals. Those other countries who spend less than they do not ration care. They ration cash. They ration care costs by controlling care prices and fees…and not by rationing the actual delivery or volumes of care.

We could use a similar model here, for the Medicare recipients who are not enrolled in a track one Medicare Advantage plan. As noted earlier, local targets are far better than a national target. Using a macro one-size-fits-all national target doesn't make sense if we really want to encourage local care improvement. It really isn't fair to police and penalize providers in lower cost parts of the country for the higher costs that can be generated by the most abusive high cost parts of the country.

So the people who enroll in a Medicare Advantage plan will have costs approved for the government by the fixed payment per month -- and the people who stay with the fee-based care would have their costs capped by adjusting the fees.

Interestingly, having a two-path approach also could allow local providers who put in place successful ACOs to have their own cash flow reality. That new reality might lend itself to some very creative care delivery and care financing inventions and collaborations.

There could actually basically be three tracks of Medicare funding. Track one would be the Medicare Advantage track. Track two would be the traditional Medicare providers who decide to participate in ACOs or medical homes. Track three would be the stand-alone fee-for-service providers who deliver separate and unconnected piecework care with no alliances, no alignments, and no collaborations and whose fees would be annually adjusted if local spending levels exceed spending targets.

That multi-track approach could -- if done well -- achieve the same targeted macro cost per beneficiary down each Medicare funding track for this country.

Using a two track approach allows the Medicare program to continue to support both ACOs and medical homes, as well experimenting with various forms of bundled purchases of care. Every effort could and should be made by creative people in the care delivery infrastructure and in Washington, D.C., itself to make that portion of Medicare both successful and sustainable.

SGR Wasn't a Strategy -- It Was a Hope

It will seem strange to some people that this two track proposal involves a reuse of the SGR approach that had been both unsuccessful and remarkably unpopular.

The SGR idea had some merit. It was just badly done.

The old SGR approach failed, in large part, because no one did anything at any level to help it succeed. It was an orphaned program. The SGR strategy was connected to absolutely nothing real relative to any kind of cost constraints or cost mitigation of any kind. The idealists who proposed the initial SGR hoped when they wrote that law that actual caregivers in this country would all know that the new SGR approach existed and that knowledge would somehow inspire many of the caregivers to do some kinds of good things that would keep care costs down -- doing those good things simply because the SGR program existed. That was well meaning as a theory, but, as noted, earlier, it really was magical thinking. Pure magical thinking. No one had any real assignments or real strategies or any real visions or plans to do any part of that cost constraint work. There were no tools of any kind for any Medicare providers to work with to achieve the SGR goals. The government set the SGR targets and then let them hover in the economy unconnected to any cost controls or cost mitigation functionality. That approach could not have been less connected to care decisions. No one was really changing care in any way to help meet that first set of SGR targets. That's why SGR-one failed. There was no accountability anywhere for anyone hitting SGR targets at any level in any place.

The first generation SGR approach wasn't a strategy. It was a hope -- a macro target based on wishful thinking and not on any kind of actual cost mitigation or care improvement agendas or strategies. It was both magical thinking and a blend of a voodoo economics with a touch of earnest idealism thrown in to make the approach feel good and politically correct at the time.

Today, we simply spend too much money on Medicare, and we are ducking the real issues and the costs we are creating are forcing our kids and our grandkids to pay for our care. This blended approach can allow us to stop using borrowed money to pay for today's cost of care for Medicare patients. The goal of the two-track approach should be to set up real spending targets that work financially to meet the budget goals of the government.

We Need Dependable, Long-Term Targets To Enable Reengineering

We will also want the new cash flow approach to set up real and dependable multiyear revenue targets that will give providers of care a sense of stability about future revenue plans and cash flows. Stability should be a key priority for this entire strategy. Ask anyone who runs an actual care site why that is true. Stability of cash flow empowers and enables future actual reengineering of real processes at real care sites. We should set up the new Medicare cost targets for three to five years at a time -- we should not move the targets, payment levels or rate sets around annually. Assuring stability for future cash flows is actually very important in the real world for providers of care because it is a lot easier to do the really hard work that is involved in reengineering care in actual care sites if you know what the total cash flow will be for your care site when you are done doing the reengineering.

Very few people who have not been actually involved in the direct delivery of care understand how important it can be for care sites to have some stability for future cash flows to enable reengineering of care processes.

People underestimate the value of stability for triggering and funding the reengineering process for care. If the heart transplant programs mentioned in the last chapter had been encouraged to reengineer that care -- but if the buyers said that they might not actually pay the restructured package price for future heart transplants for more than one year, very little reengineering would have happened in those care sites. We need multiyear goals for Medicare costs. Knowing what future cash flows will be for Medicare patients will give providers a secure revenue stream to use as the core of the reengineering process.

Five Years Rolling Goals Could Achieve Multiple Results

The very best way of achieving overall success for Medicare and the infrastructure of care delivery in America would probably be to set specific total cost goals for the country for five years in advance and then to advance the five year goal annually and roll the full set of goals forward each year to create a new five year goal set.

Some people will object to having the macro cost cap numbers for Medicare presented as five-year rolling goals instead of having annually bid processes of some kind that could change prices annual or even sooner.

Remember -- the goal we want to achieve for Medicare stability and Medicare affordability is met if we achieve a defined multiyear Medicare spending level. Setting multiyear term goals that meet Medicare needs for a defined spending level is preferable to a process where financial goals for Medicare change annually -- and therefore the cash flow coming from Medicare could change annually.

Volatile Cash Flow Undermines Care Reengineering

That need for revenue stability for future cash flow might not make sense to some people who haven't tried to redesign the functional processes of care in the real world. People who don't know much about managing the actual functionally and operational structure of care delivery might advocate for a much more volatile cash flow model -- with prices and capitation levels for plans and caregivers varying year to year -- creating some real risk of year-by-year instability for the projected cash flow for care sites and health plans. Some people might suggest that the Medicare Advantage capitation levels should be set on an annual basis -- maybe even have the capitation levels set by some kind of annual market-based bidding process in each market.

One approach, for example, might be to have local bidding of some kind done each year with the annual bids from local vendors somehow creating the payment level for local Medicare Advantage plans for the next year or two.

There are a couple of problems with that short-term bid-based model. One problem is that the process steps that would be involved in using those bids to determine the actual annual cash flow for each plan is more complex than we need at this point to simply meet our goals. We should be entirely satisfied if a solid multiyear number built into the multiyear plan already achieves the Medicare's functional cost targets. Bidding processes can move costs up or bidding process could move costs down. Medicare doesn't need variable costs. Medicare needs guaranteed and affordable costs. "Good enough" should be "good enough" for achieving the cost targets. For the next few years, to fully meet our immediate financial goals for Medicare we just need a multiyear guarantee that Medicare overall costs will go up no more than a target number for each year -- say, three percent.

We don't actually need the prices involved in Medicare funding to jump around. We just need the cost increases to meet our spending goal. And by declaring that fixed annual price increase to be the basis of the actual cash flow number, down each track, we will create whole new business model reality for the providers of care and for the health plans.

Cash Flow Stability Can Make Innovation Safe

Why is that true? This is an important reality to understand.

If providers and health plans both know three years in advance what Medicare advantage cash flow level they will have available as revenue each year, then every care site and health plan in America could start doing multiyear plans to work within that goal. Reengineering would be incented, triggered, and safely rewarded by that multiyear goal. Reengineering is the key. We very much want care sites to reengineer care costs for long-term success. If we change the cash flow package target for Medicare every year and if there is a significantly variability to the process that will create significant future cash flow instability concerns for the people who run the business units of care -- both up and down -- then it will be much harder for most care sites and health plans to do both long-range planning and process reengineering.

Some people want to put the process up for bids of some kind every year.

Doing bids of some kind each year seems superficially like a good economic model -- and in some other markets, for some other products it often can be good economic model -- but health care needs a few years of cash flow stability to adjust to the new cash flow model. Using a bid process now to create variable cash flow levels each year isn't needed to achieve the cost goals for Medicare, and it adds both an uncertainty and a potentially unhealthy, perverse and counterproductive element of pricing gamesmanship to the planning process that could seriously distract and derail the process-based thinking of health system leaders and discourage multiple levels of structured innovation.

Predatory Pricing Could Be Dysfunctional

A business model and an annual bid approach might allow some local organizations to do predatory pricing. Building new levels of annual competition based product gamesmanship around variable annual cash flow levels would also be less effective for creating massive process restructuring than setting up a more secure cash flow model with multiyear stability that lets people who run care sites do long-range planning in a very productive way.

That stability in the government stream of cash does not eliminate market forces from the model or the strategy.

Market forces will still be involved in this track one approach in a major way because the Medicare Advantage plans each have a direct price to consumers that faces consumers very directly. That price varies from plan to plan, and plans compete now based on those prices. Plans all charge a premium to patients on top of their government capitation payment. The variable pricing part of the market agenda that triggers and rewards market forces should be the premiums that face the consumers and that are charged to the members. The variables pricing should not be the capitation levels paid by the government to the plans. Capitation based on variation would involve actuarial gameship. Consumers facing pricing trigger the benefits of consumer focused gameship. We want competition between the plans for consumers. Competition between plans for consumers at the premium level should be encouraged.

Likewise, for the rest of the Medicare members, variable pricing by the various Medicare supplemental plans should be encouraged. The Medicare supplemental plans under that approach can set their local prices knowing what the new SGR-two approach will do to basic costs in each geography.

We Could Also Raise the Eligibility Age or Means Test Medicare

This book recommends using the two-track systems of Medicare advantage and SGR-two to get control over the costs of Medicare. A number of people have offered other approaches to solving the Medicare cost issues. A couple of those other proposed approaches to reducing Medicare spending levels deserve discussion and need to be understood.

Several possible solutions to Medicare costs have been proposed.

No one believes that the status quo approach is affordable for Medicare. Very bright people have been wrestling with those issues and some very good thinkers have been proposing a number of solution sets and strategies for making Medicare more affordable.

Covering fewer people would reduce costs.

One set of those proposed solutions to Medicare costs simply involves taking some type of steps to reduce the number of Medicare-eligible people. Clearly, Medicare costs would go down if fewer people had Medicare coverage. There are a couple of ways that have been proposed to reduce the number of people who have Medicare coverage. One way of reducing the number of Medicare enrollees would be to use some level of income or "means testing" to take Medicare benefits away from some higher income people. The argument for using that approach is that higher income people don't really need the Medicare benefit payments anyway. Removing higher income people from Medicare would, by definition, mean that fewer propel would have Medicare coverage.

The Medicare Edibility Age Could Be Involved

Changing the age of Medicare eligibility could also reduce the number of people with Medicare coverage.

Another approach to reduce the number of Medicare-eligible people would simply be to increase the age of Medicare eligibility. Cover older people. Currently, everyone who reaches the age of 65 is eligible for Medicare. That age trigger could be raised to 66 or 67 or even 68 at some point in time. That eligibility age change would also obviously work to bring down Medicare program costs simply because there would be fewer Medicare enrollees.

Each of those proposals can work mathematically to reduce the number of Medicare eligible people. Neither approach solves the basic cost trend problems for Medicare and neither approach does anything to improve the quality of care for Medicare patients. The truth is that forcing people to stay in the private insurance market longer when they are at age 66 and 67, will force those people who don't get Medicare coverage to buy expensive private health insurance. Insurance costs are very high for 66 and 67 year old people. Many of those people who would not be Medicare-eligible would end up buying their insurance in the new insurance exchanges. Based on income, many of them would be eligible for the government subsidy. That new subsidy expense paid by government money would eliminate some of the savings for the government for those people. Adding older people to the risk pools would raise the average cost of care quite a bit for the other people who would also be buying their coverage from those same private insurance risk pools. The higher average cost of care for those pools that would result from adding people in their mid-sixties to the pool would make the pools and the premiums less attractive to younger people. The new actuarial realties that would result for those risk pools are easy to project and easy to predict. Adding people who are 66 and 67 years old to those private insurance risk pools would make coverage even less affordable for the people who are 40 or even 60 years old, and who have been paying their premiums based on the average cost of care in those risk pools.

Similar problems happen if Medicare eligibility becomes income-based. Having higher income people suddenly ineligible for Medicare would also force those higher income people into the new private insurance risk pools to buy their own insurance. The higher income people joining the private risk pools could be 70 or 80 or 90 years old. That migration to that buying private non-Medicare insurance by much older high income people could do even more damage to the existing risk pool expenses for the 40-year-old people. Premiums would again go up if those risk pools would need to accept significant numbers of 80-year-old wealthy people who join and buy that private insurance because they were no longer eligible for Medicare coverage.

So both of those approaches could reduce the number of people with pure Medicare coverage -- and each approach would create unintentional consequences for other people who buy personal health insurance.

Flat Payments -- or Defined Contributions -- Are Also Being Proposed

This book is recommending the use of Medicare Advantage as a key part of the solution set for Medicare costs because Medicare Advantage has a cash flow that is based on a per enrollee per month guaranteed and fixed payment amount. Some policy advocates in Washington, D.C., have also been advocating recently for another kind of flat payment approach with a fixed payment per month that could also be used for Medicare patients. Those flat payment approaches have had multiple labels -- premium subsidies, premium support, Medicare vouchers, etc. Advocates for that flat payment/voucher approach basically recommend that we give all seniors a fixed amount of money to buy health insurance and then allow all seniors to use that fixed amount of money to buy a basic package of private health insurance from a private health plan. Seniors who wanted to buy more coverage could use their own money to buy the additional coverage.

That premium support approach could very clearly put a cap on government expenses for Medicare coverage per person because the total government expense for each senior would be the fixed subsidy payment -- not the cost of care for each senior. That approach looks very similar to Medicare Advantage in a sense that Medicare Advantage cash flow currently is also based on a form of flat payment from the government. The Medicare Advantage approach difference from the premium support proposals in that Medicare Advantage uses a more limited set of health insurance plans and Medicare Advantage has a more defined set of care benefits and performance standards and regulations. Some of the premium support plans that have been proposed have included a wider and more open market approach that might allow any licensed insurance companies to sell coverage to Medicare beneficiaries. Some of the basic premium subsidy approaches that have been proposed would allow seniors to make a free choice of any and all licensed health insurers who want to sell insurance to seniors. The goal of that open market provision would be basically to encourage competition for seniors among a very wide range of health insurers and to encourage maximum flexibility relative to product design and benefit approaches.

Some of the economic goals that are embedded in proposals for that premium support/voucher approach would be very similar to the existing Medicare Advantage cash flow and cost constraints. The Medicare Advantage program pays plans a fixed amount per senior per month. Seniors can only choose between Medicare Advantage-approved plans, however, to determine which plan gets their designated cash flow from Medicare. The premium support advocates generally recommend that each senior in the country be given a fixed amount of money that each senior can spend with any licensed insurer from any state to subsidize each senior's individual purchase of health insurance. Any licensed health insurer could be chosen as their insurance vendor by any consumer. Each senior could take their voucher amount and could use it to help purchase Medicare coverage from any of the competing plans in the private insurance market.

Both Approaches Create Plan Competition

One key goal of the premium support strategy is to have an increasing number of competing health plans in the market who will all offer Medicare coverage -- hopefully in creative and innovative ways. Ideally, seniors who had their premium support vouchers in hand could use their premium support money to purchase Medicare-equivalent coverage in an active marketplace of many competing insurers.

The premium support advocates say that their approach would and could cap future Medicare cost increases. That could be accurate. That voucher cap approach -- if used for all seniors -- could and would create a major level of future cost control for the U.S. Treasury.

The people who make that claim are correct. That flat payment aspect of their proposal and that cash flow model would, in fact, accomplish that cost control goal for the government as a payer. If every senior in America was on a "Premium Support" plan for Medicare on January 1 of next year, the total government expense for Medicare for next year would be the total amount of those fixed "premium support" payments -- and the cost increase for the following year for the government would be capped by whatever number the government chose as the next year's voucher level increase. It is a very basic and logical approach. That approach does raise several concerns, however, in a couple a key areas.

Seniors Could Use the Vouchers to Help Buy Insurance

Proponents of that model believe that the new voucher marketplace should be geared to allow any willing health plan who can meet minimal license requirements to be eligible as voucher recipients.

That is a relatively low barrier to participation in the program. Some states have relatively low requirements for health plans to be licensed. Quality and operational oversight varies from state to state. Some health insurers fail financially. Not having higher standards for inclusion in the voucher edibility could create some problems for both stability and program quality.

Depending on the structure of the new market, some level of the competition between the new sets of voucher-eligible health plans would probably be based on product design. Insurers in a less regulated market context might offer an array of benefit approaches. That opportunity to design products could enhance creativity but it could create confusion and generate excessive complexity. Senior products can be very confusing now. Basing future competition on a wider range of benefit design options might not be optimal for the goal of achieving fully informed purchasing decisions by seniors. An open marketplace for the new premium support vouchers with multiple benefits designs offered by multiple plans could be incredibly complex -- with product choices made available that are far beyond the capability of any senior to make an informed decision about relative to either quality or product elements.

That same open marketplace for any willing insurer could also lend itself to gamesmanship at several levels. Without some key structure and data flow setup relative to quality issues -- that approach could end up creating market forces and competitions between dueling actuaries rather than creating choices for consumers between competing care systems. The other chapters of this book would argue that having the competition for seniors taking place only at the level of the insurance structure and infrastructure rather than having competition based on care delivery performance would also probably be suboptimal. We really do need care systems to compete rather than having our actuaries compete -- because the cost of care is really what creates premiums in every setting -- not sophisticated actuarial tables.

Those issues could all be addressed. Several aspects of those premium support proposals could be improved. To make sure that seniors can make informed choices and to ensure that accountability exists for care plans, any voucher model that was set up probably could be made more robust by adding some practical and functional structure in the areas of benefit design clarity and quality reporting for care delivery. Since Medicare Advantage has clearly done a huge amount of that work, it might make sense to tie the premium support model market requirements and data flow in some way to that in place set of rules, processes and infrastructure. Using proven in place infrastructure to get a job done is often a good business decision as well as making pure administrative sense.

Patient Rollout and Rollout Delays Undermine the Savings Potential

Even if we deal effectively with those quality and complexity issues, there is still another major reason why that particular premium support approach and model might not meet our Medicare cost control needs today. The key proponents of those voucher-based plans have tended to become very cautious in their proposed timeframes for plan rollout and implementation. Most of the proponents of those premium support plans are now proposing a significantly delayed implementation timeframe for Medicare. The advocates for the premium support approach are now recommending very slow and significantly extended implementation schedules for the premium support plan. That set of delays in achieving any cost benefits creates an obvious cost control problem. We need solid cost answers for Medicare quickly. The cost control needs for Medicare could operationally be met relatively quickly if all seniors on Medicare bought their care next year using those premium support vouchers, but that isn't the proposed schedule.

That is not the schedule and the scope of eligibility that the current versions of those proposals recommend. Next year is neither their recommended timeframe or their proposed eligibility level. Key advocates of that approach have also pulled quite far back from the original goal of using the model for all seniors. The most recent versions being proposed for the premium support plans seems to have a significantly delayed implementation timeframe, and they have clearly limited eligibility levels to exclude probably the majority of seniors for at least a decade or more. So it we are looking for short-term Medicare cost savings, the reality is that most seniors won't ever use the premium support approach as it is now being proposed and the program will start relatively slowly for the smaller number of seniors who actually will be affected.

Why has the proposal been limited in those ways?

Those changes are political –- not economic or operational.

To avoid having any direct impact on any current Medicare enrollees, the current premium support proposals all now have start dates that have been significantly delayed –- with current seniors staying on their current Medicare program indefinitely and only newly eligible seniors beginning to receive the premium support subsidies and vouchers at some future point in time as their personal cash flow model for Medicare coverage.

It's easy to understand why those delays in timeframes and those reductions in the eligible seniors have been proposed.

The delays in the proposals have been done so that the political impact can keep all current seniors from being directly affected by the impact of the vouchers. The politics of that delayed time frame and limited enrollment makes complete political sense. The economic impact of those changes is, however, less positive. Those restrictions and those delays create a very expensive set of compromises and time changes relative to our goal of keeping us as a government from having to borrow money now to pay for current Medicare expenses.

In that time-delayed implementation version, cash flow only evolves very slowly to a model where inter-plan competition and care system competition can logically have any significant impact on the marketplace.

That is economically unfortunate.

Premium support proposals -- in their purest form and if they were implemented broadly and quickly -- could have exactly the massive impact on Medicare costs that their proponents advocate. Each delay in timeframes and each reduction in the scope of the affected seniors obviously proportionately reduces that desired impact.

Medicare Advantage and a Two-Track Program Could Start Now

That brings us back to the first proposal in this chapter of this book. If we really want to stop having our kids and our grandkids pay with their taxes for today's Medicare expenses, then we should take a hard look at using the working tool kits we have in place right now to buy care for Medicare enrollees and we should use the best tools we have more broadly and more quickly. We could solve our primary cost problems for Medicare by simply broadening fairly quickly the use of the current Medicare Advantage program for the vast majority of seniors. We can also decide to have the seniors who do not choose to join Medicare Advantage receive their care from the independent care infrastructure and care sites that will be paid for Medicare patients based on the SGR-two approach. That blended model could achieve the cost targets we need to meet immediately and that combined approach could be done very quickly.

From a purely functional and logistical perspective, that two-track approach works with tools we already know how to use.

Medicare Advantage is here now. It could be used tomorrow to do this work. The challenge is to extend that program in a politically viable and acceptable way to more seniors. In many markets where Medicare Advantage has been available for multiple years, the majority of seniors have already voluntarily gone down that path and most eligible seniors in those existing markets have already joined Medicare Advantage plans. Satisfaction levels for those enrollees are high and both satisfaction level and quality levels improve every year.

The Government Could Encourage Medicare Advantage Enrollment

If our government set a goal of having upwards of 80 percent of seniors in Medicare Advantage plans in five years, and if the government achieved that goal -- the government could then control Medicare costs for all those people based on the amount that would set each year as the per person Medicare Advantage payment level. That approach would achieve the full cost control levels of a full premium support voucher for 80 percent of seniors. For the other seniors, the SGR-two approach would encourage the use of team care, accountable care, medical homes and packages of care.

We Can Meet the Medicare Cost Goals With That Blended Approach

So that approach -- combining Medicare Advantage per capita payments with a modified regional SGR approach -- could meet our overall Medicare costs goals while improving care for both tracks of Medicare financing. That would be a wonderful achievement. Fixing Medicare would, of course, still leave a massive part of the federal health care budget unaddressed. We also need to fix Medicaid. We spend a huge amount of money on Medicaid and we will now be expanding that cash flow and cost burden for Medicaid hugely, as well. So how can we also take steps to bring the costs of Medicaid into line while improving service levels and the quality of care?

That work also needs to be done. That is the next chapter of this book.

We need to stop passing today's healthcare costs for both Medicare and Medicaid down to our children and our grandchildren through debt financing. It is a fiscal and even ethical sin for us to duck the key care delivery cost issues for political reasons and inflict that major burden on our kids and our grandkids when we have functional answers today that can eliminate that intergenerational cost burden and improve care at the same time.

Rationing care is absolutely the wrong answer. We need to reengineer, repackage, and reprice care. For Medicaid, we need to make care better and more accessible so that we can make it cost less. We need to reengineer that care in the context of a cash flow that enables, empowers and rewards reengineering. When that cash flow is put in place, and when it has enough longitudinal stability so that providers can count on it so they can reengineer care around it -- then we can alleviate the burden of those costs to state budgets and we can keep those budgets dollars free to spend the money on streets, roads and schools and appropriate local services.

It is time to improve our skill sets both as purchasers of care and as pure providers of care.

Both are entirely possible to do. We can do that work for our non-governmental markets by using the purchasing models outlined in the prior chapter. We need to buy care by the package, and not by the piece. We need care teams for our patients who consume over 75 percent of the costs of care[245] and really need team care.

We need electronic medical records for all patients and we need tools to connect the data for those patients. We need to make meaningful use of our patient data to improve care, support care, track care and study the results of care.

We should be on the cusp of a golden age for medical research using the new database. As an earlier chapter of this book pointed out, one recent study showed how to cut the death rate for stroke patients nearly in half with one change in procedure.[246] We need that research to be done and we need tools to get the results of those kinds of research quickly to all relevant caregivers.

All of those goals are entirely achievable. We can use the new tool set for connectivity to provide remote monitoring, in home care, patient care plan coordination and continuously improving care processes. We just need a cash flow for care that encourages use of those tools instead of crippling the use of those tools. Vertically integrated care systems that sell packages of care have the business model needed to use and enhance those tools. So do well-designed Accountable Care Organizations, and well-designed medical homes, and appropriately paid health insurers and health plans who sell care by the package to employers and the government as Medicare Advantage or capitated Medicare programs.

We could be on the cusp of a golden age for care. We also need to be on the cusp of a golden age for health. That is the topic of the final chapter of this book -- improving our total health.

Medicare Advantage has continuously improving quality scores and very high patient satisfaction levels prove the approach model is viable and can get the job done of stabilizing costs and improving both service and quality. A plan to migrate seniors to Medicare Advantage plans -- coupled with a well-designed multiyear SGR-two cap for the annual payment increases for the providers and patients who are not enrolled in those plans -- can easily meet the CBO scoring standards for cost savings. That approach to Medicare funding could remove our dependence on borrowed money to buy Medicare claims in two years. Depending on where Congress sets the annual increase percentage, that blended approach could cut the Medicare cost increases to a fixed three percent each year and save the Medicare trust fund that is now scheduled to go broke in ten years from now. Saving the trust fund can be done. We should be deeply ashamed of ourselves if we don't choose to save the fund when we have the tool kit needed to save it and that tool kit will improve care in the process.

Chapter Eight

=================

WE NEED TO MAKE MEDICAID BETTER, SMARTER, AND MORE AFFORDABLE AS WELL

More than 45 percent of the babies who were born in this country last year were born to mothers who were covered by Medicaid.[247]

For a number of states, including California, the majority of babies who were born were the children of Medicaid enrollees.[248]

Medicaid is clearly at a key logistical position relative to the future of this country. Our children are our future, and very soon a majority of our children will now have their births financed by our Medicaid Program.

Medicaid is -- at multiple levels -- growing in importance as a mechanism for purchasing care in this country. It is such a huge factor in the purchase and the delivery of care that we very much need to become wise and skilled users of that purchasing mechanism. To use Medicaid well, we will need states to play a major and changing role as an informed purchaser. Medicaid is basically a state program. To improve Medicaid, states will need to become highly skilled purchasers of both care and coverage, using Medicaid as a conduit for cash and as a template for care effectiveness and care delivery efficiency in multiple ways.

Medicare and Medicaid are two different programs.

Medicare and Medicaid are not two identical programs with different but similar names. There are a number of major differences between the two programs that we need to understand.

As noted above, Medicaid is basically a state-run program. Medicare, as was noted in the last chapter of this book, is a pure Federal program. Medicare is run directly by our national government and primarily administered by its intermediaries who are hired by the federal government to do basic administrative services. Medicaid is run by each state. Each state creates its own model for Medicaid administration.

The two programs have very different eligibility for participants. Medicare eligibility is based, by law, on the age of the person. The age that creates Medicare eligibility is the same in every state -- 65 years old. Medicare is our basic and standard national health financing program that provides basic health care coverage for all of our older Americans.

By contrast, Medicaid is not age-based. Medicaid eligibility is primarily income-based. Very poor older people can actually have both Medicare and Medicaid coverage. Those people are referred to as "dual eligible". The states and federal programs do almost nothing to coordinate the programs for those dual-eligible people.

Medicaid eligibility is primarily based on people's income levels, with some eligibility for some people based on individual people's health status. Until recently, the vast majority of Medicaid enrollees have been young and poor families -- and that helps explain why half of the births in the U.S. are now being paid for by Medicaid.

States have historically been able to have some flexibility in determining what income level and what health status levels will trigger Medicaid eligibility in each state.

The Medicare benefit package is set by the Federal Government. That benefit package is basically the same for all seniors across the country. The Medicaid benefit package has been more flexible. It has a minimum level set by the Federal Government -- but the States have also had some flexibility in creating state-specific variations for their Medicaid enrollees.

The state's flexibility is due, in large part, to the shared-funding approach that is used for the Medicaid program. States and the Federal government jointly share the costs of Medicaid. States do not pay in any way for Medicare. The States have no cash flow involved at any level in the Medicare program for our older Americans, but the states basically pay half of the costs of Medicaid. Those are two very different funding streams. Federal money pays for Medicare. A combination of state and federal money pays for Medicaid.

That state cost-sharing approach means that Medicaid is a major cost item in all state budgets. When states figure out their spending each year, they have to factor in the costs of Medicaid coverage as a direct expense for each state. Medicaid is actually a major component of all state budgets. States have to wrestle every year with the funding levels for Medicaid.

The federal government, now, in effect, borrows money to buy care for all seniors -- as the last chapter of this book pointed out.

States tend not to be able to borrow money to pay for any current expenses, so states have had to take significant steps to try to manage their Medicaid spending without using debt financing to supplement their cash flow. The attempts to keep Medicaid costs down have not been uniformly successful. Medicaid costs are increasing in almost every single state.[249] Because those Medicaid costs have been growing at a fairly rapid level, the states have responded by trying to reduce care expenses. The easiest way to reduce care expenses has been to set very low fees for the care delivered by hospitals and by doctors for Medicaid patients. States have also been forced to cut other areas of state spending in order to create cash that can be used to pay for growing Medicaid expenses.

Fee cuts for both physician and hospital care have been used extensively. Chapter Three of this book discusses that fee-setting process for both Medicaid and Medicare.

As Chapter Three pointed out, the Medicaid fee levels paid by the states tend to be significantly below the fees that are paid by the federal government for Medicare patients and even further below the fees that are charged to private paying patients in our clinics and hospitals. The Medicaid fee levels in some states now look very much like the fee schedules that are paid today by the governments in Canada to Canadian caregivers to buy care there.

Some of the California Medicaid fee levels are actually now lower than the fees paid by some of the Canadian provinces.

In addition to the fee-reduction approaches, states have been experimenting with other purchasing mechanisms for Medicare patients. Some states have decided to, in effect, outsource Medicaid -- both for administration and for the delivery of care. A number of states now use vendors to provide Medicaid coverage for designated groups of patients. As noted below, that trend of using vendors to provide Medicaid coverage will probably increase and probably will include almost all states in the next few years.

The most painful response to growing Medicaid spending has been, at a very basic level, to reduce state spending in other areas of state budgets. The next chart shows the impact of those cuts on various state budget expense categories for our states a year ago.

Figure 8.1

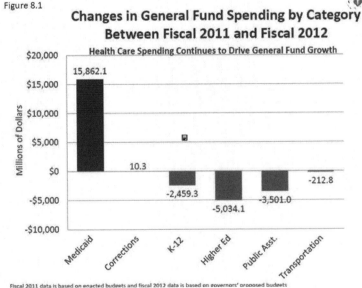

Changes in General Fund Spending by Category Between Fiscal 2011 and Fiscal 2012

Health Care Spending Continues to Drive General Fund Growth

Fiscal 2011 data is based on enacted budgets and fiscal 2012 data is based on governors' proposed budgets

The chart shows the decrease in state level spending by expense category for several other areas of state expenses where spending was cut because growing Medicaid costs simply absorbed the available state dollars and forced states to make those cuts.

Clearly, a number of other areas of state budgets have been adversely affected by the Medicaid cost increases. That has created some functional problems in some of those areas for a number of states.

The obvious fact is -- Medicaid has been and continues to be a major cost factor for states. The new Affordable Care Act will actually expand our total spending for Medicaid by increasing the number of people who are eligible for Medicaid coverage. States can choose to expand Medicaid eligibility to include more people, and that expanded set of costs will be paid entirely with federal government dollars. Those expansions will not create additional state expenses.

The federal government will directly absorb most of the increased spending incurred by those newly eligible people. Some states are agreeing to the expansion, and others are exercising their rights as states to reject the expansion plans. Some of the states who have chosen not to expand have stated that they believe that even though the federal government pays for those expansion costs now, that cash flow arrangement may change at some future point in time.

The eligibility rules for Medicaid were addressed by the ACA law because the current Medicaid program eligibility rules have excluded many of our poorest Americans for coverage.

People point out that we are the only industrialized county in the world that does not provide subsidized coverage for all of our lowest income and poorest citizens.

As a result of not covering all of our poorest people, we have low income people with significant health problems who don't get needed care. We also currently do not have an extensive infrastructure of care that is funded by the cash flow that is needed to provide care to our poorest populations. Our infrastructure in some areas is underdeveloped because we have had over 30 million uninsured Americans and they have typically not been good revenue sources for all caregivers.

That issue of not covering our poorest people will change significantly in the states where the Medicaid eligibility changes happen next year. As noted above, some states are agreeing to the new Medicaid eligibility expansion, and some states are deciding not to expand their Medicaid eligibility rules. These states have a number of ideological and financial reasons for making their decisions. In any case, because many states will do the expansions, Medicaid enrollment will grow for the country next year. Based on the states that have decided to expand Medicaid eligibility, the number of additional people with Medicaid coverage by the end of the next year will grow by roughly 10 million additional covered people.[250] Those newly covered people, by definition, will all be people with lower income levels. Some will be very poor and some will be simply poor. The expanded eligibility formula calls for Medicaid to cover people from 0 income up to about 140 percent of the federal poverty level.[251]

The old eligibility level was 100 percent of Medicaid in many states, and there were family state requirements that ended up having Medicaid function as a program for low income women and children in those states.

Whether or not we expand Medicaid in any setting, a key part of the health care strategy agenda for each state at this point in time should be to significantly improve the care that is being delivered to people in the Medicaid program.

There is some very good care being delivered to some of our Medicaid-eligible people in some care settings. However, but the vast majority of the Medicaid care delivered across the country is now delivered as individual pieces of care -- pieces of care sold with no care oversight, no quality monitoring, and usually no care coordination. As this book has pointed out multiple times, we have an unstructured and often functionally deficient set of care delivery mechanisms and sites in this country. Those mechanisms tend to be even more deficient for our low income patients. We deliver inconsistent care to low income patients, and we don't keep track of the care we do deliver. Functional databases about care for the low income, uninsured, and newly insured Medicaid enrollees are almost nonexistent.

Caregivers who share patients usually have no way of knowing at any level what care is being delivered to their patients in other care settings, and the ability of caregivers who treat the same patients to coordinate care on behalf of the patients they share is almost nonexistent. That is a problem for many patients, and it is a particular problem for low income patients. Low income people with limited means and significant access challenges actually need care coordination even more than high income patients -- and low income patients can benefit significantly when caregiver and care coordination happens.

Care for children with asthma, for example, lends itself to care coordination and to careful and skillful care management. The number of asthma crises for children can be cut by half or more with good care coordination and with accessible patient-centered care data.[252]

Children who are on Medicaid tend to have very high rates of asthma, as a group. So coordinated asthma care makes particular logistical sense at a very high level for many of those patients.

States should decide that the next generation of care delivery and care financing approaches for Medicaid should include a focus on team care and carefully collected patient data and patient-focused care coordination.

That can all be done. It all will be done if the states that pay for Medicaid coverage very deliberately include team care in their care specifications and then choose wisely in selecting and supporting their Medicaid program care delivery vendors.

States are already realizing the obvious need to move past the piecework model for buying care. The piecework payment model is particularly flawed when there are no national care linkages for most of the low income patients.

Many states are moving away from buying all care for Medicaid patients by the piece directly from individual caregivers, and those states are moving to buying care for their Medicaid patients by the package. States are increasingly purchasing that care from care systems and from health plans that sell care and deliver care by the package.

That approach of buying a complete package of care can make care significantly better, more transparent, and more accessible for Medicaid patients. It can also reduce the costs of care. Coordinated care is usually less expensive than uncoordinated piecework care. When prenatal mothers get better prenatal care and then have fewer problem births, costs go down. When low income adults with chronic conditions and acute comorbidities get team care instead of having to find their own care site for each piece and individual incident of care, costs go down.

Better care -- when that care is well engineered -- costs less money. The strategy for Medicaid programs should be to reengineer care -- not ration care. Rationing kidney transplants is a clearly inferior strategy to implementing a set of care delivery improvements that can cut the number of needed transplants by half or more.

Done well, purchasing care by the package should improve care for Medicaid patients, and it should make care more affordable for Medicaid payers. Data will be needed to make that strategy successful. A key to the success of that process will include competent, consistent, and well-designed quality of care monitoring.

The purchasing specifications used by the states need to include care quality and service levels reporting and oversight.

We need to make full use of the new sets of tools available to support care delivery. The purchasing specifications for Medicaid programs should also strongly encourage electronic care-support tool use -- like e-visits and e-monitoring for patients. We need to use those new connectivity tools to increase the effectiveness of care delivery and to make care more efficient, accessible, and affordable.

Some states have used medical homes extensively for their Medicaid patients. Those programs have tended to be very successful. They significantly improve the competence and availability of team care. The Medicaid medical homes have improved care, reduced emergency room visits, and significantly reduced the need for hospital admissions and decreased crisis care needs for the people that medical homes treat.

Those homes tend to have good computerized databases about each of their patients. They also tend to rely on the full set of available caregivers to meet patient needs. Nurses and doctors both work directly with patients in medical home settings to monitor care plans and help the patients with the therapies and the preventive care that is needed to improve care outcomes.

The Medicaid programs need to encourage flexible use of the Medical home team members and flexible use of various connectivity tools to monitor care and create electronic contacts between patients and caregivers.

Significant care reengineering is possible if the full set of available tools is used -- and the cost of care can be reduced if they are used well. Reengineering is a much more ethical, effective, and affordable set of solutions for medical costs than care rationing.

Medicaid needs to evolve from being an incident-based care delivery approach with no quality monitoring and no care coordination into an approach that creates both patient-centered care data and patient-centered care.

States Need to Purchase Wisely

The easiest and most functional way to achieve those goals is for the states to hire health plans or to create health-plan equivalent functions that can perform all the needed levels of data collection and also have the in-house competencies and capabilities needed to perform those key levels of care oversight and those care-monitoring roles.

Being a smart buyer is very important for state governments at this point in history. Smart buying needs to become a core competency for states. If the states create clear specifications for Medicaid care delivery and if states enter into well-designed contracts with health plans or with health plan equivalent organizations to do that Medicaid care delivery work, and if the health plans then do that work for a preset premium payment instead of doing that work and billing for each piece of care on a piecework payment basis -- then each state can save money by getting a fixed package price for all needed care. If that process is done well, each state can also improve care quality and service levels by officially assigning someone who has the tools to do the work providing oversight for quality to actually do that work.

Again -- as with the early versions of some Medicare programs -- there have been some historical reasons for some people to be cautious about relying on this strategy to solve today's Medicaid problems. A number of states have gone down an outsourcing path for Medicaid before -- some with success and some with unfortunate results.

In the early days of states assigning Medicaid members to health plans, there were some abuses by some plans in the process. The basic concept should be a good thing to do, but not all plans who initially took on capitated Medicaid patients actually did that work well.

There were some plans who took on more Medicaid members than they could serve. Some plans had inadequate and badly located provider networks. Data monitoring was not a very robust expertise or skill set for both states and many health plans at that earlier point in time.

So some abuses happened. Some states were not particularly competent buyers in those early times in some settings. The idea of "outsourcing" Medicaid coverage was new at that point and the buyer skill set and tool kits were often both relatively thin in many places.

The model worked really well in some sites. It can work really well. But some of the early versions created some real problems. Policy people with good memories remember that it is possible to go down this path of buying Medicaid coverage as a package and do it badly and wrong.

The skill sets of the states as buyers are now much better. The product is more clearly defined. Multiple levels of quality oversight are in place. Data needs are understood -- and the available data tools are for both. Those days and that set of consequences should never return.

We Need Accountable Parties To Continuously Improve and Reengineer Care

The truth is we need this set of tools for Medicaid patients at this point in time. Buying care by the piece has clearly failed. Piecework care delivery is inflexible and far too often entirely inadequate to meet the needs of Medicaid patients. Low income people need team care. Low income people need care plans and care follow-up. Low income people need care sites that follow quality tracking and improvement agendas.

Health Improvement Is Also Needed

In that overall approach and strategy, actual health improvement for people also needs to be a major Medicaid priority. It is better for any population or sets of people to take effective steps to prevent a disease or an adverse medical condition instead of just taking steps to respond -- often in crisis mode -- to medical problems and issues often they have occurred. Prevention is better than remediation as a basic strategy. We actually need both. But an optimal strategy for the care of a population relies on prevention efforts very heavily, because it is better to avoid a disease than it is to cure that disease. Medicaid is no exception to that general guideline.

The next chapter of this book deals very directly with the issues of obesity and inactivity as major causes of both bad health and excessive health care costs. Both of those behavior issues can be addressed. Both need to be addressed. The chapter discusses that in detail. Activity levels for Medicaid patients actually provide a major potential health improvement asset and offer an opportunity that needs to be included as part of purchasing specifications for the states when they change health plans and when they implement health systems for the new levels of Medicaid care.

Neuron Connectivity Is Also Extremely Important

Another prevention and intervention area that needs to be a particular focus for our Medicaid program is the neuron connectivity levels of our youngest children. Neuroconnectivity is a major medical challenge and a major opportunity for our children. It is a pure, biological fact that the brains of our very young children are making massive numbers of neuron connectivity linkages in the earliest years of their lives. Ages zero to three are actually extremely important times for that development.[253] If the children's brains receive the right level of input in the very early years, the neuron connectivity levels for a child can be very high. Each child is on his or her own individual and personal path relative to neuron connectivity. If the right level of input does not happen for a child in those very early years, then most of those children will never be able to achieve their full potential in society.

Studies show much lower levels of performance in school and lower success levels in other life areas for the children who have the most significant linkage deficits. Those children who have neuron linkage deficits will directly add to the direct costs of Medicaid at multiple levels. Drug use, for example, tends to be 60 percent higher for those children.

This is an area where care delivery can help by guiding parents in best behaviors. The care system now teaches the value of vitamins, healthy eating, and healthy activity levels. Our caregivers also need to teach parents about neuron connectivity.

Measuring vocabulary at the kindergarten level is an excellent mark to get a sense of the neuron connectivity success that has happened for a child. The children with the lowest vocabulary counts -- children who know under 1,000 words in comparison to other children in kindergarten who know 5,000 to 10,000 words -- those children with lower word knowledge also end up with lower reading skills in early grades.

The children who have the lower reading skills in very early grades are 40 percent more likely to become pregnant, 60 percent more likely to drop out of schools and nearly 80 percent more likely to go to jail.[254]

For people who are in jail, more than 70 percent of the prisoners came from the group of people who had those low levels of reading skills in those early years.[255]

For the children who have fallen behind their peers at that early point in life, fewer than 10 percent can ever catch up. More than 90 percent of these children cannot catch up with other students -- and those children end up in a statistical category with higher high school dropout rates, higher pregnancy rates, much higher drug use, increased health problems, and higher levels of being incarcerated.

Clearly, Medicaid could save money relatively quickly at multiple levels if all children had the right neuron stimulation input from age zero to age three or four that could put all children on a different and better life trajectory and reduce the risk of school failure, drug use, and even incarceration as adults.

Physicians and care teams who see Medicaid mothers and who treat the youngest of our children need to make that information available to mothers and their families. Medicaid should require care systems to teach that information to the mothers. Mothers invariably want to do the right things for the children -- but that can be hard to do if mothers do not know what the right thing to do is.

When mothers know that they can and should do things with their children that can significantly increase their children's ability to learn and ability to succeed, then those things are obviously more likely to happen for their children. They will not and do not happen in many settings when the mothers do not have that basic knowledge base.

That information is particularly important to this country at this point in time and important to this chapter of this book because several studies have shown that the children born to mothers on Medicaid tend to have lower levels of these inputs in their lives. Studies have also shown that when these children with lower input levels receive higher input levels, their lives change. The number of babies being born in these situations is increasing. The first sentence in this chapter addressed that issue.

We will soon have half of babies born in this country born to Medicaid mothers. We are at 48 percent today[256] -- an increase from roughly 25 percent twenty years ago.

We already have more people in jail than any industrialized country in the world.[257] We also have one of the highest levels of high school dropouts.[258] We need to change those trajectories, or the situation we face as a country in these areas will get even worse.

So we need to add neuron connectivity to obesity and inactivity as part of the health agenda and the health improvement strategy for the children who are covered by Medicaid. Medicaid obviously can't provide the neuron-triggering input that each of those children need, but Medicaid caregivers can teach the issues as well as teaching obesity and inactivity issues to all people with Medicaid coverage.

Overall, for Medicaid, we need to take advantage of this time of change in health care delivery and health care financing to put Medicaid on an entirely new and better path.

It could be a major waste of an opportunity if we did not take these steps, and take them well.

The next chapter deals with two more key areas where we can change the trajectory of American health care if we do a couple of key things and do them well.

Now that we know what we know, it would be criminal not to use that knowledge to improve our health and significantly reduce the amount of money we spend on care.

CHAPTER NINE

LET'S CUT COSTS BY
IMPROVING HEALTH

We would spend a lot less money of health care in this country if people were healthier. That is pure common sense. The cost of care is created by the need for care. If we didn't need care, we wouldn't need to spend our money getting and using care.

Those are very basic points to consider. They are simple truths that we too often overlook as we focus on how to make care better and more affordable.

When we think very deeply and seriously about how we could truly reduce the total costs of care in this country, sheer logic and basic arithmetic both tell us that we could reduce those care costs if we needed less care.

Is that possible to do? Is there anything we can actually do that has any significant likelihood of success in reducing our need for care?

The answer to that question -- to most people's surprise -- is yes.

When you look at the goal of cutting health care costs in this country from that specific perspective...when you look to see if and how we can actually reduce those costs by significantly improving people's health -- and when you then look in very practical ways for the functional approaches and achievable and actionable things we can do that will actually work in the real world to significantly improve people's health status -- yes is actually the answer to that question.

Why is yes the answer? Behaviors are the key to yes.

We know for an absolute fact that our behaviors create and trigger the chronic conditions that drive 75 percent of care costs in our country.[259] We also know for a fact that the two basic behaviors that trigger almost all of the chronic diseases are identical for all of those diseases that create all of those expenses. The two behaviors that trigger diabetes, heart disease, asthma, hypertension, and significantly increase the risk levels for a couple of key cancers are 1) unhealthy eating, 2) Inactivity.[260]

Those two very basic behaviors create, drive and exacerbate almost all of the chronic health problems that create more than 75 percent of health care cost in America.

Two Behaviors Are the Key to Population Health

These two behaviors are the keys to population health. They are transformational. If we could somehow persuade people to practice healthy eating and if we could just get people to be physically active, we could cut the rate of those chronic conditions by half or more. That would have a massive and very real impact on the costs of care.

The problem is, of course, that behavior change can be very hard. Healthy eating has almost magical impacts on health -- but it has been very hard to get people to eat well and to eat at levels that do not trigger obesity. Obesity is an epidemic of its own at this point. The next chart shows the explosion of obesity in this country over the last two decades.

The obesity story is a sad and frustrating history of behavior change failure. We have been trying as a country to make obesity a higher visibility issue and encourage healthy eating. There are some good and well-meaning programs that are attempting to achieve those goals. Those programs have been almost entirely ineffective. We have made some progress in some areas, but we are losing the overall weight war primarily because food intake triggers neurochemical rewards in people that make most weight control programs ineffective.

Figure9.1

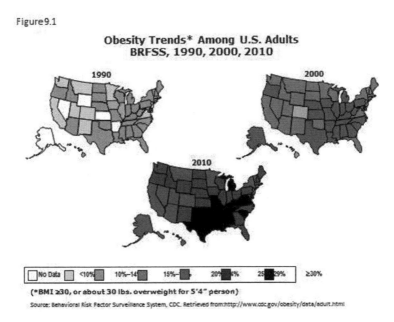

Obesity Trends* Among U.S. Adults
BRFSS, 1990, 2000, 2010

(*BMI ≥30, or about 30 lbs. overweight for 5'4" person)

Source: Behavioral Risk Factor Surveillance System, CDC. Retrieved from:http://www.cdc.gov/obesity/data/adult.html

Does that mean that the situation is helpless?

No, not at all. We need to regroup, reassess and refocus our efforts. We need to shift our focus as a primary public health intervention from obesity to activity. Activity is the key. Improving activity levels actually can have a positive impact on health that exceeds the benefits of reducing obesity. People have not known that to be true until relatively lately. We know that we are dangerously inactive in this country. The number of dangerously inactive people exceeds the number of people who are obese. [261]The Lancet medical journal called inactivity levels among the top health risk for humans today.[262] They made their point convincingly, clearly, and well. The risk levels for inactive people exceeds the risk levels for obese people[263] -- and unhealthy eating and inactivity lead to a similar set of chronic conditions.[264] We can have a major impact on reducing each of those diseases if we can just get people to be physically active.

So if it is extremely difficult to successfully address obesity, is there any hope that we might deal successfully with inactivity?

The answer is, yes.

The key strategy is to get people to walk.

Walking Is a Therapeutic Activity

Walking is a therapeutic activity.

Walking works amazingly well to restore, maintain and improve health.

Most people do not appreciate the incredible value of walking.

The human body is made to walk and the human body is much healthier when we walk.

The good news is, we now know from a rich array of new science that walking is the single most effective behavior that can be used by human beings to improve individual and collective health. The new science is robust and clear. The opportunities for using walking to improve health are becoming increasingly obvious to everyone who looks at population health issues. We are finally coming to understand that the human body really does need to walk to be healthy. Walking, alone, has huge benefits. People who walk are literally half as likely to become diabetic.[265] Walkers are also much less likely to have strokes or heart disease[266] -- and people who walk even have significantly lower levels of cancer.[267]

Walking is a high leverage, achievable, and very practical activity. Walking doesn't need to be just one component of a long-term, complex multilevel solution to health improvement. Walking works well all by itself. Walking can have almost immediate impact for most people. The new science of walking is almost unbelievable. Look at the statistics and the growing body of incredibly powerful research results. The appendix of this book lists several of studies. Our bodies clearly need to walk to be healthy.

Cutting the Number of New Diabetes by Half Is Possible

When people walk just 30 minutes a day, five or more days per week, the number of new diabetics can be reduced by more than half.[268] Reducing the number of new diabetics by half is obviously a massive opportunity for both health improvement and cost reduction.

People with diabetes currently consume over 40 percent of the cost of care for Medicare.[269] Diabetes is the fastest growing disease for Americans.[270] Look at the next chart.

Figure 9.2

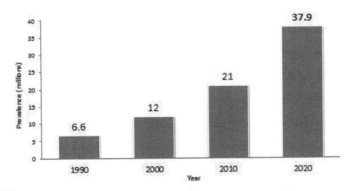

Prevalence of diagnosed type 2 diabetes in the United States:

We are seeing an explosion in the number of people with diabetes in this country.

Cutting the number of new diabetics by half could be the single most powerful thing that could be done to cut Medicare costs for our government. That is not unachievable. That goal of reducing the number of new diabetes by half could be reached simply by increasing the activity level of our Medicare beneficiaries and getting seniors to walk. It would be a very good thing to have fewer people with diabetes in our population. Walking, all by itself massively reduces the number of people who become diabetic. We need people who are pre-diabetic to know that fact of medical reality.

If our caregivers, our communities, and our leadership in various settings all successfully encouraged walking for seniors, the impact on population health and on the health of the seniors who walk could be almost immediate and very effective.

Walking Reduces Multiple Diseases -- Significantly

That's the good news. The even better news is that diabetes isn't the only chronic disease that can be impacted significantly and very quickly by walking.

Walking 30 minutes a day, five days a week also cuts the number of strokes and heart attacks by nearly 40 percent.[271] Hypertension levels improve for walkers.[272] Walking actually has a huge impact on the frequency and risk levels for multiple diseases. Walking cuts the rate of congestive heart failure by over 30 percent.[273] Walking lowers blood pressure, makes the blood vessels more supple, and helps lower cholesterol levels.[274] Walkers are significantly less likely to catch colds and walking reduces the recovery time for the people who do get colds by over 30 percent.[275]

Walking helps the body resist cancer. People who walk 30 minutes a day, five days a week, are 30 percent or more less likely to get colon cancer, prostate cancer, pancreatic cancer and breast cancer.[276]

Walking helps the body resist diseases and walking has an amazingly beneficial impact on helping people recover from diseases.

Breast cancer patients who walk regularly while under medical treatment actually have up to a 50 percent lower mortality rate from that cancer compared to non-walking breast cancer patients.[277]

One amazing study looked at the brain deterioration of a group of patients who's DNA showed them to be at high risk of Alzheimer's disease. The high risk people who were inactive had high levels of brain plaque buildup over the course of the study. By contrast, there was very little additional buildup in the brains of the high risk for Alzheimer's patients who walked.[278]

The Science of Walking Is Highly Encouraging

All of these data points about the benefits of walking come from legitimate, controlled medical trials where the walkers and the non-walkers are appropriately matched for various other factors. Many studies are being done. The studies are all coming up with very similar conclusions. The science of walking is becoming increasingly clear. Walking works. The human body clearly needs to walk and our bodies benefit significantly when walking is part of our lives.

Many of the studies that prove those points to be true are listed in the endnotes to this book. Physicians and medical researchers in multiple settings are beginning to understand the huge positive impact of walking. And the very real dangers of not walking. Those same researchers are also beginning to understand the frightening and debilitating health risks that result from being inactive and not walking at all. As noted above, The Lancet medical journal in Great Britain just did an eighty-page special report that called inactivity the biggest single health risk on the planet for humans today. A recent American study showed that being inactive cuts years off our lives.[279] The Lancet studies shared that conclusion and extended it to multiple countries.

Walking Has Physiological Benefits As Well

Walking doesn't just improve physical health -- preventing diseases and helping people recover more quickly and more successfully from their diseases. Walking also has both psychological and emotional benefits. People who walk tend to experience significant mental health improvements as well.

The mental health benefits are even easier to understand than the physical disease-related benefits.

Walking usually creates positive neurochemicals in the brains of people who walk. Medical experts have known for decades that positive neurochemicals enhance people's emotional health. Walking generates those positive neurochemicals. Several studies have shown that walking can help prevent and alleviate and even help cure depression for some people.[280] People who walk regularly tend to feel good about walking. Positive neurochemicals are a very natural and effective way of dealing with stress, tension, and depression. In effect, walking is a powerful antidepressant and anti-anxiety medication. Walking 30 minutes a day, five days a week actually outperformed the standard pharmaceutical treatments used for depression in several studies.

In addition, depressed people who took their medication and who also walked that same 30 minutes a day significantly increased the effectiveness of their antidepressant medications.[281] Walking has reversed depression in some people.

Walking Sometimes Reverses Early Stages of Diabetes As Well

Walking has not only reversed depression in some people, but it has also been able to actually reverse early-stage diabetes in a number of patients.[282] That is another extremely important piece of information. Walking can not only help prevent diabetes -- it can also be used to help some people who have become diabetic actually reverse the disease and improve their health to the point where those people are no longer diabetic. That was startling information. Many people have believed that type two diabetes is irreversible. That turned out not to be true for some people with early diabetes when they walk a significant amount of time. Reversing diabetes for these patients is a huge win for them and that finding is another great enforcement for the benefits of walking.

The Impact of Walking Can Be Remarkably Quick

The beneficial results are also, often, remarkably quick.

One of the most commonly held beliefs in health care policy circles about various traditional health improvement strategies and programs has been that it always takes a very long time to see any positive economic impact and any beneficial biological returns from healthy behaviors. People in policy circles who have been focused on costs tend to avoid even looking at health improvement strategies as a possible tool for real-world, short-term cost reductions on the theory that the health improvement agendas all will take years or even decades to achieve any significant positive results.

That is, in fact, true of many traditional health improvement agendas. It is, however, absolutely not true of walking. Walking doesn't just create a set of long-term paybacks of good heath over some extended period in time. In many cases, the benefits of walking are realized very quickly.

Depression results are also often fairly immediate. The benefits of walking can be realized in days and weeks. Reversing or improving diabetes, for example, can be an almost immediate payback from walking...both, changing the need for care and reducing the cost of care very quickly.

Positive results for patients with depression often happen in less than a month. Walking reverses some chronic diseases and prevents others and the impact of walking on significant and expensive conditions can often be seen in weeks or months -- not decades.

Walking Gives Us a New Way of Thinking About Costs

The practical benefits we can derive from walking are so significant and so immediate that they sometimes seem to be almost unbelievable. That set of information about how our bodies need to walk gives us a whole new way of thinking about the explosion in chronic diseases and their escalating costs.

We need to get people to walk. We need to figure out how to make walking an easy thing to do.

Why Hasn't Walking Been a Top Population Health Prevention Strategy?

So why haven't we used this strategy earlier? We were not this smart about the full impact of walking even a relatively short time ago. We actually did not know until relatively recently how many benefits can result from walking. The new data and the expanding science relative to walking is actually a relatively new set of information and therapeutic insights. Those new studies and their findings were not part of the thinking for most traditional health improvement agendas. The lack of walking strategies in the population health planning process in past years makes sense today because the science of medicine is just now beginning to understand the multiple benefits that can result from walking. Again -- the good news is that we do know this information now. Those benefits of walking are increasingly clear. Our bodies obviously -- on average -- function better in many ways when we walk. The human body clearly needs to walk to be healthy. The physiology of the human species clearly needs walking to happen to optimize blood flow, optimize resistance to disease and to balance and refresh internal chemistry. So it is a very good thing that we are finally beginning to understand that very useful fact to be true because once we understand those issues, we can start to do important things that help encourage, facilitate and enable walking in multiple sites and settings. Doing important things now should be our focus today.

Walking Doesn't Require a Lot of Special Equipment or Very Much Time

Walking strategy work can be relatively easy to do.

One of the very best things about walking, itself, is that it is relatively easy to do. Walking doesn't require a lot of special equipment or specially engineered physical settings. Walking can happen almost everywhere. Walking can happen in multiple contexts and walking can be done in a vast array of physical environments. The only equipment needed for most people to walk is walkable shoes. Because it can be done in many places with a minimum amount of equipment, we can be relatively efficient in creating strategies that can be used in almost every setting where we live, work, or congregate. We don't need to build swimming pools or ski slopes to support walking.

Walking Benefits Do Not Take a Lot of Time

The other huge impact factor that we need to know to build our future walking support strategies is that walking also does not need to talk a lot of time.

One of the very best things that we are learning about walking is that it doesn't take each of us a lot of walking time each day to realize high level of benefits. It does take some time -- but it actually doesn't take a lot of time. We don't need to walk for hours every day to benefit from walking. We don't even need to walk for a full hour. Walking 30 minutes a day five to seven days a week is generally enough walking to trigger major health benefits. Longer walking times are beneficial, but extremely high levels of benefits are triggered by those 30 minutes.

Half an hour is real time but 30 minutes isn't a really long time. And, new studies are showing, less than 30 minutes is a lot better for our heart than being totally inactive.[283] Even a relatively small level of motion is beneficial. The new science also tells us that the difference between being fully inert and moving around throughout the course of the day has huge health consequences all by itself. New science tells us that being inert and motionless creates major health risks for each inert person. So any activity is good -- and just walking -- for only half an hour a day -- seems to be enough time to get the body mechanisms that are triggered by walking into positive gear and beneficial functionally for most people.

The 30 Minutes Can Be Done in Two Fifteen-Minute Increments

There is even better news about the timeframes.

The 30 minutes a day doesn't even have to be done in one uninterrupted 30 minute stretch. That is -- once again -- wonderful news.

We don't need to find a full 30 minutes of uninterrupted walking time each day. The health advantages of walking also seem to exist if the walking is done in two fifteen-minute increments.[284] Some recent indications are that walking twenty minutes at a time might actually be a very high value -- almost optimal -- walking time.[285] It is possible that two twenty-minute walks each day could give most people the best health results and that walking agenda of two twenty-minute walks might have the best impact on our mental health as well. Two fifteen-minute walks seem to be enough to trigger that whole array of benefits mentioned above.

That ability to break the 30 minutes into pieces is another piece of very important information. Why? Because for many busy people, it can be relatively hard to find an uninterrupted 30-minute time slot that can be used for walking every single day. It can be a lot easier for busy people to find two 15- or two 20-minute walking times at different points in the day.

Fifteen minutes of walking time for an individual can happen going to and from work or going to and from school. Fifteen minutes can even be scheduled and achieved during coffee breaks or during lunch times. Fifteen-minute intervals can happen often and very naturally at different points in our day. That flexibility relative to the timeframes creates a lovely world of walking opportunities for both individuals and for community leaders who want to support walking to improve health. Devoting a couple of basic 15-minute intervals to walking each day can have a major positive impact on our health and on our sense of well-being, and those 15-minute time slots can be logistically very achievable.

Walking Can Reduce the Role of Chronic Disease

So, at the macro level, walking takes minimal equipment. It can be conveniently scheduled. And it can have a huge impact on both individual and population health.

All of those facts tell that walking should be a key part of our overall cost reduction strategy for this country. That is true because walking reduces the rate of the chronic conditions that create most health care costs.

Remember what this book has said several times about the origin of care costs.

Chronic conditions currently create 75 percent of the cost of care in this country.[286] Cancer creates roughly another 5 percent of our total care costs.[287] Walking alleviates the incidence of all major chronic diseases and walking even reduces the incidence of several cancers. Preventions and cures are both relevant to walking strategies. Walking can help cure a variety of chronic diseases, and walking can help improve the survival rates for a couple of cancers.[288] Reductions in the need for care obviously reduces the cost of care. Cutting the cost of several of our most expensive diseases by 10 percent or more could be absolutely achievable for the entire country if we could get a number of people to walk a reasonable amount of time on a regular basis.

Walking Could Reduce the Total Cost of Care

That is a very important point for us to understand and utilize.

If we could get large percentages of the American people to walk a reasonable amount of time, we could have a massive impact on both the incidence of care and the cost of care. People would be healthier, happier, and more productive. It seems too good to be true, but we could all spend less money on health care and we could improve people's lives if we could just get more people to walk.

We clearly need to encourage basic activity levels for Americans.

Unfortunately, we are not doing that very well now. We tend to be a culture of inactivity, and we have engineered physical activity out of our lives and our children's lives. Our school children have never been so inactive. The number of adults in our country who have dangerous levels of inactivity now exceeds 50 percent.[289]

Obesity –– the other major health risk –– only affects 30 percent of America.[290] The next section of this chapter deals with the issues of obesity. As noted above, unhealthy eating and obesity are both real problems. Obesity also needs to be addressed as a key health issue for our country.

We Need To Help People Be More Active

So how can we help people make walking part of their life?

This is a time for creative thinking. Now that we understand the amazing benefits of walking, we need to think creatively in multiple settings about how we can get people to walk.

Workplaces and communities and schools all offer significant opportunities to us.

We obviously need walking friendly work environments. We need walking friendly communities. We need walking friendly schools and we need walking friendly routes to schools. Multiple studies have shown that school children who walk to school get better grades and are less restless in the classroom than non-walking kids.[291]

We Need People To Understand the Benefits of Walking

It is clear that if we are going to do something meaningful to improve the health of our population, we should build a formal, well thought through national agenda, strategy and program around walking. Education and learning is a key first step. We need to teach everyone the basic benefits of walking. All Americans should understand this very basic set of issues. When people individually come to understand the major and very real benefits of walking, people are much more likely to walk. So we need teaching and learning to be a key point of the American strategy. We need to teach everyone in this country the benefits and values of walking -- and we need to make walking easy to do...because when people are ready to walk, we need to make it possible to walk.

Teaching is a key first step. We need our leaders in this country and in every community to teach all of the rest of us the benefits of walking. Culture change is led by leaders and our leaders need to actually lead on this incredibly important issue. We need to explain to all Americans why walking is the right thing to do and we need to explain to everyone the likelihood of a real personal gain for most walkers. The science that proves that gain to be true for people individually and for population health grows every day. That study that was mentioned earlier about Alzheimer's patients needs to be known by a lot of people. The study of high risk Alzheimer's patients showed that when the high risk people were entirely inert, the rate of plaque buildup in the brain was much higher than the buildup in the brain of high risk people who had normal activity levels. But when those same high risk people simply increased their activity levels and when those high risk patients walked 30 minutes a day, the level of additional buildup in their brains stopped entirely.[292]

That is an amazing result. That is amazing science. That really tells us that simple walking gives us benefits both for our physical health and our mental health. We need to help all Americans understand the impact of all of those studies that prove the clear benefit of walking to us all. People need to know the science, so that people can make better informed decisions about their own lives.

Smoking and Obesity Are Also Problems and Opportunities

We need to also address both smoking and obesity if we are going to have an optimal impact on people's health. Smoking does more direct damage than any other behavior. We need to make smoking hard to do. We need to encourage people not to smoke and we need to make smoking inconvenient to do.

Smoking campaigns need to be run and supported. This book doesn't need to reinforce that agenda because it exists today and it is the right thing to do. Smoking is a major behavior problem and we need to help people not smoke.

We also need to deal very directly and effectively with the issues of obesity. Obesity is very much a major health problem for our country. Obesity also creates another major health opportunity. We have an explosion of obesity in our country. We can and should also reduce the rate of obesity in this country. The numbers are staggering. Over a third of our population is now obese.[293] The following charts show another view of the increase in obesity in this country. As most people know, obesity is also connected to heart disease, diabetes, increased rates of cancers and a wide array of chronic conditions.

Figure 9.3

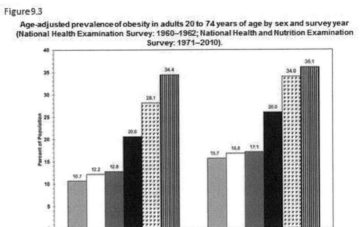

Age-adjusted prevalence of obesity in adults 20 to 74 years of age by sex and survey year (National Health Examination Survey: 1960–1962; National Health and Nutrition Examination Survey: 1971–2010).

Go A S et al. Circulation 2013;127:e6-e245

American Heart Association

Learn and Live

Figure 9.4

Trends in the prevalence of obesity among US children and adolescents by age and survey year (National Health and Nutrition Examination Survey: 1971–2010).

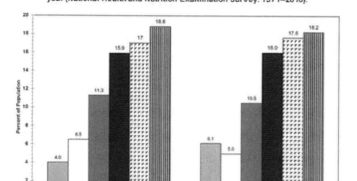

Go A S et al. Circulation 2013;127:e6-e245

American Heart Association

Learn and Live

Copyright © American Heart Association

We need to help people be active and we very much need to help people deal with the issues of obesity. Most people who write about the impact of behaviors on chronic diseases lead with obesity as the focus of their work and mention activity levels lightly or not at all. Some health care pieces about behaviors and chronic disease actually mention activity levels for people only as a factor that can help some people fight obesity. This book takes the exact opposite approach. This book focuses on activity levels first because of the new science about the health improvement opportunities that are presented by activity and about the massive health risks that are created by inactivity. We need to do better with both obesity and inactivity -- and the easiest and highest leverage strategies relative to inactivity.

Walking Is a Tool That Can Transform Community Health

Walking is a major focus of this book because walking is a clear tool that can transform community health. That absolutely does not mean we should ignore obesity. Obesity is a huge health risk and obesity needs does need to be addressed as well. A number of studies have shown that when people start walking regularly, weight loss often follows. Appetites change. People who are not as depressed also often eat less.

We need to take practical steps and achieve education programs to help prevent and reduce obesity as well as increase activity if we are going to achieve better levels of population health.

So what can we do to help people who are now obese?

And what can we do to keep people from becoming obese?

Obesity -- like inactivity -- results from individual choices that people make about personal behaviors. Obesity is also very much behavior-linked. We need to help people understand and use behaviors, approaches, and strategies that prevent and help reduce obesity.

Make the Right Thing Easy To Do

Healthier eating is an important first step.

We definitely need to help obese and overweight people with healthier eating. When people eat healthier foods and avoid unhealthy foods, the problems stemming from obesity are much easier to resolve. So we need to help people eat healthy food. We need to figure out how to do that in practical ways. We need to make the right thing easy to do by making healthy food cheaper and easier to obtain than unhealthy food.

If we want to think in terms of process improvement and not just think in terms of lecturing people about obesity or scolding people about being overweight, we need to take practical steps to make healthy eating easier to do for people who need to practice healthy eating. The very best care and health-improvement strategies are often those strategies that figure out the right thing and then make the right thing easy to do.

Make the Right Thing Easy To Do for Obesity

So how can we do that for obesity? We need to start with the food supply. We need to make healthier food available more broadly. We know what unhealthy foods are. It isn't a secret. We should avoid those foods. We need to cut way back on consuming saturated fats, for example. We clearly need to entirely eliminate transfats from our diets. Fat intake can be a kind of dietary poison. Fat intake clogs arties and increases heart attack risk. Overweight and normal weight people both need convenient access to healthier, lower fat foods.

We also need to reduce our sugar intake. Multiple studies show that weight and health can be improved when people reduce their intake of sugar.[294] We very much need vegetables, we need foods with natural sugars, and we need lean proteins to be easily available.

Tofu and other protein substitutes can be worked creatively into diets. We need to teach people how to integrate those foods into their diets to improve health. Most people do not know how to add tofu to a diet other than by going to an Asian restaurant and ordering their tofu curry. That strategy isn't useful for home cooking. We need to educate people about the value and benefits of healthy eating -- and then we need to facilitate access to healthier food in our workplaces, schools, and communities.

Clearly, we need to teach, preach, enable, and support healthy eating. We need to create access to healthier foods and we need to help people with the volume of food intake. High volumes of food intake obviously help make people overweight and obese. We need people to eat less. We need people to eat less sugar and to avoid saturated fat entirely. That will only happen if people believe that there is a value to be achieved by eating less that will exceed the downsides that people often experience when trying to eat lower volume of food.

Dieting Can Trigger Negative Neurochemicals

One major challenge that we obviously face for our healthy eating strategies is that dieting and food intake reduction can both trigger negative neurochemicals in many people's brains. Stress levels and stress chemicals can be triggered in people's brains by various diets and by food intake reductions.[295] It's hard to maintain any level of weight loss as a personal agenda or as a set of consistent behavior choices for an individual when the process of reducing food volume intake increases stress and generates negative neurochemicals in people's brains.

By contrast, activity levels generate positive neurochemicals in most people's brains. That negative neurological impact that can result from reducing food intake and the positive impact and neurochemicals that can result from activity levels is one of the key reasons why increasing activity levels and improving activity agendas to get people walking regularly and often has a higher likelihood of success for actually improving both population health and individual health compared to health improvement strategies that are built around reducing people's eating levels. That is an important biological difference. Walking creates positive neurochemicals. Dieting can create negative neurochemicals. To enhance the likelihood of success for any behavior change strategies, it is better and easier when our neurochemicals support our strategy. It is obviously harder to follow a plan when our neurochemicals actually resist our strategy. Walking and dieting have very different neurochemical impacts. Walking generates positive neurochemicals much of the time. Some people even become somewhat addicted to walking. Almost no one becomes addicted to diets or to food deprivation and the few people who do have that addiction to food derivation often have other significant difficulties.

So when we look at the agendas available to us for reducing obesity and compare them to the agendas involved in reducing inactivity, the solution set that has the highest likelihood of working well in the real world to improve population health in the immediate future involves increasing activity levels -- specifically walking.

That's why the opening pages of this chapter on health improvement were focused on walking and not on obesity. That probably surprised some readers. Obesity usually gets a lot more attention than inactivity in health-related publications. Most people understand the risks of obesity. Relatively few people appreciate the risks of inactivity.

Fit Beats Fat for Many People

Interestingly, when you look at the relative risks to an individual that result from inactivity versus obesity -- fit actually beats fat as a risk reduction focus for most people. Being inert is very high risk.

If you have to choose between being thin and being active, thin loses to active as a risk reduction strategy. Thin people who are inert are often at a higher health-risk level than overweight people who are active. Overweight people who walk -- who choose to be active -- have risk levels equal to or better than inactive people who are much thinner.[296]

So another very important point to keep in mind as we set up our highest priority agendas for better health for our work places, our communities and our schools is that being inert is a higher health risk than being obese for most people. The risk is higher for inactivity and the frequency of inactivity is greater. We actually have more inactive people as we have obese people in this country.[297] That information actually gives us a huge opportunity to add value to a lot of lives. Look at the real numbers earlier in this chapter. About 30 percent of Americans are measurably obese.[298] About 60 percent of Americans are inactive.[299] So we need to make some serious decisions about our health improvement agendas going forward. We need to work on both obesity and inactivity. Healthier eating and active living create a very good overall strategy. In each area, it makes sense to focus our energy on the behaviors of highest risk and on the highest likelihood of putting strategies in place that actually work.

Diabetes Is a Disease of Urbanization

We Americans are not alone in facing this set of behavior-related health issues. The whole world is facing similar problems relative to behaviors and chronic disease. The rate of diabetes is growing across the planet. Diabetes is now common in countries where it was once rare. Why is that happening? Why is diabetes becoming common in countries that used to have almost no diabetics? There is no germ that carries diabetes as a disease across national boundaries. So why are we seeing a worldwide epidemic of diabetes?

Cities are the problem.

Figure 9.5

Top World Cities by Population

	1950			2012	
Rank	Country	Population	Rank	Country	Population
1	New York, United States	12,463,000	1	Tokyo-Yokohama, Japan	37,126,000
2	London, United Kingdom	8,860,000	2	Jakarta, Indonesia	26,063,000
3	Tokyo, Japan	7,000,000	3	Seoul-Incheon, South Korea	22,547,000
4	Paris, France	5,900,000	4	Delhi, DL-HR-UP, India	22,242,000
5	Shanghai, China	5,406,000	5	Manila, Philippines	21,951,000
6	Moscow, Russia	5,100,000	6	Shanghai, SHG, China	20,860,000
7	Buenos Aires, Argentina	5,000,000	7	New York, NY-NJ-CT, United States	20,464,000
8	Chicago, United States	4,906,000	8	Sao Paulo, Brazil	20,186,000
9	Ruhr, Germany	4,900,000	9	Mexico City, Mexico	19,463,000
10	Kolkata, India	4,800,000	10	Cairo, Egypt	17,816,000

Source: Four Thousand Years of Urban Growth: An Historical Census by Tertius Chandler. 1987. St. David's University Press. 2012. http://www.demographia.com/db-worldua.pdf

Diabetes is a disease of urbanization. We are urbanizing in country after country. We have more megacities on the planet today than at any time in the history of the world. The following chart shows to top ten cities 30 years ago by size and the top ten cities today. We humans are massively urbanizing. Why does urbanization trigger diabetes? Look at how people live in cities. Urbanization triggers some significant behavior changes. When people in many countries used to live in the countryside (instead of in the new megacities), people in those countries walked extensively. They also ate a lot of fruits and very local agricultural products. There was almost no diabetes in those rural communities and there were relatively lower levels of diabetes in those countries.

So why is urbanization a cause of diabetes?

When people move to those large cities, many end up in inadequate housing situations, in slums and various settlement areas. In those settings they tend to walk very little. Entire days can be almost motionless for a jobless person living in a slum. Many people who live in the new, large urban slums stay very close to their hut or shelter. Their food and the food eaten by other people in those countries has switched from locally grown foods to eating mass-produced imported foods. Those newly urbanized countries now import cheap food in large quantities. The new diets of the people in those megacities are now dangerously white. Their food base tends to be white sugar, white grain, and white rice. White food in those three categories of food can create a level of nutritional poison. Diabetes is the common result from the intake of eating only those processed white foods...and eating them in large quantities...and then being inactive to the point of being almost inert.

There are now large numbers of people who are diabetic in each of those countries. The urban dwellers in those countries face the double blow of bad and unhealthy food and inactivity. The people who live in those new urban settings are increasingly obese and in some settings they are literally almost entirely inert.

So what can be done about that problem in those countries? Now that we know what the problem is and also now that we know what can be done to mitigate the problems, the leaders in those countries need to go to some obvious next steps and turn that medical science into political, functional, and societal realities. Those countries need to create movement and activity in those urban settings -- getting people on their feet daily in ways that will help restore health. Food supplies need to be improved. It's time for practical solutions to those very basic and fundamental problems. The issues are just as basic as having safe water to drink. Activity levels and safe water are both basic conditions of better health.

It's time for practical solutions to those very basic and fundamental problems. The issues are just as basic as having safe water to drink. Activity levels and safe water are both basic conditions of better health.

We Did Not Knowingly Support Inactivity

So why are we just beginning to take steps to support walking and better levels of activity?

We did not do practical things to solve those problems in the past in part because we did not expect the problem to get this bad. We also, to be honest, did not know any practical things to do. The obesity epidemic was obvious to everyone, but no one knows how to deal effectively with obesity. When people live on a diet of processed food that can trigger the biological result of obesity, it's pretty hard to simply change the food supply of a great array of people. The white sugar, flour, and rice diets are all cheap, seductive, and tasty. They are particularly attractive and dangerous to people who are inactive.

To have an impact on the epidemic of diabetes today, all of the countries facing those issues will need to get people on a healthy eating agenda to restore them to normal weight levels. Increasing activity levels actually can help. We basically do need a universal HEAL agenda -- Healthy Eating Active Living -- to be the collective, widely supported strategy for multiple countries. All of those countries need to help people increase their activity levels and learn about the damage created by our current diets.

We Very Much Need a National Culture of Health

In this country, we need our national government and our national leaders to take a lead role in helping us create, aspire to, adopt, and adapt to a culture of health. There is no reason for our national leaders not to make building a culture of health for this country into a major priority for us all. We need clear, national leadership from the White House, the Secretary of Health, the Surgeon General, and from the U.S. Congress to explain to the American people why we will all be much better off if we achieve a culture of health.

We need to teach healthy behaviors and we need to create a national belief system that says healthy behaviors are desirable, and those behaviors are what we all should choose to do. At this point in our history, we need our leadership at multiple levels to be helping all of us -- people in communities, people in schools, and people in working settings -- to understand and appreciate both the new science of health and the behavioral choices we each have.

Diabetes isn't inevitable and it isn't a communicable disease. It is a biological result that is incurred by the behavioral choices we make. We now need to teach people that their risk of cancer, stroke, heart disease, diabetes, and depression can all be impacted by our behaviors. We need people to collectively believe in a culture of health so that we all help each other and reinforce each other's healthy choices.

We Need To Make Healthy Behaviors Easy To Do

As people decide to make healthy behaviors the way we live, we will need to set up ways of making those healthy behaviors easy to do. We very much need our local governments to help make that agenda of health real in practical and very local ways.

Why do local governments need to be part of that health improvement agenda?

Walking is a very local thing to do. Eating healthy local foods is also an inherently local thing to do. We can only walk where we are. We need local governments to create and maintain safe places to walk, and we need local government to facilitate wide-spread access to healthy -- often locally grown -- foods.

Improving our collective health is obviously the best single strategy we can have to bring down the costs of care in this country. In prior years, some people made that statement, but the people who made that statement generally did not have any actual strategy or practical steps in mind to help achieve that goal. This book is about practical steps -- for both care improvement and improved health.

We are a lot smarter now. We are better informed. Our tool kit is better. The science of health and prevention is very clear and has definitely gotten better. When people stop smoking the health benefits for those people begin very quickly. We also now know that there is also an almost immediate positive financial return from improving people's activity levels. We know that walking is a sufficient, efficient, and an entirely effective way of achieving our health goal of better levels of activity.

We also know that there are very quick financial returns from helping people lose weight. So we need to apply that new wisdom in our communities and our workplaces. We need workplaces that sponsor, encourage, and enable walking for their workers. That is possible to do. It isn't hypothetical, theoretical, ideological, or philosophical. It is purely practical.

Employers prefer practical solutions to real problems, so we should do practical things in work settings to help improve our workers health.

On a large scale, we need laws that make smoking expensive and inconvenient. We need food laws that restrict the worst kind of dietary fats and discourage use of the unhealthy processed sugar. Unhealthy foods should be more expensive and harder to obtain, while healthy foods should be the cheapest and most readily available option. We need people to understand the true negative health impact of unhealthy foods so they can make the right choices.

Knowledge is power. We need people with the power to change their own lives. We need support for healthy eating at multiple levels and we need laws that restrict access to unhealthy foods. Those efforts can all be an effective part of our overall health improvement agenda.

Finland Proved That a Culture of Health Is Possible

Health care costs now consume roughly 18 percent of our total economy.[300] We are on a path to expand that 18 percent to more than 20 percent.[301] Twenty percent will be financially crippling. If we create a true culture of health and people increase the levels of healthy behaviors -- we can keep that from happening. We can significantly improve health outcomes, reduce the need for health care services, and bring down the total cost of care by having healthier people. That's how this chapter began. It is the truth. It would be irresponsible of us -- now that we know the science and understand the actual impact of the health agenda -- not to create an activity friendly culture of health and put in place a community infrastructure that supports, enables, and facilitates health.

Finland actually went down that road to create a culture of health as a country. Finland went from being probably the least healthy country in Europe to being the healthiest country in just a few years by very deliberately creating a culture of health.

The next chart shows the success levels in Finland. We can replicate those results here.

Figure 9.6

Age-adjusted Mortality Rates of Coronary Heart Disease in North Karelia and the Whole of Finland Among Males Aged 35-64 Years from 1969 to 2006

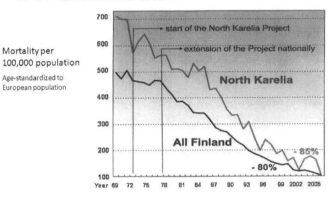

Source: Pekka Puska; The North Karelia Project, 30 years successfully preventing chronic diseases.

We have been both ignorant and passive about those issues for too long. We need to transform ourselves into a nation of people who make more healthy choices and we need to take health to the next agenda.

It isn't rocket science.

It may, however, involve some political science. These recommendations are definitely well supported by medical science. Now it is a matter of values. It is both unethical and economically stupid not to do the right thing now that we know the right things to do.

We Can Keep Health Care from Bankrupting America

We need to improve our care delivery in this country. We need to improve the safety of care in this country. We need to create a rich and comprehensive data flow that gives us all the data we need to deliver care and improve care in this country.

We need to make care better and we need to make care more affordable. We need to directly address both the quality and the costs of care.

That can all be done. We will need to change a few key things we do -- but those goals are within our grasp.

This book is intended to offer a path to achieving those goals and achieving them quickly enough that we can keep health care from bankrupting this country.

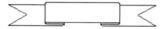

Kaiser Permanente Awards and Recognitions for Quality, Service, Creativity and Functionality

2013

- University of St. Thomas, Minneapolis, Minnesota, Lifetime Achievement Award, November 2013
- AHIP Lifetime Achievement Award. America's Health Insurance Plans June 2013
- "Foundation of the Year" Award. Gov. Edmund G. Brown Jr.'s 2013 Volunteer Service Awards. June 2013.
- Twenty-nine Environmental Excellence Awards. Practice Greenhealth. May 31, 2013.
- Platinum Award for Best Employer for Healthy Lifestyles. National Business Group on Health. May 22, 2013.
- Leapfrog Award for Kaiser Permanente Hospitals Rated Among Safest in the Nation. The Leapfrog Group. May 9, 2013.
- Highest ranking in J.D. Power and Associates Member Satisfaction Study. J.D. Power and Associates. May 3, 2013.
- Worksite Innovation Award for KP Walk! and Platinum Fit-Friendly Companies Program Company Award. American Heart Association. May 2013.
- AHA Award of Honor. The American Hospital Association (AHA) Award of Honor to George C. Halvorson, chairman and chief executive officer (CEO), Kaiser Permanente.
- Pharmacy Quality Alliance's annual Quality Award for health plans achieving excellence in medication safety and quality. Pharmacy Quality Alliance. April 2, 2013.
- Guinness World Record for Most Colorectal Cancer Screenings. Guinness World Records. March 31, 2013.

- Highest rating on California's Annual Clinical Quality Report Card for overall quality of care for fifth consecutive year. Healthcare Quality Report Card from the California Office of the Patient Advocate. March 28, 2013.
- Highest rating in HMO category, which measures members' satisfaction with their total care and service. Healthcare Quality Report Card from the California Office of the Patient Advocate. March 28, 2013.
- Kaiser Permanente Health Plans Named eValue8's 2012 Top Performers, including awards for creativity and innovation in health care. National Business Coalition on Health. The March 11, 2013.
- 2013 HIStalk Health Care IT Lifetime Achievement Award. Health Care IT News and Opionion. March 4, 2013.
- Eisenberg Award for Patient Safety and Quality Efforts. The Joint Commission. March 2, 2013.
- Kaiser Permanente's Medicare Plans Earn Top NCQA Health Insurance Rankings. National Committee for Quality Assurance. 2012–2013.

2012

- Six eHealthcare Leadership Awards for the use of the Internet and technology to support the commitment to total health. Strategic Health Care Communications. November 30, 2012.
- Leapfrog Award for Kaiser Permanente Hospitals being among the safest in the nation. The Leapfrog Group. June 2012.
- Highest rating in the nation in 13 Medicare Measures. The 5-Star Star Quality rating system for Medicare Advantage Plans. Centers for Medicare and Medicaid Services (CMS). October 2012.
- Highest rating in the nation, Six 5-Star Medicare Health Plans. The 5-Star Star Quality Rating System for Medicare Advantage Plans. CMS. October 2012.

- Highest scores in the nation in 16 NCQA/HEDIS Effectiveness of Care Measures. National Committee for Quality Assurance (NCQA)/The Healthcare Effectiveness Data and Information Set (HEDIS). October, 2012.
- 20 hospitals ranked Top Performer in Quality. The Joint Commission. September 19, 2012.
- Leadership in Energy & Environmental Design (LEED) Platinum certification awarded to Napa Data Center. U.S. Green Building Design Council. July 2012.
- Highest in Customer Satisfaction among Mail-Order Pharmacies for fourth consecutive year. J.D. Power and Associates as. July 2012.
- Platinum Award for Best Employer for Healthy Lifestyles. National Business Group on Health. July 2012.
- Top 20 in Computerworld's 2012 List of 100 Best Places to Work in IT. International Data Group Network. July 2012
- Highest ranking in 2012 J.D. Power and Associates Employer Satisfaction Study for Second Year in a Row. J.D. Power and Associates. July 20, 2012.
- Leapfrog Awards. Kaiser Permanente Hospitals among the Safest in the Nation. The Leapfrog Group. July 2012.
- No. 1 in Customer Loyalty in the 2012 Satmetrix Net Promoter® Benchmark Study. The Net Promoter Company. March 2012.
- Laboratory of the year. The Medical Laboratory Observer. March 2012
- Stage 7 Awards. Healthcare Information and Management Systems Society (HIMSS). February, 2012.

2011

- Four eHealthcare Leadership Awards for the use of the Internet and technology to support the commitment to total health. Strategic Health Care Communications. December 7, 2011.

- Leapfrog Awards 18 Kaiser Permanente Hospitals as Top Hospitals for their outstanding success in such areas as infection rates, safety practices, mortality rates for common procedures and measures of efficiency. The Leapfrog Group. December 2011.
- Named No. 1 Green-IT Organization by Computerworld for excellence in IT practices that benefit the environment. International Data Group Network. October 2011.
- Recognized by J.D. Power and Associates as Highest in Customer Satisfaction among Mail-Order Pharmacies for Third Consecutive Year. J.D. Power & Associates. October 2011.
- 10 Kaiser Permanente Hospitals Honored as 'Top Performer' in Quality and Safety. The Joint Commission. September 2011.
- HIMSS Davies Award Presented for Organizational Excellence for Electronic Health Record Implementation. HIMSS Davies Award. September 2011.
- Pharmacy Quality Alliance's annual Quality Award for health plans achieving excellence in medication safety and quality. Pharmacy Quality Alliance. June 2011.
- U.S. News & World Report gives 13 Kaiser Permanente hospitals highest ranking for reputation, mortality, patient safety and other areas, including nurse staffing and technology. U.S. News & World Report. March 2011.

END NOTES

[1] C. Schoen, R. Osborn, D. Squires, M. M. Doty, R. Pierson, and S. Applebaum. "New 2011 Survey of Patients with Complex Care Needs in 11 Countries Finds That Care Is Often Poorly Coordinated." *Health Affairs Web First*, November 9, 2011.

[2] OECD. "Health at a Glance 2011: OECD Indicators."

[3] U.S. Bureau of Labor Statistics. "100 Years of U.S. Consumer Spending Data for the Nation, New York City, and Boston." May 2006.

United States Department of Agriculture. "The 20th Century Transformation of U.S. Agriculture and Farm Policy." *Economic Information Bulletin*, Number 3. June 2005.

[4] U.S. Bureau of Labor Statistics. "Consumer Expenditures 2011." September 25, 2012. http://www.bls.gov/news.release/cesan.nr0.htm.

United States Department of Agriculture. "The 20th Century Transformation of U.S. Agriculture and Farm Policy." *Economic Information Bulletin*, Number 3. June 2005.

[5] MedPac. "Hospital Payment Basics Acute Inpatient Services Payment System." *Payment Basics*. October 2009. http://www.medpac.gov/documents/medPAc_payment_Basics_09_hospital.pdf.

[6] Centers for Disease Control. "Chronic Diseases The Power to Prevent, The Call to Control: At A Glance 2009." http://www.cdc.gov/chronicdisease/resources/publications/AAG/chronic.htm.

[7] M. O'Grady, P. John, and A. Winn. "Substantial Medicare Savings May Result If Insurers Cover 'Artificial Pancreas' Sooner For Diabetes Patients." *Health Affairs*. August 2012, vol. 31, 8:1822-1829.

[8] G. Anderson. "Chronic Care: Making the Case for Ongoing Care." *Robert Wood Johnson Foundation*. February 2010. www.rwjf.org/pr/product.jsp?id=50968.

[9] R. Mangione-Smith and others. "The Quality of Ambulatory Care Delivered to Children in the United States." *The New England Journal of Medicine*. 2007:357(15):1515-1523.

[10] F. Booth, S. Gordon, C. Carlson, and M. Hamilton. "Waging war on modern chronic diseases: primary prevention through exercise biology." *Journal of Applied Physiology*. 2000:88:774-787.

Centers for Disease Control. "Chronic Diseases The Power to Prevent, The Call to Control: At A Glance 2009." http://www.cdc.gov/chronicdisease/resources/publications/AAG/chronic.htm.

[11] American Diabetes Association. "Diabetes Fact Sheet." http://main.diabetes.org/stepup/diabetes_facts.pdf.

[12] M. O'Grady, P. John, and A. Winn. "Substantial Medicare Savings May Result If Insurers Cover 'Artificial Pancreas' Sooner For Diabetes Patients." *Health Affairs.* August 2012, vol. 31, 8:1822-1829.

[13] Ibid.

[14] J. Torpy, C. Lynm, and R. Glass. "Diabetes." *Journal of the American Medical Association.* 2009:301(15):1620.

[15] G. Coldlitz. "Economic Costs of Obesity and Inactivity." *Medicine and Science in Sports Exercise.* 1999:11(Suppl):S663-667..

[16] G. Coldlitz. "Economic Costs of Obesity and Inactivity." *Medicine and Science in Sports Exercise.* 1999:11(Suppl):S663-667.

Centers for Disease Control. "Chronic Diseases The Power to Prevent, The Call to Control: At A Glance 2009." http://www.cdc.gov/chronicdisease/resources/publications/AAG/chronic.htm.

[17] American Diabetes Association. "Diabetes FAQ." http://www.diabetes.org/diabetes-basics/prevention/pre-diabetes/pre-diabetes-faqs.html.

[18] United States Department of Health and Human Services. "HHS Targets Efforts on Diabetes." January 13, 2006. http://www.hhs.gov/news/factsheet/diabetes.html.

[19] J. Huerta and others. "Physical Activity and Risk of Cerebrovascular Disease in the European Prospective Investigation into Cancer and Nutrition-Spain Study." Stroke. 2013:44:111-118.

M. Tully and others. "Randomised controlled trial of home-based walking programmes at and below current recommended levels of exercise in sedentary adults." *Journal of Epidemiology & Community Health.* 2007:61(9):778-83.

[20] RSNA Press Release. "Walking Slows Progression of Alzheimer's." *Radiological Society of North America.* November 29, 2010. http://www2.rsna.org/timssnet/media/pressreleases/pr_target.cfm?ID=508.

[21] J. Lee. "5 Ways Activity Helps to Reverse Depression." *ChooseHelp.com.* http://www.choosehelp.com/depression/5-reasons-why-getting-active-reduces-feelings-of-depression/5-ways-activity-helps-to-reverse-depression.

[22] E. Giovannucci and others. "Physical Activity, Obesity, and Risk for Colon Cancer and Adenoma in Men." *Annals of Internal Medicine.* 1995:122:327-334.

[23] M. Holmes, W. Chen, D. Feskanich, C. Kroenke, and G. Colditz. "Physical Activity and Survival After Breast Cancer Diagnosis." *JAMA.* 2005; 293(20):2479-2486.

[24] S. Heffler and others. "Health Spending Projections for 2001–2011: The Latest Outlook." *Health Affairs.* 2002:21(2):207-218.

[25] E. Emanuel. "Spending More Doesn't Make Us Healthier." New York Times. October 27, 2011. http://opinionator.blogs.nytimes.com/2011/10/27/spending-more-doesnt-make-us-healthier/.

[26] OECD. "Health at a Glance 2011: OECD Indicators."

[27] U.S. Bureau of Labor Statistics. "The Employment Situation – October 2012." November 2, 2012. http://www.bls.gov/news.release/pdf/empsit.pdf.

[28] Philadelphia Enquirer. "100 Biggest Non-Governmental Employers." *The Top 100 Businesses in the Philadelphia Region.* 2009. http://www.philly.com/philly/business/top100/12255951.html.

[29] PWC Medical Technology. "The Race for Global Leadership." *Medical Technology Innovation Scorecard.* January 2011. http://download.pwc.com/ie/pubs/2011_medical_technology_innovation_scorecard_the_race_for_global_leadership_jan.pdf.

[30] Ibid.

[31] P. Hussey, S. Wertheimer, A. Mehrotra. "The Association Between Health Care Quality and Cost: A Systematic Review." *Annals of Internal Medicine.* 2013:158(1):27-34.

[32] T. Lagu and others. "The Relationship Between Hospital Spending and Mortality in Patients With Sepsis." *Archives of Internal Medicine.* 2011:171(4):292-299.

[33] Kaiser Family Foundation and Health Research Educational Trust. "Employer Health Benefits 2012 Annual Survey." September 11, 2012. http://ehbs.kff.org/.

[34] Kaiser Family Foundation. "Health Care Costs: Key Information on Health Care Costs and Their Impact." May 2012. http://www.kff.org/insurance/upload/7670-03.pdf.

[35] U.S. Senate Special Committee on Aging Hearing: "A Prescription for Savings: Reducing Drug Costs to Medicare" July 21, 2011. http://aging.senate.gov/events/hr236opt.pdf.

[36] International Federation of Health Plans. "2011 Comparative Price Report Medical and Hospital Fees by Country." http://www.ifhp.com/documents/2011iFHPPriceReportGraphs_version3.pdf.

[37] Ibid.

[38] Ibid.

[39] Ibid.

[40] Ibid.

[41] Centers for Disease Control. "Chronic Diseases The Power to Prevent, The Call to Control: At A Glance 2009." http://www.cdc.gov/chronicdisease/resources/publications/AAG/chronic.htm.

[42] Health Grades. "American Hospital Quality Outcomes 2013." *Healthgrades Report to the Nation.* 2012.

[43] California Office of Statewide Health Planning and Development. "The California Report on Coronary Artery Bypass Graft Surgery, 2009 Hospital Data." April 2012.

[44] T. Lagu and others. "The Relationship Between Hospital Spending and Mortality in Patients With Sepsis." *Archives of Internal Medicine.* 2011:171(4):292-299.

[45] Centers for Disease Control. "Cancer Rates by State." *Cancer Prevention and Control.* http://www.cdc.gov/cancer/dcpc/data/state.htm.

[46] Committee on Quality of Health Care in America (L. Kohn, J. Corrigan, and M. Donaldson, Editors). "To Err Is Human: Building a Safer Health System." *Institute of Medicine.* November 1, 1999.

[47] Ibid.

[48] Ibid.

[49] Committee on Quality of Health Care in America. "Crossing the Quality Chasm: A New Health System for the 21st Century." Institute of Medicine: Shaping the Future for Health. March 2001.

[50] "Institute of Medicine's Roundtable on Value & Science-Driven Health Care." Institute of Medicine. July 2011. http://www.iom.edu/Activities/Quality/~/

media/Files/Activity%20Files/Quality/VSRT/Core%20Documents/Background.pdf.

[51] Ibid.

[52] S. Sidney and others. "Closing the Gap Between Cardiovascular and Cancer Mortality in an Integrated Health Care Delivery System, 2000-2008: The Kaiser Permanente Experience." *Circulation.* 2011:124(A13610).

[53] R. Dell, D. Greene, S. Schelkun, and K. Williams. "Osteoporosis Disease Management: The Role of the Orthopedic Surgeon." *The Journal of Bone & Joint Surgery.* 2008:90(4):188-194.

[54] California Office of Statewide Health Planning and Development. "The California Report on Coronary Artery Bypass Graft Surgery, 2009 Hospital Data." April 2012.

[55] National Institute of General Medical Sciences. "Sepsis Fact Sheet." November 2012. http://www.nigms.nih.gov/Education/factsheet_sepsis.htm.

[56] Centers for Disease Control. "Estimating Health Care-Associated Infections and Deaths in U.S.Hospitals, 2002." *Public Health Reports.* March-April 2007.

[57] Agency for Healthcare Research and Quality. "Pressure Ulcer Risk Assessment and Prevention: Comparative Effectiveness." *Comparative Effectiveness Review.* May 2013.

[58] Ibid.

[59] Internal KP data.

[60] National Cancer Institute. "Map Story: Breast Cancer." https://gis.cancer.gov/mapstory/breast/.

[61] L. Stannard. "Breast Cancer & Brain Metastases Life Expectancy." Livestrong.com, April 26, 2011. http://www.livestrong.com/article/21919-breast-cancer-brain-metastases/.

Taussig Cancer Institute. "2011 Outcomes." Cleveland Clinic. 2011.

Internal KP data.

[62] Internal KP data.

[63] National Quality Measures Clearinghouse. "Pressure ulcer prevention and treatment protocol: percentage of inpatients with pressure ulcers whose medical record contains documentation of a partial wound assessment with every dressing change." *Agency for Healthcare Research and Quality.* http://qualitymeasures.ahrq.gov/content.aspx?id=36735.

[64] CALNOC. "The CALNOC Overview." http://calnoc.affiniscape.com/associations/13337/files/01.20.2011%20CALNOC%20Overview.pdf.

[65] Internal KP data.

[66] D. Berlowitz and others. "Preventing Pressure Ulcers in Hospitals." *Agency for Healthcare Research and Quality.* http://www.ahrq.gov/professionals/systems/long-term-care/resources/pressure-ulcers/pressureulcertoolkit/putoolkit.pdf.

[67] M. Eber, R. Laxminarayan, E. Perencevich, and A. Malani. "Clinical and Economic Outcomes Attributable to Health Care–Associated Sepsis and Pneumonia." *Archives of Internal Medicine,* 2010; 170(4); 347-353.

[68] Ibid.

[69] Global Sepsis Alliance. "International Organizations Declare Sepsis a Global Medical Emergency." October 1, 2010. http://www.globalsepsisalliance.org/about/merinoff/press_release.pdf.

[70] National Institute of General Medical Sciences. "Sepsis Fact Sheet." November 2012. http://www.nigms.nih.gov/Education/factsheet_sepsis.htm.

[71] California Office of Statewide Health Planning and Development "In-Hospital Mortality, 2006." *OSHPD Research Brief.* November 2008.

[72] A. Whippy and others. "Kaiser Permanente's Performance Improvement System, Part 3: Multisite Improvements in Care for Patients with Sepsis." *Joint Commission Journal on Quality and Patient Safety.* 2011:37(11):483.

[73] M. Raghavan and P. Marik. "Management of sepsis during the early 'golden hours." *The Journal of Emergency Medicine.* 2006: 31(2):185-199.

[74] A. Whippy and others. "Kaiser Permanente's Performance Improvement System, Part 3: Multisite Improvements in Care for Patients with Sepsis." *Joint Commission Journal on Quality and Patient Safety.* 2011: 37(11): 483.

[75] Ibid.

[76] A. Bessent. "Health care waste, fraud and abuse -- all true." *Newsday.* September 12, 2012. http://www.newsday.com/opinion/viewsday-1.3683911/bessent-health-care-waste-fraud-and-abuse-all-true-1.3996503.

[77] J. Aleccia. "Look-alike, sound-alike drugs trigger dangers." *NBC News.* May 28, 2010. http://www.msnbc.msn.com/id/37386398/ns/health-health_care/t/look-alike-sound-alike-drugs-trigger-dangers/.

[78] "F as in Fat: How Obesity Threatens America's Future." *Robert Wood Johnson Foundation Issue Report.* September 2012.
OECD. "Health at a Glance 2011: OECD Indicators."

[79] Lancet Physical Activity Series Working Group. "Effect of physical inactivity on major non-communicable diseases worldwide: an analysis of burden of disease and life expectancy." *The Lancet,* July 21, 2012, Vol. 380, Issue 9838; 219-229.

[80] M. O'Grady, P. John, and A. Winn. "Substantial Medicare Savings May Result If Insurers Cover 'Artificial Pancreas' Sooner For Diabetes Patients." *Health Affairs,* August 2012, Vol. 31, 8:1822-1829.

[81] W. Konrad. "Protecting Yourself From the Cost of Type 2 Diabetes." *New York Times.* November 12, 2010. http://www.nytimes.com/2010/11/13/health/13patient.html.

[82] Centers for Disease Control and Prevention. "National Diabetes Fact Sheet: National Estimates and General Information on Diabetes and Prediabetes in the United States." 2011. http://www.cdc.gov/diabetes/pubs/pdf/ndfs_2011.pdf.

[83] Ibid.

[84] W. Bogdanich and J. Craven McGinty. "Medicare claims show overuse for CT scanning." *New York Times.* June 17, 2011. http://www.nytimes.com/2011/06/18/health/18radiation.html?pagewanted=all&_r=0.

[85] D. Cosgrove and others. "A CEO Checklist for High-Value Health Care." *Institute of Medicine Discussion Paper.* June 5, 2012. http://www.iom.edu/Global/Perspectives/2012/CEOChecklist.aspx.

[86] R. Dell, D. Greene, S. Schelkun, and K. Williams. "Osteoporosis Disease Management: The Role of the Orthopedic Surgeon." *The Journal of Bone & Joint Surgery.* 2008:90(4):188-194.

[87] Editorial. "Simple Treatments, Ignored." *New York Times.* September 8, 2012. http://www.nytimes.com/2012/09/09/opinion/sunday/simple-treatments-ignored.html?_r=2&.

[88] D. Cosgrove and others. "A CEO Checklist for High-Value Health Care." *Institute of Medicine Discussion Paper.* June 5, 2012. http://www.iom.edu/Global/Perspectives/2012/CEOChecklist.aspx.

[89] R. Dell, D. Greene, S. Schelkun, and K. Williams. "Osteoporosis Disease Management: The Role of the Orthopedic Surgeon." *The Journal of Bone & Joint Surgery.* 2008:90(4):188-194

[90] Committee on Quality of Health Care in America (L. Kohn, J. Corrigan, and M. Donaldson, Editors). "To Err Is Human: Building a Safer Health System." *Institute of Medicine.* November 1, 1999.

[91] National Institute of Health, Subcommittee on Courts, the Internet, and Intellectual Property. "NIH's Public Access Policy." *NIH Director's Report.* February 5, 2008.

[92] B. Meier. "Maker Aware of 40% Failure in Hip Implant." *New York Times.* January 22, 2013. http://www.nytimes.com/2013/01/23/business/jj-study-suggested-hip-device-could-fail-in-thousands-more.html?_r=0.

Associated Press. "FDA gives heart implant recall highest warning." *NBC News.* July 1, 2005. http://www.nbcnews.com/id/8434931/ns/health-heart_health/t/fda-gives-heart-implant-recall-highest-warning/.

[93] A.C. Flint and others. "Inpatient Statin use Predicts Improved Ischemic Stroke Discharge Disposition." *Neurology.* 2012:78(21):1678-1683.

[94] Ibid.

[95] Ibid.

[96] Ibid.

[97] National Institute of Health, Subcommittee on Courts, the Internet, and Intellectual Property. "NIH's Public Access Policy." *NIH Director's Report.* February 5, 2008.

[98] S. Young and others. "Sharing Clinical Knowledge." Care *Management Institute.* July 10, 2012. http://www.iom.edu/~/media/Files/Activity%20Files/Quality/VSRT/IC%20Meeting%20Docs/ICD%2007-10-12/Scott%20Young.pdf.

[99] Editorial. "Simple Treatments, Ignored." *New York Times.* September 8, 2012. http://www.nytimes.com/2012/09/09/opinion/sunday/simple-treatments-ignored.html?_r=2&.

[100] S. Heffler and others. "Health Spending Projections for 2001–2011: The Latest Outlook." *Health Affairs.* 2002:21(2):207-218.

[101] American Lung Association. "Asthma." http://www.lung.org/associations/states/colorado/asthma/Asthma.html.

[102] N. Pheatt, R. Brindis, and E. Levin. "Putting Heart Disease Guidelines into Practice: Kaiser Permanente Leads the Way." *The Permanente Journal.* 2003:7(1):18-23.

[103] National Institute of General Medical Sciences. "Sepsis Fact Sheet." November 2012. http://www.nigms.nih.gov/Education/factsheet_sepsis.htm.

[104] Health Grades. "American Hospital Quality Outcomes 2013." *Healthgrades Report to the Nation.* 2012.

[105] Internal KP data.

[106] Kaiser Permanente. "2012 Annual Report."

[107] Ibid.

[108] International Federation of Health Plans. "2011 Comparative Price Report Medical and Hospital Fees by Country." http://www.ifhp.com/documents/2011iFHPPriceReportGraphs_version3.pdf.

109 Ibid.

110 Ibid.

111 Ontario Regulation 856/93Professional Misconduct. "Section 1 (1) 22." Medicine Act. 1991. http://www.e-laws.gov.on.ca/html/regs/english/elaws_regs_930856_e.htm.

112 International Federation of Health Plans. "2011 Comparative Price Report Medical and Hospital Fees by Country." http://www.ifhp.com/documents/20 11iFHPPriceReportGraphs_version3.pdf.

113 Ibid.

114 Ibid.

115 International Federation of Health Plans. "Who we Are." http://www.ifhp.com/who.html.

116 International Federation of Health Plans. "2011 Comparative Price Report Medical and Hospital Fees by Country." http://www.ifhp.com/documents/20 11iFHPPriceReportGraphs_version3.pdf..

117 Transforming Maternity Care. "Average Charges for Giving Birth: State Charts." http://transform.childbirthconnection.org/resources/datacenter/chargeschart/statecharges/.

118 International Federation of Health Plans. "2011 Comparative Price Report Medical and Hospital Fees by Country." http://www.ifhp.com/documents/20 11iFHPPriceReportGraphs_version3.pdf.

119 Centers for Medicare and Medicaid Services. "National Health Expenditure Data Fact Sheet." https://www.cms.gov/Research-Statistics-Data-and-Systems/Statistics-Trends-and-Reports/NationalHealthExpendData/NHE-Fact-Sheet.html.

120 California Department of Health Care Services. "Medi-Cal Rates as of 11/15/2012." http://files.medi-cal.ca.gov/pubsdoco/Rates/rates_download.asp.

121 International Federation of Health Plans. "2012 Comparative Price Report Medical and Hospital Fees by Country." http://www.ifhp.com/documents/20 11iFHPPriceReportGraphs_version3.pdf.

122 International Federation of Health Plans. "2011 Comparative Price Report Medical and Hospital Fees by Country." http://www.ifhp.com/documents/20 11iFHPPriceReportGraphs_version3.pdf.

123 Ibid.

124 Ibid.

125 Office of Massachusetts Attorney General Martha Coakely. "Examination of Health Care Cost Trends and Cost Drivers Pursuant to G.L. c. 118G, sec 6 ½ (b)." Report for Annual Public Hearing. June 22, 2011. http://www.mass.gov/ago/docs/healthcare/2011-hcctd-full.pdf.

126 International Federation of Health Plans. "2011 Comparative Price Report Medical and Hospital Fees by Country." http://www.ifhp.com/documents/20 11iFHPPriceReportGraphs_version3.pdf.

127 "Heart Surgery in India - The Cost and Quality Factor." Heart Consult's Blog. February 10, 2011. http://www.heart-consult.com/content/heart-surgery-india-cost-and-quality-factor.

128 T. Lagu, M. Rothberg, B. Nathanson, P. Pekow, J. Steingrub, P. Lindenauer." The Relationship Between Hospital Spending and Mortality in Patients With Sepsis." Archives of Internal Medicine. 2011:171(4):292-299.

129 S. Brill. "Bitter Pill: Why Medical Bills Are Killing Us." Time. March 4, 2013. http://healthland.time.com/why-medical-bills-are-killing-us/.

[130] "Illinois hospital prices vary widely, Medicare data show." *Chicago Tribune.* May 08, 2013. http://articles.chicagotribune.com/2013-05-08/business/chi-medicare-hospital-charges-20130508_1_health-care-overhaul-law-major-joint-replacement-hospitals.

[131] Ibid.

[132] C. Terhne. "Medicare charges vary widely at California hospitals, new data show." *Los Angeles Times.* May 08, 2013. http://articles.latimes.com/2013/may/08/business/la-fi-mo-medicare-hospital-costs-20130508.

[133] Ibid.

[134] M. Booth. "Colorado hospitals charge up to 10 times Medicare's rates, data show." The Denver Post. May 8, 2013. http://www.denverpost.com/ci_23198935/some-hospitals-charge-vastly-more-same-care-including.

[135] Ibid.

[136] S. Brill. "Bitter Pill: Why Medical Bills Are Killing Us." *Time.* March 4, 2013. http://healthland.time.com/why-medical-bills-are-killing-us/.

[137] C. Schoen, M. M. Doty, R. H. Robertson, and S. R. Collins, "Affordable Care Act Reforms Could Reduce the Number of Underinsured U.S. Adults by 70 Percent," *Health Affairs,* Sept. 2011 30(9): 1762–71.

[138] International Federation of Health Plans. "2011 Comparative Price Report Medical and Hospital Fees by Country." http://www.ifhp.com/documents/2011iFHPPriceReportGraphs_version3.pdf.

[139] Ibid.

[140] Ibid.

[141] Ibid.

[142] R. Bazell. *HER-2: The Making of Herceptin, a Revolutionary Treatment for Breast Cancer.* New York (NY): Random House. 1998.

[143] "Guideline Summary: American Society of Clinical Oncology/College of American Pathologists Guideline Recommendations for Human Epidermal Growth Factor Receptor HER2 Testing in Breast Cancer." *Journal of Oncology Practice.* 2007:3(1):48-50.

[144] N. Kresge. "Study Questions Current use of Herceptin." *San Francisco Chronicle.* September 24, 2012. http://www.sfgate.com/default/article/Study-questions-current-use-of-Herceptin-3890947.php.

[145] Price Waterhouse Coopers. "The Factors Fueling Rising Health Care Costs." December 2008.

[146] Virginia Mason Institute. "Advanced Imaging: Evidence-based Decision Rules Used at Virginia Mason Medical Center." http://www.virginiamasoninstitute.org/advanced-imaging.

[147] International Federation of Health Plans. "2011 Comparative Price Report Medical and Hospital Fees by Country." http://www.ifhp.com/documents/2011iFHPPriceReportGraphs_version3.pdf.

[148] Ibid.

[149] "2012 Medicare Physician Fee Schedule Payment Rates Computed Tomography." www.usa.siemens.com/healthcare.

[150] California Department of Health Care Services. "Medical Rates." January 15, 2013.

[151] "That CT scan costs how much?" *Consumer Reports.* July 2012. http://www.consumerreports.org/cro/magazine/2012/07/that-ct-scan-costs-how-much/index.htm.

[152] St. Luke's University Health Network. "St. Luke's Becomes First Hospital in the Region to Offer a Lung Cancer Screening Program for Long-Term Current and Former Smokers." July 7, 2011. http://www.slhn.org/News/2011/CT-Scans-Screen-Smokers.aspx.

[153] "Radiation Dose in X-Ray and CT Exams." RadiologyInfo.org. http://www.radiologyinfo.org/en/safety/?pg=sfty_xray.

[154] International Federation of Health Plans. "2011 Comparative Price Report Medical and Hospital Fees by Country." http://www.ifhp.com/documents/2011iFHPPriceReportGraphs_version3.pdf.

[155] Ibid.

[156] Ibid.

[157] D. Squires. "The U.S. Health System in Perspective: A Comparison of Twelve Industrialized Nations." *The Commonwealth Fund, Issues in International Health Policy.* 2011:16.

[158] OECD. "Health at a Glance: Europe 2012."

[159] D. Squires. "The U.S. Health System in Perspective: A Comparison of Twelve Industrialized Nations." *The Commonwealth Fund, Issues in International Health Policy.* 2011:16..

[160] Ibid.

[161] Ibid.

[162] C. Schoen and R. Osborn. "The Commonwealth Fund 2011 International Health Policy Survey of Sicker Adults in Eleven Countries." *Commonwealth Fund.* November 2011.

[163] Central Intelligence Agency. "The World Factbook." https://www.cia.gov/library/publications/the-world-factbook/rankorder/2102rank.html.

[164] J. Arvantes. "'Solid Investments in Primary Care Workforce' Needed, AAFP Member Tells Congressional Committee." *American Academy of Family Physicians.* April 26, 2013. http://www.aafp.org/online/en/home/publications/news/news-now/government-medicine/20130426rusttestimony.html.

[165] International Federation of Health Plans. "2011 Comparative Price Report Medical and Hospital Fees by Country." http://www.ifhp.com/documents/2011iFHPPriceReportGraphs_version3.pdf.

[166] G. Anderson, U. Reinhardt, P. Hussey and V. Petrosyan. "It's The Prices, Stupid: Why The United States Is So Different From Other Countries." *Health Affairs.* 2003:22(3):89-105.

[167] Texas State Historical Association. "Justin Ford Kimball." The Handbook of Texas Online. http://www.tshaonline.org/handbook/online/articles/fki09.

[168] D. Cosgrove and others. "A CEO Checklist for High-Value Health Care." *Institute of Medicine Discussion Paper.* June 5, 2012. http://www.iom.edu/Global/Perspectives/2012/CEOChecklist.aspx.

[169] Kaiser Permanente. "Interregional HIV Treatment Practice Resource." 2011.

Centers for Medicare and Medicaid Services. "Physician Fee Schedule." http://www.cms.gov/apps/physician-fee-schedule/.

[170] R. Dell, D. Greene, S. Schelkun, and K. Williams. "Osteoporosis Disease Management: The Role of the Orthopedic Surgeon." *The Journal of Bone & Joint Surgery.* 2008:90(4):188-194

[171] R. Dell, D. Greene, S. Schelkun, and K. Williams. "Osteoporosis Disease Management: The Role of the Orthopedic Surgeon." *The Journal of Bone & Joint Surgery.* 2008:90(4):188-194.

Centers for Medicare and Medicaid Services. "Physician Fee Schedule." http://www.cms.gov/apps/physician-fee-schedule/.

[172] "Heart disease and stroke deaths drop significantly for people with diabetes." Centers for Disease Control and Prevention. May 22, 2012. http://www.cdc.gov/media/releases/2012/p0522_heart_disease.html.

[173] Kaiser Permanente. "2011 Annual Report."

[174] CALNOC. "The CALNOC Overview." http://calnoc.affiniscape.com/associations/13337/files/01.20.2011%20CALNOC%20Overview.pdf.

National Quality Measures Clearinghouse. "Pressure ulcer prevention and treatment protocol: percentage of inpatients with pressure ulcers whose medical record contains documentation of a partial wound assessment with every dressing change." *Agency for Healthcare Research and Quality*. http://qualitymeasures.ahrq.gov/content.aspx?id=36735.

[175] Kaiser Permanente. "Reducing Pressure Ulcers in Kaiser Foundation Hospitals." *Measuring Patient Safety in our Hospitals*. May 2012. https://healthy.kaiserpermanente.org/static/health/pdfs/quality_and_safety/multi/multi_pressure_ulcers.pdf.

[176] D. Berlowitz and others. "Preventing Pressure Ulcers in Hospitals." *Agency for Healthcare Research and Quality*.

[177] CALNOC. "The CALNOC Overview." http://calnoc.affiniscape.com/associations/13337/files/01.20.2011%20CALNOC%20Overview.pdf.

[178] D. Berlowitz and others. "Preventing Pressure Ulcers in Hospitals." *Agency for Healthcare Research and Quality*.

[179] CALNOC. "The CALNOC Overview." http://calnoc.affiniscape.com/associations/13337/files/01.20.2011%20CALNOC%20Overview.pdf.

[180] Centers for Medicare and Medicaid Services. "National Health Expenditure Data Fact Sheet." https://www.cms.gov/Research-Statistics-Data-and-Systems/Statistics-Trends-and-Reports/NationalHealthExpendData/NHE-Fact-Sheet.html.

[181] S. Heffler and others. "Health Spending Projections for 2001–2011: The Latest Outlook." *Health Affairs*. 2002:21(2):207-218..

[182] "Quality Improvement Program Leads To Better Asthma Outcomes And Saves $1.46 For Every Dollar Spent." *Medical News Today*. February 21, 2012. http://www.medicalnewstoday.com/releases/241931.php.

[183] Centers for Disease Control and Prevention. "Asthma in the U.S." *Vital Signs*. May 2011. http://www.cdc.gov/vitalsigns/asthma/.

[184] Internal KP data.

[185] National Quality Measures Clearinghouse. "Pressure ulcer prevention and treatment protocol: percentage of inpatients with pressure ulcers whose medical record contains documentation of a partial wound assessment with every dressing change." *Agency for Healthcare Research and Quality*. http://qualitymeasures.ahrq.gov/content.aspx?id=36735.

[186] "Wal-Mart's Keys to Successful Supply Chain Management." *University of San Francisco Online Education Resources*. http://www.usanfranonline.com/wal-mart-successful-supply-chain-management/.

[187] H. Tu and J. May. "Self-Pay Markets in Health Care: Consumer Nirvana or Caveat Emptor?" *Health Affairs*. 2007:26(2):217-226.

[188] Ibid.

[189] OECD. "Health Data 2012 - Frequently Requested Data; Health Care Activities, Average length of stay, all causes, days." October 2012 update.

[190] R. Hauboldt and N. Ortner. "2002 Organ and Tissue Transplant Costs and Discussion." *Milliman Research Report*. July 2002.

[191] D. Kamerow. "Great health care, guaranteed." *BMJ*. 2007:334:1086.

[192] Kaiser Permanente. "Fast Facts About Kaiser Permanente." http://share.kaiserpermanente.org/article/fast-facts-about-kaiser-permanente/.

[193] Kaiser Permanente. "2012 Annual Report."

[194] Kaiser Permanente News Center. "Healthy Bones Program Reduces Hip Fractures by 37 Percent, Kaiser Permanente Study Finds." November 4, 2008. http://xnet.kp.org/newscenter/pressreleases/nat/2008/110408healthybones.html

[195] Internal KP data.

[196] Internal KP data.

[197] Editorial. "Simple Treatments, Ignored." *New York Times*. September 8, 2012. http://www.nytimes.com/2012/09/09/opinion/sunday/simple-treatments-ignored.html?_r=2&.

[198] Internal KP data.

[199] D. Cosgrove and others. "A CEO Checklist for High-Value Health Care." *Institute of Medicine Discussion Paper*. June 5, 2012. http://www.iom.edu/Global/Perspectives/2012/CEOChecklist.aspx.

[200] Ibid.

[201] R. Dell, D. Greene, S. Schelkun, and K. Williams. "Osteoporosis Disease Management: The Role of the Orthopedic Surgeon." *The Journal of Bone & Joint Surgery*. 2008:90(4):188-194.

[202] Kaiser Permanente. "2012 Annual Report."

[203] S. Heffler and others. "Health Spending Projections for 2001–2011: The Latest Outlook." *Health Affairs*. 2002:21(2):207-218.

[204] National Committee for Quality Assurance. "HEDIS & Performance Measurement." http://www.ncqa.org/HEDISQualityMeasurement.aspx

[205] Centers for Disease Control and Prevention. "NCHS Data on Health Insurance and Access to Care," November 2012. http://www.cdc.gov/nchs/data/factsheets/factsheet_hiac.htm.

[206] Joint Commission Center for Transforming Healthcare. "Reducing Sepsis Mortality." June 28, 2012. http://www.centerfortransforminghealthcare.org/projects/detail.aspx?Project=8.

[207] CALNOC. "The CALNOC Overview." http://calnoc.affiniscape.com/associations/13337/files/01.20.2011%20CALNOC%20Overview.pdf.

[208] National Quality Measures Clearinghouse. "Pressure ulcer prevention and treatment protocol: percentage of inpatients with pressure ulcers whose medical record contains documentation of a partial wound assessment with every dressing change." *Agency for Healthcare Research and Quality*. http://qualitymeasures.ahrq.gov/content.aspx?id=36735.

[209] D. Berlowitz and others. "Preventing Pressure Ulcers in Hospitals." *Agency for Healthcare Research and Quality*. http://www.ahrq.gov/professionals/systems/long-term-care/resources/pressure-ulcers/pressureulcertoolkit/putoolkit.pdf.

[210] Internal KP data.

[211] Centers for Disease Control. "Chronic Diseases The Power to Prevent, The Call to Control: At A Glance 2009." http://www.cdc.gov/chronicdisease/resources/publications/AAG/chronic.htm.

[212] D. Muhlestein. "Continued Growth Of Public And Private Accountable Care Organizations," *Health Affairs Blog*. February 19, 2013. http://healthaffairs.org/blog/2013/02/19/continued-growth-of-public-and-private-accountable-care-organizations/.

[213] Centers for Disease Control. "Chronic Diseases The Power to Prevent, The Call to Control: At A Glance 2009." http://www.cdc.gov/chronicdisease/resources/publications/AAG/chronic.htm.

[214] California Association of Public Hospitals and Health Systems. "Medical Homes in the Safety Net: Spotlight on California's Public Hospital Systems." *Policy Brief*. March 2010. https://www.caph.org/content/upload/AssetMgmt/PDFs/Publications/MedicalHomePolicyBriefMarch2010.pdf.

[215] H. Pham and others. "Care Patterns in Medicare and Their Implications for Pay for Performance," *New England Journal of Medicine*. 2007:356:1130-1139.

[216] V. Arora and others. "Improving Inpatients' Identification of Their Doctors: Use of FACE™ Cards," *Joint Commission Journal on Quality and Patient Safety*. 2009:35(12):613–619.

[217] Centers for Disease Control. "Chronic Diseases The Power to Prevent, The Call to Control: At A Glance 2009." http://www.cdc.gov/chronicdisease/resources/publications/AAG/chronic.htm.

[218] Kaiser Permanente. "2012 Annual Report."

[219] Ibid.

[220] Kaiser Permanente. "Fast Facts About Kaiser Permanente." http://share.kaiserpermanente.org/article/fast-facts-about-kaiser-permanente/.

[221] Editorial. "Simple Treatments, Ignored." *New York Times*. September 8, 2012. http://www.nytimes.com/2012/09/09/opinion/sunday/simple-treatments-ignored.html?_r=2&.

[222] D. Cosgrove and others. "A CEO Checklist for High-Value Health Care." *Institute of Medicine Discussion Paper*. June 5, 2012. http://www.iom.edu/Global/Perspectives/2012/CEOChecklist.aspx.

[223] Kaiser Permanente News Center. "Healthy Bones Program Reduces Hip Fractures by 37 Percent, Kaiser Permanente Study Finds." November 4, 2008. http://xnet.kp.org/newscenter/pressreleases/nat/2008/110408healthybones.html.

[224] Internal KP data.

[225] B. Crawford, M. Skeath, and A. Whippy. "Kaiser Permanente Northern California sepsis mortality reduction initiative." *Critical Care*. 2012:16(Suppl 3):12.

[226] Internal KP data.

[227] National Quality Measures Clearinghouse. "Pressure ulcer prevention and treatment protocol: percentage of inpatients with pressure ulcers whose medical record contains documentation of a partial wound assessment with every dressing change." *Agency for Healthcare Research and Quality*. http://qualitymeasures.ahrq.gov/content.aspx?id=36735.

[228] D. Berlowitz and others. "Preventing Pressure Ulcers in Hospitals." *Agency for Healthcare Research and Quality*. http://www.ahrq.gov/professionals/systems/long-term-care/resources/pressure-ulcers/pressureulcertoolkit/putoolkit.pdf.

[229] T. Lagu, M. Rothberg, B. Nathanson, P. Pekow, J. Steingrub, P. Lindenauer." The Relationship Between Hospital Spending and Mortality in Patients With Sepsis." *Archives of Internal Medicine*. 2011:171(4):292-299.

[230] S. Heffler and others. "Health Spending Projections for 2001–2011: The Latest Outlook." *Health Affairs*. 2002:21(2):207-218.

[231] C. Schoen and R. Osborn. "The Commonwealth Fund 2011 International Health Policy Survey of Sicker Adults in Eleven Countries." *Commonwealth Fund*. November 2011.

[232] D. Cutler, K. Davis, and K. Stremikis. "The Impact of Health Reform on Health System Spending." *Commonwealth Fund*. May 2010.

[233] C. DeNavas-Walt, B. Proctor, and J. Smith. "Income, Poverty, and Health Insurance Coverage in the United States: 2011." *United States Census Bureau Current Population Reports*. September 2012.

[234] S. Cohen and N. Uberoi. "Differentials in the Concentration in the Level of Health Expenditures across Population Subgroups in the U.S., 2010." *Agency for Healthcare Research and Quality*. Statistical Brief #21. August. 2013. http://meps.ahrq.gov/mepsweb/data_files/publications/st421/stat421.shtml.

[235] MedPac. "The Medicare Advantage program: Status Report." Report to the Congress: *Medicare Payment Policy*. March 2012. http://www.medpac.gov/chapters/Mar12_Ch12.pdf.

[236] R. Moffit. "The Second State of Medicare Reform: Moving to a Premium-Support Program." *The Heritage Foundation Executive Summary Backgrounder*. November 28, 2011. http://thf_media.s3.amazonaws.com/2011/pdf/bg2626.pdf.

[237] "AHIP Statement on Medicare Advantage." *America's Health Insurance Plans*. September 19, 2012. http://www.ahip.org/News/Press-Room/2012/AHIP-Statement-on-Medicare-Advantage.aspx.

[238] Centers for Medicare & Medicaid Services. "Choose Higher Quality for Better Health Care." October 2012. http://www.medicare.gov/Publications/Pubs/pdf/11226.pdf.

[239] Centers for Disease Control and Prevention. "National Diabetes Fact Sheet: National Estimates and General Information on Diabetes and Prediabetes in the United States." 2011.

[240] Ibid.

[241] M. O'Grady, P. John, and A. Winn. "Substantial Medicare Savings May Result If Insurers Cover 'Artificial Pancreas' Sooner For Diabetes Patients." *Health Affairs*. 2012:31(8):1822-1829.

[242] Kaiser Permanente News Center. "Kaiser Permanente Leads the Nation with Six 5-Star Medicare Health Plans." October 15, 2012. http://xnet.kp.org/newscenter/pressreleases/nat/2012/101512_medicare_stars_final.html.

[243] Ibid.

[244] Ibid.

[245] Centers for Disease Control. "Chronic Diseases The Power to Prevent, The Call to Control: At A Glance 2009." http://www.cdc.gov/chronicdisease/resources/publications/AAG/chronic.htm.

[246] Editorial. "Simple Treatments, Ignored." *New York Times*. September 8, 2012. http://www.nytimes.com/2012/09/09/opinion/sunday/simple-treatments-ignored.html?_r=2&.

[247] A. Rossier Markus and others. "Medicaid Covered Births, 2008 Through 2010, in the Context of the Implementation of Health Reform." *Women's Health Issues*. 2013:23 (5):273-280.

[248] Ibid.

[249] C. Truffer and others. "2012 Actuarial Report on the Financial Outlook for Medicaid." *Office of the Actuary, Centers for Medicare & Medicaid Services* 2012.

[250] V. Smith and others. "Medicaid in a Historic Time of Transformation: Results from a 50-State Medicaid Budget Survey for State Fiscal Years 2013 and 2014." *Kaiser Family Foundation*. October 2013.

[251] Centers for Medicare and Medicaid Services. "Medicaid Eligibility." http://www.medicaid.gov/Medicaid-CHIP-Program-Information/By-Topics/Eligibility/Eligibility.html.

[252] "Quality Improvement Program Leads To Better Asthma Outcomes And Saves $1.46 For Every Dollar Spent." *Medical News Today*. February 21, 2012. http://www.medicalnewstoday.com/releases/241931.php.

[253] National Center for Infant Toddlers and Families. "Brain Development." *Zero to Three*. http://www.zerotothree.org/child-development/brain-development/.

[254] Ounce of Prevention Fund. "Why Investments in Early Childhood Work." http://www.ounceofprevention.org/about/why-early-childhood-invest-ments-work.php.

[255] National Institute for Literacy, 1998.

[256] A. Markus and others. "Medicaid Covered Births, 2008 Through 2010, in the Context of the Implementation of Health Reform." *Women's Health Issues*. 2013: 23(5):e273-e280.

[257] R. Walmsley. "World Prison Population List." *International Centre for Prison Studies*. Ninth Edition.

[258] OECD. "Education at a Glance 2013: OECD Indicators."

[259] Centers for Disease Control. "Chronic Diseases The Power to Prevent, The Call to Control: At A Glance 2009." http://www.cdc.gov/chronicdisease/resources/publications/AAG/chronic.htm.

[260] World Health Organization. "Noncommunicable Diseases Fact Sheet." March 2013. http://www.who.int/mediacentre/factsheets/fs355/en/.

[261] Centers for Disease Control and Prevention. "FastStats" Exercise or Physical Activity." National Center for Health Statistics. http://www.cdc.gov/nchs/fastats/exercise.htm.

Centers for Disease Control and Prevention. "Adult Obesity Facts." Overweight and Obesity. http://www.cdc.gov/obesity/data/adult.html.

[262] The Lancet. "Physical Activity." July 2012. http://www.thelancet.com/series/physical-activity.

[263] C. Williams. "Fit and Fat Beats Lean and Lazy in Survival." ABC News. Dec. 4, 2007. http://www.abcnews.go.com/Health/BeautySecrets/story?id=3952052.

[264] M. Cecchini and others. "Tackling of Unhealthy Diets, Physical Inactivity, and Obesity: Health Effects and Cost-Effectiveness." *The Lancet*. 2010:376 (9754): 1775-1784.

[265] American Diabetes Association. "Diabetes FAQ." http://www.diabetes.org/diabetes-basics/prevention/pre-diabetes/pre-diabetes-faqs.html.

[266] J. Huerta and others. "Physical Activity and Risk of Cerebrovascular Disease in the European Prospective Investigation into Cancer and Nutrition-Spain Study." Stroke. 2013:44:111-118.

M. Tully and others. "Randomised controlled trial of home-based walking programmes at and below current recommended levels of exercise in sedentary adults." *Journal of Epidemiology & Community Health. 2007:61(9):778-83.*

[267] Arnold School of Public Health. "Study involved studying data from exams, treadmill tests at Cooper Clinic in Houston." *University of South Carolina.* March 23, 2009. http://www.sph.sc.edu/news/breastcancer.htm.

K. Wolin and others. "Leisure-time physical activity patterns and risk of colon cancer in women." *International Journal of Cancer.* 2007:121: 2776–2781.

J. Antonelli and others. "Exercise and prostate cancer risk in a cohort of veterans undergoing prostate needle biopsy." *Journal of Urology.* 2009:182(5):2226-31.

E. Giovannucci and others. "Physical Activity, Obesity, and Risk for Colon Cancer and Adenoma in Men." *Annals of Internal Medicine.* 1995:122:327-334.

[268] American Diabetes Association. "Diabetes FAQ." http://www.diabetes.org/diabetes-basics/prevention/pre-diabetes/pre-diabetes-faqs.html.

[269] M. O'Grady, P. John, and A. Winn. "Substantial Medicare Savings May Result If Insurers Cover 'Artificial Pancreas' Sooner For Diabetes Patients." *Health Affairs,* August 2012, vol. 31, 8:1822-1829.

[270] Agency for Healthcare Research and Quality. "Diabetes Disparities Among Racial and Ethnic Minorities." http://www.ahrq.gov/research/findings/factsheets/diabetes/diabdisp/index.html.

[271] BMJ Open. "Walking for Heart Health? Speed It Up, Study Suggests." *Health Day.* October 8, 2012. http://consumer.healthday.com/Article.asp?AID=669394.

[272] M. Tully and others. "Randomised controlled trial of home-based walking programmes at and below current recommended levels of exercise in sedentary adults." *Journal of Epidemiology & Community Health.* 2007:61(9):778-83.

[273] J. Boone-Heinonen and others. "Walking for prevention of cardiovascular disease in men and women: a systematic review of observational studies." *Obesity Reviews.* 2009:10(2): 204–217.

[274] J. Myers. "Exercise and Cardiovascular Health." *Circulation.* 2003:107: e2-e5.

[275] D. Nieman, D. Henson, M. Austin. "Upper respiratory tract infection is reduced in physically fit and active adults." *British Journal of Sports Medicine.* 2011:45(12):987-92.

[276] Arnold School of Public Health. "Study involved studying data from exams, treadmill tests at Cooper Clinic in Houston." *University of South Carolina.* March 23, 2009. http://www.sph.sc.edu/news/breastcancer.htm.

K. Wolin and others. "Leisure-time physical activity patterns and risk of colon cancer in women." *International Journal of Cancer.* 2007:121: 2776–2781.

J. Antonelli and others. "Exercise and prostate cancer risk in a cohort of veterans undergoing prostate needle biopsy." *Journal of Urology.* 2009:182(5):2226-31.

E. Giovannucci and others. "Physical Activity, Obesity, and Risk for Colon Cancer and Adenoma in Men." *Annals of Internal Medicine.* 1995:122:327-334.

[277] M. Holmes, W. Chen, D. Feskanich, C. Kroenke, and G. Colditz. "Physical Activity and Survival After Breast Cancer Diagnosis." *JAMA.* 2005:293(20):2479-2486.

278 D. Head and others. "Exercise Engagement as a Moderator of the Effects of APOE Genotype on Amyloid Deposition." *Archives of Neurology*. 2012:69(5):636-43.

279 P. Katzmarzyk, I-Min Lee. "Sedentary behaviour and life expectancy in the USA: a cause-deleted life table analysis." *BMJ Open*. 2012:2:e00082.

280 J. Blumenthal et al. "Effects of Exercise Training on Older Patients With Major Depression." *Archives of Internal Medicine*. 1999:159(19):2349-2356.

J. Sieverdes and others. "Association between Leisure Time Physical Activity and Depressive Symptoms in Men." *Medicine and Science in Sports & Exercise*. 2012:44(2):260-265.

281 J. Blumenthal et al. "Effects of Exercise Training on Older Patients With Major Depression." *Archives of Internal Medicine*. 1999:159(19):2349-2356.

J. Mota-Pereira et al. "Moderate exercise improves depression parameters in treatment-resistant patients with major depressive disorder." *Journal of Psychiatric Research*. 2011:45(8):1005-1011.

R. Robertson, A. Robertson, R. Jepsona, M. Maxwell. "Walking for depression or depressive symptoms: A systematic review and meta-analysis." *Mental Health and Physical Activity*. 2012:5(1):66–75.

J. Blumenthal and others. "Exercise and pharmacotherapy in the treatment of major depressive disorder." *Psychosomatic Medicine*. 2007:69(7):587-96.

282 E. Lim and others. "Reversal of type 2 diabetes: normalisation of beta cell function in association with decreased pancreas and liver triacylglycerol." *Diabetologia*. 2011: 54(10): 2506–2514.

283 J. Sattelmair and others. "Dose Response Between Physical Activity and Risk of Coronary Heart Disease." *Circulation*. 2011: 124: 789-795.

284 M. Murphy, S. Blair, E. Murtagh. "Accumulated versus continuous exercise for health benefit: a review of empirical studies." *Sports Medicine* (Auckland, N.Z.). 2009:39(1):29-43.

285 T. Parker-Pope. "The Surprising Shortcut to Better Health." *New York Times*. May 4, 2012. http://well.blogs.nytimes.com/2012/05/04/the-surprising-shortcut-to-better-health.

286 Centers for Disease Control. "Chronic Diseases The Power to Prevent, The Call to Control: At A Glance 2009." http://www.cdc.gov/chronicdisease/resources/publications/AAG/chronic.htm.

287 T. Marsland and others. "Reducing Cancer Costs and Improving Quality Through Collaboration With Payers: A Proposal From the Florida Society of Clinical Oncology." *Journal of Oncology Practice*. 2010:6(5):265-269.

288 Arnold School of Public Health. "Study involved studying data from exams, treadmill tests at Cooper Clinic in Houston." *University of South Carolina*. March 23, 2009. http://www.sph.sc.edu/news/breastcancer.htm.

K. Wolin and others. "Leisure-time physical activity patterns and risk of colon cancer in women." *International Journal of Cancer*. 2007:121: 2776–2781.

J. Antonelli and others. "Exercise and prostate cancer risk in a cohort of veterans undergoing prostate needle biopsy." *Journal of Urology*. 2009:182(5):2226-31.

E. Giovannucci and others. "Physical Activity, Obesity, and Risk for Colon Cancer and Adenoma in Men." *Annals of Internal Medicine*. 1995:122:327-334

[289] Centers for Disease Control and Prevention. "FastStats - Exercise or Physical Activity." *National Center for Health Statistics*. http://www.cdc.gov/nchs/fastats/exercise.htm.

[290] Centers for Disease Control and Prevention. "Adult Obesity Facts." Overweight and Obesity. http://www.cdc.gov/obesity/data/adult.html

[291] A. Singh and others. "Physical activity and performance at school: a systematic review of the literature including a methodological quality assessment." *Archives of Pediatrics & Adolescent Medicine*. 2012:166(1):49-55.

[292] D. Head and others. "Exercise Engagement as a Moderator of the Effects of APOE Genotype on Amyloid Deposition." *Archives of Neurology*. 2012:69(5):636-43.

[293] Centers for Disease Control and Prevention. "Adult Obesity Facts." Overweight and Obesity. http://www.cdc.gov/obesity/data/adult.html.

[294] R. Johnson and others. "Dietary Sugars Intake and Cardiovascular Health: A Scientific Statement From the American Heart Association." *Circulation*. 2009:120:1011-1020.

[295] A. Tomiyama and others. "Low Calorie Dieting Increases Cortisol." *Psychosomatic Medicine*. 2010:72 (4): 357-364.

[296] F. Ortega And Others. "The Intriguing Metabolically Healthy but Obese Phenotype: Cardiovascular Prognosis and Role of Fitness." *European Heart Journal*. 2013:34 (5):389-397.

[297] Centers for Disease Control and Prevention. "FastStats" Exercise or Physical Activity." National Center for Health Statistics. http://www.cdc.gov/nchs/fastats/exercise.htm.

Centers for Disease Control and Prevention. "Adult Obesity Facts." Overweight and Obesity. http://www.cdc.gov/obesity/data/adult.html.

[298] Centers for Disease Control and Prevention. "Adult Obesity Facts." Overweight and Obesity. http://www.cdc.gov/obesity/data/adult.html.

[299] Centers for Disease Control and Prevention. "FastStats - Exercise or Physical Activity." National Center for Health Statistics. http://www.cdc.gov/nchs/fastats/exercise.htm.

[300] Centers for Medicare and Medicaid Services. "National Health Expenditure Data Fact Sheet." https://www.cms.gov/Research-Statistics-Data-and-Systems/Statistics-Trends-and-Reports/NationalHealthExpendData/NHE-Fact-Sheet.html.

[301] Centers for Medicare and Medicaid Services. "National Health Expenditure Data Fact Sheet." https://www.cms.gov/Research-Statistics-Data-and-Systems/Statistics-Trends-and-Reports/NationalHealthExpendData/NHE-Fact-Sheet.html.